Ethical Competence in Nursing Practice

Catherine Robichaux, PhD, RN, CNS, Alumna CCRN, is an adjunct assistant professor at the University of Texas Health Science Center in San Antonio, Texas, and the University of Mary in Bismarck, North Dakota. Her clinical background is adult critical care and she has taught ethics at the undergraduate and graduate levels. Dr. Robichaux serves as the Nursing Ethics Council faculty advisor and research mentor at University Health System in San Antonio, Texas. She has conducted and published funded research on ethical issues in end-of-life care in adult and pediatric/neonatal intensive care units and moral distress and ethical climate in acute care settings. She has also explored the quality of dying and death in rural and border hospitals in the Southwest. Dr. Robichaux has been a contributing editor for ethical issues for *Critical Care Nurse* and serves on the editorial board of *Clinical Nursing Studies* and the editorial advisory board of the *Online Journal of Issues in Nursing*. She was a member of the steering committee to revise the American Nurses Association's (ANA) 2015 Code of Ethics and is currently a member of the ANA Center for Human Rights and Ethics Advisory Board. Dr. Robichaux is a recipient of the Circle of Excellence Award from the American Association of Critical Care Nurses for her work in promoting ethical work environments.

Ethical Competence in Nursing Practice

COMPETENCIES, SKILLS, DECISION MAKING

CATHERINE ROBICHAUX, PhD, RN, CNS, ALUMNA CCRN

EDITOR

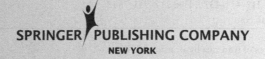

SPRINGER PUBLISHING COMPANY
NEW YORK

Springer Publishing Company, LLC
11 West 42nd Street
New York, NY 10036
www.springerpub.com

Acquisitions Editor: Elizabeth Nieginski
Senior Production Editor: Kris Parrish
Composition: Westchester Publishing Services

ISBN: 978-0-8261-2637-5
e-book ISBN: 978-0-8261-2638-2
Instructor's Test Bank: 978-0-8261-2624-5
Instructor's PowerPoints: 978-0-8261-2629-0

Instructor's materials are available to qualified adopters by contacting textbook@springerpub.com

16 17 18 19 20 / 5 4 3 2 1

The author and the publisher of this Work have made every effort to use sources believed to be reliable to provide information that is accurate and compatible with the standards generally accepted at the time of publication. Because medical science is continually advancing, our knowledge base continues to expand. Therefore, as new information becomes available, changes in procedures become necessary. We recommend that the reader always consult current research and specific institutional policies before performing any clinical procedure. The author and publisher shall not be liable for any special, consequential, or exemplary damages resulting, in whole or in part, from the readers' use of, or reliance on, the information contained in this book. The publisher has no responsibility for the persistence or accuracy of URLs for external or third-party Internet websites referred to in this publication and does not guarantee that any content on such websites is, or will remain, accurate or appropriate.

Library of Congress Cataloging-in-Publication Data

Names: Robichaux, Catherine, author, editor.
Title: Ethical competence in nursing practice : competencies, skills, decision making / Catherine Robichaux.
Description: New York, NY: Springer Publishing Company, LLC, [2017] | Includes bibliographical references.
Identifiers: LCCN 2016015602 | ISBN 9780826126375 | ISBN 9780826126382 (e-book)
Subjects: | MESH: Ethics, Nursing | Clinical Competence
Classification: LCC RT85 | NLM WY 85 | DDC 174.2/9073—dc23
LC record available at https://lccn.loc.gov/2016015602

Printed in the United States of America by Bradford & Bigelow.

To my husband, Hugh,

and my family

Contents

PART I
FOUNDATIONS OF ETHICAL NURSING PRACTICE

PART II
SKILLS AND RESOURCES FOR ETHICAL DECISION MAKING

Contributors

Barbara L. Chanko, RN, MBA, is a nurse and health care ethicist. Over almost three decades, she has provided ethics consultation and worked to improve ethical health care practices within the Department of Veterans Affairs (VA). In particular, she participates in improving the quality of ethics consultation at 140 VA medical centers through the development of standards for performing ethics consultation and the creation of tools and educational materials aimed at supporting these standards and improving the knowledge and skill of VA ethics consultants. She completed the certificate program in bioethics and the medical humanities from the Montefiore Medical Center/New York University (NYU) in 2003, and presents regularly at the American Society for Bioethics and Humanities (ASBH) and the International Conference on Clinical Ethics Consultation (ICCEC). She is also an associate of the Division of Medical Ethics, Department of Population Health, NYU School of Medicine, and serves as ethics faculty for the medical school.

Maryanne M. Giuliante, DNP, GNP, RN, ANP-C, is the Nurse Practitioner Program Manager for the Hartford Institute for Geriatric Nursing (HIGN) at New York University (NYU). She received her doctorate in nursing practice (DNP) at Rutgers University in New Jersey. She received both her geriatric and adult nurse practitioner degrees from Hunter College in New York. Dr. Giuliante was a pioneer in advocating and helping to develop one of the first oncology nurse practitioner residency programs in the United States at Memorial Sloan-Kettering Cancer Center (MSKCC). She has spent the last 20 years in acute care, most recently as an oncology nurse practitioner at MSKCC, where her work focused on adult and geriatric patients with melanoma, sarcoma, and head and neck cancers. She continues to maintain her clinical practice at MSKCC. In addition to her clinical work, she has dedicated her time instructing and mentoring students by serving as a clinical professor in various colleges and universities in New York. She has also served as a DNP clinical instructor while at MSKCC, and is currently a DNP faculty mentor at NYU. Over the past two decades, Dr. Giuliante's experience has led her into many areas of nursing including medicine, oncology, cardiology, kidney transplantation, and postsurgery acute care.

Douglas Houghton, MSN, ARNP, ACNPC, CCRN, FAANP, has an extensive background in critical care, spanning more than two decades. He is a national leader in advancing the role of the nurse practitioner within the critical care environment. Mr. Houghton has clinical expertise in ethics and end-of-life care, and has published and lectured on these and other topics frequently at the national and international levels. Mr. Houghton is educated as a family and acute care nurse practitioner, and holds national certification in acute care (ACNPC) and in critical care nursing. He was inducted as a fellow of the American Association of Nurse Practitioners in 2011 for recognized national contributions to the nurse practitioner profession. He has worked as a nurse practitioner in the trauma intensive care unit at Ryder Trauma Center, Jackson Health System in Miami, Florida, for more than 20 years, and has been an active member of the Center's ethics committee for more than 10 years, consulting on complex clinical ethics cases.

Carol Jorgensen Huston, MSN, MPA, DPA, FAAN, has been a professor of nursing at California State University, Chico (CSUC), since 1982 and was named the 2008/2009 Outstanding Professor for CSUC. She served as the director of that program from 2010 to 2015. She was also the 2007 to 2009 president of Sigma Theta Tau International Honor Society of Nursing and is a fellow in the American Academy of Nursing. Dr. Huston is the author of five textbooks on leadership, management, and professional issues in nursing (18 editions total) and publishes widely in leading professional journals. In addition, Dr. Huston is a frequent speaker at nursing and health care conferences and has keynoted more than 250 presentations worldwide.

Craig M. Klugman, PhD, is a professor of bioethics in the Department of Health Sciences at DePaul University. He holds master's degrees in medical anthropology and bioethics and a doctorate in medical humanities. He is the blog editor for bioethics.net and is the copresident of the Health Humanities Consortium. He serves on the ethics committee at Northwestern University Hospital and is the editor of the *MacMillan Handbook in Philosophy: Medical Ethics* and *Ethical Issues in Rural Health*. He is the creator of Texaslivingwill.org and the award-winning producer of the film, *Advance Directives*. The author of nearly 300 articles, Dr. Klugman studies end-of-life issues, public health ethics, and ethics education.

Joan Kub, PhD, MA, PHCNS-BC, FAAN, is an associate professor at Johns Hopkins University School of Nursing with joint appointments in the Bloomberg School of Public Health and Johns Hopkins School of Medicine. She coordinates the joint MSN/MPH program and MSN in public health nursing programs at Johns Hopkins. She is currently serving as Chair of the Quad Council and was president of the Association of Community Health Nursing Educators (ACHNE) from 2014 to 2016. Dr. Kub represented the American Nurses Association (ANA) and ACHNE on the workgroups that developed the *Public Health Nursing: Scope and Standards of Practice* published in 2007 and 2013, respectively. She is certified by the American Nurses Credentialing Commission (ANCC) as an advanced public health nurse and has served populations across the life span through her roles as a nurse educator, nurse researcher, and provider of care. Her career is marked by an integration of public health science, nursing, and ethics, which is reflected in her research as a coinvestigator on several National Institutes of Health (NIH) grants focused on end-of-life decision making, her publications, and her ongoing service on the clinical ethics committee for Johns Hopkins Hospital since 1992.

Mary K. Walton, MSN, MBE, RN, is the director of Patient and Family Centered Care and Nurse Ethicist at the Hospital of the University of Pennsylvania and an adjunct assistant professor of medical ethics and health policy, Perelman School of Medicine, University of Pennsylvania. She received her BSN and MSN from the University of Pennsylvania and earned a master of bioethics degree and a certificate in clinical ethics mediation from the University of Pennsylvania School of Medicine. She has practiced in academic health care settings for over 40 years and has a progressive history of leadership. Her roles of clinical nurse specialist and nurse manager included responsibility for clinical ethics committees and ethics consultation services, cultural competency training, and the establishment of evidence-based practice standards. Currently she is responsible for organizational initiatives focused on clinical ethics and improving the patient and family experience of care. As cochair of a hospital-based Patient and Family Advisory Council, she leads quality improvement efforts to support person-centered care and patient engagement. She has published in the areas of collaboration, advocacy, healthy work environment, nursing history, and patient-centered care.

SUPERVISORY EDITOR

Janet Weber, PhD, holds a BSN and MSN from St. Louis University and an EdD in curriculum and instruction from Memphis State University. She recently received the status of Professor Emerita of Nursing after teaching for 37 years at Southeast Missouri State University. During that time, she taught a variety of nursing courses in both the undergraduate and graduate programs. She served as coordinator and then director of the RN–BSN program for over 20 years, leading in the development of the RN–BSN curriculum from a face-to-face to a fully online program. She has authored and coauthored several editions of a nursing assessment handbook and textbook that has been translated into four languages, as well as numerous other book chapters and articles. In addition, she has given many national and international presentations on nursing diagnoses, nursing leadership, and teaching methods. She chaired the publications committee and serves on the editorial board for the North American Nursing Diagnosis Association International.

Contributor Acknowledgments

Katherine Brown-Saltzman, MA, RN

Codirector, Ethics Center
UCLA Health System
Los Angeles, California

Donna Casey, BSN, MA, RN, FABC, NE-BC

Vice President Patient Care Services
Cochair, Ethics Committee
Christiana Care Health System
Newark, Delaware

Jan Fortier, RN, CNCCP(C)

Staff Nurse, PICU/PCICU
Stollery Children's Hospital
Edmonton, Alberta, Canada

Kathleen Marotta, BSN, RN

Staff Nurse III
Pediatric Intensive Care Unit
University Health System
San Antonio, Texas

Carol Pavlish, PhD, RN, FAAN

Associate Professor
Prelicensure Program Director
UCLA School of Nursing
Los Angeles, California
Professor Emeritus
St. Catherine University
St. Paul, Minnesota

Jeanie L. Sauerland, BS, BSN, RN
Assistant Director Nursing Ethics Service
University Health System
San Antonio, Texas

Evelyn Swenson-Britt, PhD, RN
Adjunct Clinical Faculty
School of Nursing
University of Texas Health Science Center
San Antonio, Texas

Esther Vandermeulen, BSN, RN, CCRN
Staff Nurse III
Medical Intensive Care Unit
University Health System
San Antonio, Texas

Blas Villa, BS, BSN, RN, CCRN
Staff Nurse III
Medical Intensive Care Unit
University Health System
San Antonio, Texas

Foreword

The understanding of ethics is vital to the practice of nursing. This essential and fundamental knowledge guides nurses through their daily practice, yet across the country one sees that ethics education for nurses has often been limited. This book, in its broad scope, addresses ethical concerns through theoretical knowledge, assessment, and skill building within a range of specialty practices, enabling nurses to enrich and develop their critical thinking and ethical competency.

Having a voice in ethical concerns depends on many elements that go far beyond having an opinion. To be heard requires knowledge, self-exploration, dexterity, and a willingness to be fluent in a language of values, meaning, and moral complexity. Nursing is privileged to be grounded in caring and an ethic of care that brings to health systems a valuable perspective as it identifies and discerns how to respond to complex ethical concerns.

This book appears at a time when nurses' voices in all matters of health care ethics have become increasingly important. Ethical complexities in clinical practice are not new; indeed, a formal Code of Ethics has existed since 1950. It is also true that many nurses, throughout history and in current times, have performed courageous acts of advocacy. However, technological advances are raising new questions, the "bottom line" stretches the seams of our shared work, organizational cultures can be disheartening, and gaps in care continue to plague healthcare systems—all of which profoundly influence the patients' experiences of care, clinicians' experiences of providing care, systems that organize care delivery, and the care outcomes (often disparate) that result. The matters and practice of ethics have never been more urgent for nurses and their patients.

Provided with the opportunity to contribute to this collection of thoughtful essays and critically important lessons on ethical competence, we call upon all nurses to strengthen their engagement with ethically complex situations within the context of interdisciplinary, team-based health care. This strong voice requires each of us to reflect on our values, accept responsibility for creating ethical work environments, and attune to our own needs for self-care as we immerse ourselves in a nursing practice that fully embraces ethical complexities.

Values are an inherent part of being human. These ideals organize our daily lives, clarify our decisions, shape our relationships, and contribute to the meaning we derive from our existence. Values emerge from past experiences, influence our current experiences, and often direct our choices about future experiences. Values are personal, but they also seep into our professional lives and merge with our professional standards and codes to shape our clinical practice. Occasionally, it behooves us to pause and reflect on our unique kaleidoscope of personal values and professional ethics. This book provides the opportunity to become more thoughtful and knowledgeable about the personal and professional values that guide our daily clinical practice.

The chapters also encourage us to examine and take more responsibility for the conditions in which our nursing practice occurs. Provision 6 in the ANA Code of Ethics (2015) requires us to take action in creating "morally good environments that enable nurses to be virtuous" (p. 23). As nurses, we can no longer afford to be bystanders of climates that normalize "moral muteness" (Verhezen, 2010, p. 180). If there are risks involved in asking important questions that pertain to our care of patients, we must challenge the status quo and transition toward a culture of ethical mindfulness where interdisciplinary, ethics-based conversations become routine and comfortable. Emanuel (2000) noted that ethics is intricately woven into the "webs of interaction" that occur in our systems of care (p. 151). This suggests that relationships are the key to crafting and nurturing ethical cultures. With that in mind, this book provides philosophical and pragmatic guidance on building relational capacity and communication skills, both of which are essential during team-based ethical conversations. Once these shared deliberations become effective, trust, which forms the foundation of ethical cultures, gradually restructures our systems of care. This transformative change is never easy but seems essential if nurses are to become "full partners with . . . other healthcare professionals in redesigning health care in the United States" (Institute of Medicine, 2010, p. 4).

Finally, self-care is a moral imperative. Provision 5 in our ANA Code of Ethics (2015) refers to "duties to self," which include attending to not only patients' health and safety but also our own. An ethical practice of self-care promotes sustainability by addressing the hemorrhaging of individuals—overcome by disengagement, burnout, apathy, and a loss of meaning—from our profession. Care of oneself inoculates nurses in powerful ways to develop resiliency. It is not just the taking care of one's physical body; it provokes recognition of all the psychosocial and spiritual elements needed for durability in the face of challenges, suffering, injustices, and the demands of service. Even in an ethically sound environment, value differences will give rise to moral distress, which can escalate and exacerbate over time, depleting nurses' reserves and ability to respond. Ongoing self-assessment, maintaining a plan of self-care, recognizing the potency of healthy boundaries, and the worth of the tend-and-befriend response to stress, all promote commitment to health (Taylor et al., 2000).

Self-care is also practical, because no matter how well we prepare ourselves to deliberate and collaborate in ethically difficult situations, ethical complexities and conflicts that give rise to moral distress will remain a part of clinical practice. The keys are proactively developing a personal and professional resilience plan that includes both maintenance and distress-oriented strategies and then attuning to early signs of distress so the appropriate actions can be taken.

As part of our ethics research, we check in with ICU nurses on a fairly regular basis. At a recent check-in, nurses were debriefing from a very difficult patient situation, and one nurse commented, "I think nursing practice is sacred—not in the sense of religion, but in the sense that we share a sacred time and space with patients and their families. They trust us to do that with them, and as difficult as it is, it is also an incredible privilege." That speaks to the importance of the lessons in this book. The author has assembled chapters that provide an opportunity for us all to become more skilled and collaborative in our ethical practices, which, in turn, creates ethical environments that are conducive to our own moral integrity and the practice of safe, high-quality care for patients, their families, and our communities.

Carol Pavlish, PhD, RN, FAAN
Associate Professor
UCLA School of Nursing
Los Angeles, California

Katherine Brown-Saltzman, MA, RN
Co-Director, Ethics Center
UCLA Health System
Los Angeles, California

REFERENCES

American Nurses Association. (2015). *Code of ethics for nurses with interpretive statements.* Silver Spring, MD: Nursebooks.org

Emanuel, L. (2000). Ethics and the structure of healthcare. *Cambridge Quarterly of Healthcare Ethics, 9,* 151–168.

Institute of Medicine. (2010). *The future of nursing: Leading change, advancing health.* Washington, DC: National Academies Press.

Taylor, S. E., Klein, L. C., Lewis, B. P., Gruenewald, T. L., Gurung, R. A. R., & Updegraff, J. A. (2000). Biobehavioral responses to stress in females: Tend-and-befriend, not fight-or-flight. *Psychological Review, 107,* 441–429.

Verhezen, P. (2010). Giving voice in a culture of silence: From a culture of compliance to a culture of integrity. *Journal of Business Ethics, 96,* 187–206. doi:10.1007/s10551-010-0458-5

Preface

As with most books, the idea for this volume evolved over many years and numerous discussions with staff nurses and educators. Working primarily in adult critical care, I was initially interested in the ability of some nurses to recognize and engage in ethical situations. While other nurses may have identified ethical issues, they often appeared reluctant to initiate or participate in discussions with patient/family members and/or other providers. This reluctance and inaction did not reflect a lack of responsibility or advocacy but seemingly one of sufficient *ethical competence*: the knowledge, skills, and attitudes required to address the many ethical issues that arise daily in nursing practice. Although not as prevalent as it is today, these nurses expressed emotions associated with moral distress such as regret, anger, and thoughts about leaving the profession. This book was written to provide a framework to assist nurses in achieving this ethical competence. It presents a framework that incorporates the cognitive and affective processes that form an understanding of ethical competence in nursing practice: sensitivity, judgment, motivation, and action. Beginning with a brief overview of ethical theories and principles and building on the experiences of readers who are practicing nurses, each chapter includes one or more evolving case scenarios. Questions posed with each case scenario encourage ethical sensitivity, awareness of personal values, and use of a decision-making model that integrates elements of virtue and care ethics. Recognizing the challenges that arise when attempting to implement a justifiable decision, strategies to maintain ethical motivation, or moral courage, are also presented. A distinguished panel of thought leaders and educators in nursing ethics has authored chapters relating to their particular areas of clinical specialty. The content incorporates the American Association of Critical-Care Nurses Essentials of Baccalaureate Education for Professional Nursing Practice, as well as the relevant Institute of Medicine (IOM) and the Quality and Safety Education for Nurses (QSEN) competencies for patient care. The content of the book also incorporates the most updated (2015) version of the Code of Ethics for Nurses. Questions for discussion are included at the end of each chapter as well as PowerPoint slides and additional questions and answers provided for classroom use by instructors. *Qualified instructors may obtain access to ancillary materials by contacting textbook@springerpub.com.*

Skills to enhance the nurse's actions in everyday ethical practice with patients, family members, and peers, such as protecting autonomy, promoting safety, and speaking out against lateral violence, are discussed. As the nurse is obligated to maintain and improve the moral environment, several chapters discuss the competencies needed to recognize and address organizational and societal issues. Benner (2003) has stated, "It is probably not an exaggeration to say that in every clinical encounter there are ethical issues at the personal, provider, and social levels" (p. 375). While one book cannot encompass all potential situations, our goal is to provide a core framework and useful skills and strategies to actively engage in these issues.

REFERENCE

Benner, P. (2003). Enhancing patient advocacy and social ethics. *American Journal of Critical Care*, *12*(4), 374–375.

Acknowledgments

This book would not be possible without the chapter authors who gave their time and expertise to this project. Their collaboration and contributions exemplify the teamwork required for ethical discourse and outcomes. I am also thankful to the practicing nurses who suggested case scenarios and to those who reviewed various chapters and provided valuable insights and comments. My mentors and role models who encouraged ethical thinking and growth both personally and through their work include Angela P. Clark, PhD, RN, ACNS-BC, FAAN, FAHA; Mary C. Corley, PhD, RN; Carol Pavlish, PhD, RN, FAAN; Vicki Lachman, PhD, APRN, MBE, FAAN; and Patricia Benner, PhD, RN, FAAN. Special thanks go to Elizabeth Nieginski, executive editor at Springer, who nurtured this project from the beginning, and Janet Weber, EdD, RN, for her constructive critiques and remarkable editing skills. Finally, I am grateful daily for the support and patience of my husband, Hugh.

Ethical Competence in Nursing Practice

Foundations of Ethical Nursing Practice

1

Recognizing Ethical Terms, Theories, and Principles

CRAIG M. KLUGMAN

We all make ethical decisions every day. To walk or take public transportation. To buy organic or commercially raised food. To take an extra shift or attend a child's performance. Over a lifetime, we learn how to consider and make choices among these types of situations where we weigh values, consider outcomes, and make choices with consequences. In life, ethics is about being a good person, thinking logically, and making reasoned choices. Ethics helps guide our behavior so that we can live civilly with other people in society.

As a registered nurse, one studies ethics because the everyday ethics we spend a lifetime developing often do not consider the kind of life-and-death decisions that nursing practice requires. Nurses often encounter competing interests/conflicts between their own beliefs, what the profession asks, what the patient wants and needs, what the institution requires, and what other health professionals demand. Studying nursing ethics and bioethics helps one develop tools to navigate the ethical labyrinth of the professional environment.

Examining topics and issues that one is likely to encounter helps the nurse consider how she or he would act in a situation. Having considered varied cases, one has a better idea of how to act when confronted with a real-life dilemma.

In short, ethical nursing is good nursing. As a registered nurse you need to understand that ethics is the process of moral deliberation, of asking and reflecting on questions about how one ought to act or decide in a given situation. Ethics is an essential part of nursing that forms the backbone of how we treat our patients, our health care colleagues, our profession, and each other. You will need to understand Rest's four components of moral competence that includes moral sensitivity, moral judgment, moral motivation, and moral character. Finally, it is important that you clearly understand six tenets of nursing ethics: virtue, caring, beneficence, nonmaleficence, and autonomy.

CASE SCENARIO

Jonathan Garcia has been a nurse for 8 years in labor and delivery. He is currently assisting Mrs. Jackson who is in labor with her third child, at 36 weeks gestation. She has placental previa and has refused to consent for blood transfusion if it should be necessary. On several occasions, Mrs. Jackson presented the team and her obstetrician with information from her church on why she rejects blood and blood products and has shared a copy of her blood refusal card. Dr. McComb is the physician on call and believes that Mrs. Jackson needs a C-section immediately. However, Dr. McComb declines to do surgery with the blood refusal in place.

"Don't you want your baby to live?" Jonathan overhears Dr. McComb saying, "How would you feel if your baby doesn't have a mother?" Mrs. Jackson is in tears and finally relents, "Enough. Please stop talking. Okay do the surgery. Save my baby." During the C-section, Mrs. Jackson hemorrhages and Dr. McComb orders Jonathan to hang 4 units of blood.

Questions to Consider Before Reading On

1. What should Jonathan do?

2. How would the selected provisions/statements from the Code of Ethics (Box 1.1) be used to support Jonathan's actions?

WHY STUDY ETHICS?

Cases like the one Jonathan faces where you have to make decisions without a clear "right" answer are one reason why nurses should study ethics. In ethics, one learns to be aware of sensitive issues and difficult situations. Studying ethics teaches one to form and ask questions, to reflect on the situation, and to consider potential resolutions.

Box 1.1

Ethical Terms, Theories, and Principles—Provisions and Relative Statements From the Code of Ethics

PROVISION 1
The nurse practices with compassion and respect for the inherent dignity, worth, and unique attributes of every person.

FROM INTERPRETIVE STATEMENT 1.4
Respect for human dignity requires the recognition of specific patient rights, in particular, the right to self-determination. Patients have the moral and legal right to determine what will be done with and to their own person; to be given accurate, complete, and understandable information in a manner that facilitates an informed decision; and to be assisted with weighing the benefits, burdens, and available options in their treatment, including the choice of no treatment. They also have the right to accept, refuse, or terminate treatment without deceit, undue influence, duress, coercion, or prejudice and to be given necessary support throughout the decision making and treatment process. . . .

Nurses have an obligation to be knowledgeable about the moral and legal rights of patients. Nurses preserve, protect, and support those rights by assessing the patient's understanding of both the information presented and explaining the implications of decisions.

FROM INTERPRETIVE STATEMENT 2.1
The nurse's primary commitment is to the recipients of nursing and health care services—patient or client—whether individuals, families, groups, communities, or populations. When the patient's wishes are in conflict with others, nurses help resolve the conflict. Where conflict persists, the nurse's commitment remains to the identified patient.

FROM INTERPRETIVE STATEMENT 2.2
Nurses must examine the conflicts arising between their own personal and professional values and the values and interests of others who are also responsible for patient care and health care decisions, and perhaps patients themselves. Nurses address these conflicts in ways that ensure patient safety and promote the patient's best interests while preserving the professional integrity of the nurse and supporting interprofessional collaboration.

(continued)

Box 1.1

Ethical Terms, Theories, and Principles—Provisions and Relative Statements From the Code of Ethics (continued)

PROVISION 6

The nurse, through individual and collective effort, establishes, maintains, and improves the ethical environment of the work setting and conditions of employment that are conducive to safe, quality health care.

FROM INTERPRETIVE STATEMENT 6.1

- Virtues are universal, learned, and habituated attributes of moral character that predispose persons to meet their moral obligations, that is, *to do* what is right.
- There are more particular attributes of moral character, not expected of everyone, that are expected of nurses. These include knowledge, skill, wisdom, patience, compassion, honesty, altruism, and courage. These attributes describe what the nurse is to be as a morally "good nurse."

FROM INTERPRETIVE STATEMENT 6.2

- Obligations focus on what is *right and wrong* or what we are *to do* as moral agents.
- Obligations are often specific in terms of principles such as beneficence or doing good; nonmaleficence or doing no harm; justice or treating people fairly; reparations, or making amends for harm; fidelity, and respect for persons.

FROM INTERPRETIVE STATEMENT 6.3

Nurses are responsible for contributing to a moral environment that demands respectful interactions among colleagues, mutual peer support, and open identification of difficult issues, which includes ongoing professional development of staff in ethical problem solving.

Source: ANA (2015).

WHAT IS ETHICS?

At some point in their careers, most nurses encounter scenarios like the one that Jonathan faces. These challenges may be over patient care, power differentials, differing goals of treatment, or perspective on the patient and family. In this section, we will examine the difference between ethics and morality.

Questions to Consider Before Reading On

1. How would you define ethics in your current nursing practice?

2. Provide an example of how you integrate ethics in everyday practice.

Most people have heard of the concept of ethics and at some point in life, everyone has had to make ethical decisions. Ethics is a part of everyday life. Pick up a newspaper and reports of ethics issues appear regularly: "Elected Official Guilty of Ethics Violation," "CEO of Company X Dismissed on Ethics Charges," "Doctor Reprimanded for Ethics Violations," "News Agency Admits Ethics Violation in Reporting," and "Nurses Struggle with Ethical Dilemmas." Although each of these headlines uses the same word, the term ethics has a very different meaning in each situation.

In general, ethics is the "branch of knowledge dealing with moral principles" ("Ethics," 2014). One of the earliest writers of ethics was the ancient Greek philosopher Aristotle who defined ethics as the application of moral knowledge. This definition is the philosophical one, meaning the examination of how people make decisions regarding what is right and what is wrong. As demonstrated in Table 1.1, the term "ethics" has different meanings in different contexts. When looking at the headlines about ethics in government or business, ethics refers to a branch of the legal code that deals with proper behavior. When an elected official commits an ethics violation, he or she is breaking the law. A business or government ethics violation can lead to fines or imprisonment.

The news agency, physician, and nursing headlines refer to when an organization or a profession develops a code of behavior that members of the profession are expected to follow: "The codes of conduct or moral principles recognized in a particular profession, sphere of activity, relationship, or other context or aspect of human life" ("Ethics," 2014). Rather than being legal precepts, these are violations of agreed upon principles of behavior.

In the world of nursing, ethics is about what one ought to do (or ought not to do). The guide to ethical nursing conduct is the American Nurses Association's Code of Ethics for Nurses (ANA, 2015). Thus, an ethical nurse is one who follows the principles of the Code. A second sense of ethics in nursing is making decisions about right and wrong. These situations are ambiguous and are not anticipated by either law or the Code. Ethics in this sense is a process of moral deliberation where one identifies the ethical issue, collects information, performs an analysis, and makes a well-informed and reflective decision.

Morality

As mentioned previously, ethics is a process of moral deliberation. This begs the question, What are morals and morality? Morality is a personal belief

Table 1.1

Definitions of Ethics

ETHICS	DISCIPLINE	DEFINITION
	Public Policy and Law	Following the legal code that dictates appropriate behavior
	Business	Following the legal code that dictates appropriate behavior Moral principles that guide conduct
	Philosophy	Examination of how people make decisions regarding right and wrong
	Nursing	A professional code of conduct (ANA Code of Ethics) that guides nurses in what they ought to do in professional practice Making decisions about right and wrong in specific clinical situations

about what is right and what is wrong. Our morality is formed from our experiences. We learn it from our parents, our schools, religion, and popular media. Sometimes our morality is irrational and illogical. We might believe that abortion is wrong and capital punishment is acceptable even though both entail ending a potential human future.

Since morality is a belief, it does not have to be defended or explained. It is simply what you know to be true absent evidence. One's morality is individual, even if you share beliefs with others, ultimately your version of right and wrong belongs to you.

Questions to Consider Before Reading On

1. Describe a care situation in which your morality or belief(s) influenced your action(s).

2. What was the outcome of the situation?

3. Did this outcome influence your beliefs and future actions? Why? Why not?

Bioethics

Bioethics is the subfield of philosophy that looks at ethical decision making and proper conduct in the life sciences: "The broad terrain of the moral problems of the life sciences, ordinarily taken to encompass medicine, biology, and some important aspects of the environmental, population and social sciences" (Reich, 1995, 250). This field evolved in the early 1970s and has become the umbrella term for ethics of the various health care professions. Nursing ethics is a subset of bioethics.

Bioethics brings together medical ethics, nursing ethics, public health ethics, and other professionally based ethics into a single subfield as a result of four social forces. The first reason for the rise of bioethics was the rapid advance in life science and health care delivery technology since the mid-20th century. Kidney transplants, chronic dialysis, liver transplants, heart transplants, and in vitro fertilization all changed the way that health care professionals related to the human body and the possibilities for medical healing.

Second, bioethics arises from media reports on abuses in human research. A 1972 article in *The New York Times* by journalist Jean Heller introduced the public to the "Tuskegee Study of Untreated Syphilis in the Negro Male." This was a research program from 1932 to 1972 in which nearly 600 African American men were observed as part of a study in the natural progression of syphilis. Even though a cure for syphilis became widely available in the 1940s, the subjects were actively isolated from access to cure. A second article was a publication by Harvard anesthesiologist Henry Beecher in *The New England Journal of Medicine* where he outlined 22 human research studies that he felt violated ethical standards.

The third social force was engagement with the public. Physicians, nurses, lawyers, theologians, philosophers, and other scholars interested in ethical issues in the life sciences were sought by the media to comment on advances in medical technology. The U.S. government also engaged those active in these issues by recruiting scholars to serve on panels to investigate the social implications of human subjects in research and medical advances in order to guide the development of law, policy, and regulation.

Fourth, bioethics evolves out of the Civil Rights movement. Prior to the 1970s, physicians, and to a lesser extent nurses, made most patient medical decisions. During the late 1960s/early 1970s, people who had limited political voice were demanding their equal rights in the public sphere. Similarly, patients demanded the right to make their own decisions in the health care sphere. Patients and their families wanted to know the diagnosis and prognosis of disease. Rather than being a subject of health care, they wanted to be partners with health care professionals in deciding treatment and future care.

BRIEF HISTORY OF NURSING ETHICS

Since its founding, ethics has been an integral part of the nursing profession. Florence Nightingale, the recognized founder of modern nursing, was particularly concerned with the ethical conduct of her nurses. In her writings from the late 1800s, she explained that a nurse was focused foremost on the patient's recovery and comfort. The nurse is diligent, observant, concise, confident, quiet and knows her role in the health care and household hierarchy (Nightingale, 2010). These values provide guidance for behavior and action in nursing.

Mrs. Lystra E. Gretter wrote the *Florence Nightingale Pledge* in 1893. Gretter, who was at the Farrand Training School for Nurses in Detroit, modified the *Hippocratic Oath* that was followed mainly by physicians. Her pledge focuses primarily on the nurse's character, profession, confidentiality, and relationship to the physician:

> I solemnly pledge myself before God and in the presence of this assembly, to pass my life in purity and to practice my profession faithfully. I will abstain from whatever is deleterious and mischievous, and will not take or knowingly administer any harmful drug. I will do all in my power to maintain and elevate the standard of my profession, and will hold in confidence all personal matters committed to my keeping and family affairs coming to my knowledge in the practice of my calling. With loyalty, will I endeavor to aid the physician in his work, and devote myself to the welfare of those committed to my care (Gretter, 1893).

In 1926, a proposal was put forth by the ANA for a professional nurses code of ethics. This original code was created as part of the development of nursing as a profession and moved from focusing on concerns about the conduct of the nurse (in dress and comportment) to the maintenance of relationships. The 1926 code concerned itself with the nurse's relationship to the patient, to medicine, to allied health professions, to peers, and to the nursing profession. In regard to the patient, the nurse was supposed to devote his or her skill and knowledge to patient care and the patient's family. Nurses were expected to know the practice laws of their state and maintain competence in scientific medicine. This also meant that she or he should "respect the physician as the person legally and professionally responsible for the medical and surgical treatment of the sick" (ANA, 1926, p. 601). In regard to peer relationships, the code recommends following the Golden Rule.

However, it was not until 1950 that the first formal ANA Code of Ethics was adopted. Titled the Code for Professional Nurses, the code was renamed as the Code for Nurses with Interpretive Statements and was revised in 1976, 1985, 2001, and 2015. The Code has three purposes: (1) "statement of the ethical values, obligations, duties and professional ideals of nurses individually

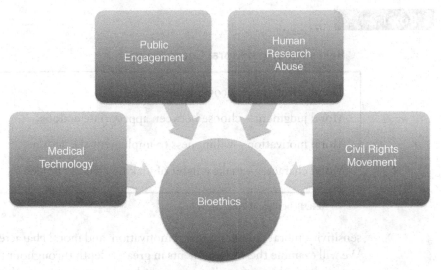

Figure 1.1 Social factors leading to bioethics.

and collectively; (2) profession's non-negotiable ethical standard; and (3) an expression of nursing's own understanding of its commitment to society" (ANA, 2015, p. viii). In its modern iteration, the code offers nine "provisions" that talk about aspirational concepts such as protecting human dignity, advocating for health as a human right, and maintaining the integrity of the profession. It focuses more on global issues and systems-level factors than on individual patients and how to get along with a physician. The Code charges the nurse with protecting the health care environment, encouraging research and scholarship, and working for social justice.

Questions to Consider Before Reading On

1. Figure 1.1 illustrates the social factors leading to the development of bioethics. Choose one factor. How did it influence the development of nursing ethics?

2. How has this, or other factors, influenced the revisions of the Code of Ethics?

ETHICAL DILEMMAS/ISSUES

When working in a clinical environment, it is common to hear someone say that there is an "ethical issue" or that an "ethics consult" is needed for a case. Our everyday ethics do not always serve well in the specific environment of the clinic. Professional scenarios are not those one encounters in the lay world and thus may require a different consideration.

Psychologist James Rest developed the idea that in order for a person to be morally mature, he or she must have four psychological components: moral

Box 1.2

Rest's Theory of Moral Competence

Moral sensitivity—recognize the issue

Moral judgment—choose between appropriate actions

Moral motivation—willingness to implement the action

Moral character—make a habit of making ethical choices

Source: Rest, Bebeau, and Volker (1986).

sensitivity, moral judgment, moral motivation, and moral character (Box 1.2). We will examine these components in greater depth throughout this chapter. Sensitivity is the notion that one must be able to recognize that an ethical dilemma exists and that our actions have implications for others (Rest et al., 1986).

An ethical dilemma is a conflict over values—where there are two competing and important goals that are in opposition to one another. For example, in Jonathan's case there is the patient's belief about blood transfusion and the physician's order to transfuse. Sometimes the members of the health care team will have different goals from each other and those may vary from the desires of the patient and his or her family. For instance, a family may want to bring a dying patient home for a hospice program but the physician wants to try additional treatments.

To identify the ethical dilemma, you can ask several questions:

- Does the situation pose a potential harm to another person?

- Has there been an inability to reach a decision on what steps to take?

- Is there a disagreement on what is important?

- Is there a disagreement on the goals of care?

If the answer to any of these questions is yes, then there may be an ethical dilemma. At the very least, an ethical perspective on the situation may provide some insight and opportunity for reflection.

Question to Consider Before Reading On

1. An ethical dilemma is a "conflict over values." Using the preceding questions, describe how you identified a recent practice situation as an ethical dilemma.

An ethical issue is when there is a question of what a person ought to do or ought not to do. These are questions about appropriate behavior and action. To identify an ethical issue, you can ask several questions:

- Is a power hierarchy influencing the freedom of people to express their opinions or to have their ideas respected?

- Would concern be raised if people outside of the institution (or in the media) knew about this?

- Is a person being asked to do something that would injure her or his personal reputation or integrity?

- Is a person being asked to do something that he or she feels is wrong (i.e., moral distress)?

For example, in the opening case, Mrs. Jackson agreed to blood products despite her stated reasons and providing evidence that she was not in favor of this. But given the power that her physician had over her and her vulnerability, did she have the freedom to speak out? Does Jonathan have the ability to express perhaps a concern about how consent was obtained without fear of losing his job or being moved to a less desirable assignment? How is he going to feel later when the physician orders blood if he believes Mrs. Jackson's beliefs and the consent process were violated? How would the hospital look if the local newspaper published an article that said the hospital let a woman die who could have been saved? Or if the headline said that the hospital bullied a woman into care she did not want? These questions suggest that there is indeed an ethical aspect to the case.

Question to Consider Before Reading On

1. Have you experienced a situation such as Jonathan's in which you felt unable to express a concern about a patient situation? What would have enabled you to express your concerns? Peer/management support? Assertiveness skills?

Once you have identified that there is an ethical dilemma or issue in a case, you have to analyze the case to determine the possible courses of ethical action.

THEORIES

The second part of Rest's theory of moral competence is the component of moral judgment—choosing between available courses of action. Most cases have multiple possible choices and outcomes. Some choices will lead to better outcomes and some to worse, but rarely is there one single correct course of action. The goal is not to find the one "right" course of action, but rather to find the "better" options. One uses reason to determine the possible choices and the implications of those choices.

In this section, we discuss ethical theories that provide perspective on how to approach finding the better answer in a case (Table 1.2). Each theory has a different notion of on what a person should base the decision. Some

Table 1.2

Ethical Theories' Notion of the Good

THEORY	WHAT IS GOOD
Ethics of care	Caring and nurturing
Deontology	Following the moral law, rules, and principles
Utilitarianism	Best outcome; greatest good for the greatest number
Principlism	Autonomy, beneficence, nonmaleficence, and justice

theories say follow the rules, others say choose what makes the best outcome. Each theory has a different notion of *the good*, which is the aim of action or the goal. Think of these theories as tools in your toolbox. You may have an idea that one will work better in the current scenario or you might need to use a couple to determine the various acceptable options.

Ethics of Care

As a psychologist, Carol Gilligan determined that men and women reason differently. Whereas men are focused on rules, principles, and justice, women are more focused on relationships, caring, and nurturing (Gilligan, 1982). This observation led to feminist ethicists developing the ethics of care. In nursing, this is the most important theory because it forms the foundation of nursing ethics.

Ethics of care states that what is good is caring and nurturing. Thus, when making a decision, the better choice is the one that cares for and nurtures the patient. Consider Jonathan. One could argue that an ethics of care would suggest he gives the blood because it is hard to care or nurture for someone who is dead. However, one could also argue that caring and nurturing is supporting a person in their desires. Mrs. Jackson changes her mind only after she is encouraged with bias to consent. An ethics of care might suggest that caring for her is maximizing her right to make her own decisions and to protect her from undue influence and a power imbalance that silences her voice.

Using this theory as a tool points out two potential choices. Choosing between the two can be difficult and that is one of the shortcomings of this theory—being based on relationships and notions of caring and nurturing means that the decision is also based on impressions and feelings internal to the relationship.

Deontology

Deon is a Greek term that means "obligation" or "necessity." Deontology is the idea that the better ethical choice is the one that adheres to a rule or moral law. This theory is also known as "duty-based ethics" since it is a belief that one has an obligation to act according to the rules. If you know the rule, then you should act to follow it.

The most famous deontologist is Immanuel Kant (1724–1804). Kant believed that an action was moral only if it was done with the intent to act out of an obligation to follow the moral law (Kant, 1995). He is a universalist thinker, which means that the rule is the same for every person, in every time, and in every place. In other words, what is right is always right and what is wrong is always wrong. For example, Kant tells us that suicide is always wrong and lying is always wrong.

Kant also believed in the idea of autonomy, that an individual who has the ability to make his or her own decisions should be permitted to do so. Autonomy means self-governance or a person gets to decide what happens to himself or herself.

In the case of Mrs. Jackson, Jonathan must follow the rules as to what is right. One rule might be that the physician makes decisions regarding the medical treatment of the patient. To determine which is the better choice under a deontological framework, one would ask whether the law is a universal one. Should a nurse always follow a physician's orders? What if the physician told the nurse to do something illegal or damaging to her or his reputation? In those situations, clearly the physician should not be followed, which means that this cannot be a rule.

Another rule could be that hospital personnel should always save a life when possible. This would require ignoring all do-not-resuscitate (DNR) orders and always resuscitating even if the patient did not want it. Since this is not a rational action, the rule cannot exist.

Or the rule might be that a patient must consent for treatment and, given Dr. McComb's hard sell, Jonathan may be questioning whether Mrs. Jackson gave informed consent or was simply coerced into signing a document. The same thinking asks whether a patient should be treated when consent may have been given under duress. That would mean that patients could never say no to any procedures. The answer, of course, is that such a rule is not rational. Therefore, Jonathan should not give the treatment because of the questionable circumstances of the consent. That Mrs. Jackson and her baby might die shows a shortcoming of this theory—outcomes are not considered.

Thus, deontology asks us to look at the rules whether those are morality, institutional rules, professional principles, or civic laws.

Utilitarianism

The philosopher Jeremy Bentham is credited with forming the theory of utilitarianism. According to Bentham, utility is an action that increases happiness and decreases pain. In order to determine if an action will indeed serve this purpose, one must look at the potential outcome. Thus, utilitarianism requires one to look at the likely outcomes of an action and choose the one that is most likely to increase pleasure and decrease pain (Bentham, 2007).

More specifically, Bentham was not interested in the benefit to the individual, but to society as a whole. Utilitarianism is the underlying principle of public health ethics where the goal is to produce *the greatest happiness for the greatest number*.

In modern ethics, utilitarianism is often used to mean the best choice is the one that leads to the best outcome for both groups, and, in a clinical setting, for individuals. Looking at the case of Mrs. Jackson, giving her blood would save her life and probably that of her baby. Not giving blood might honor her true wishes, but would also likely lead to her death. The utilitarian perspective would suggest that saving her life not only increases her chances for happiness but would also increase the happiness of her baby and family. A utilitarian would choose to give the blood even though such an action might not reflect Mrs. Jackson's desires.

Principlism

In 1977, philosopher Tom L. Beauchamp and theologian James F. Childress published *The Principles of Biomedical Ethics*. In this volume, they presented four principles to serve as guidelines for moral deliberation: autonomy, nonmaleficence, beneficence, and justice. These principles are not a fundamental theory of the good nor are they rules of behavior. Instead, they are midlevel tenets that derive from common morality—"the universal norms shared by all persons committed to morality" (Beauchamp & Childress, 2013, p. 3).

Autonomy is the notion that humans with the ability and capacity to reason have a right to self-governance. To act with autonomy means that a choice must be intentionally made by a person who has an understanding of the risks, benefits, and alternatives. Additionally, the choice must be voluntary and free from coercion. An autonomous person makes his or her own choices.

Nonmaleficence is the idea that through one's actions, one should do no harm or at the very least, not make things worse. Beneficence is an obligation to promote the welfare of another. This includes preventing harm when possible. For example, if a patient is on a gurney in the hallway underneath a weak ceiling, nonmaleficence says that you should not jump on the weak ceiling, which would harm the patient as it fell on him or her. Beneficence says you should move the patient from under the weak ceiling to prevent harm if it should fall.

Justice is the principle that looks at the community perspective. It asks about the fair distribution of benefits and burdens. Justice also states that likes should be treated alike. In other words, treat people fairly. Thus, a person should not have a lower salary based merely on an arbitrary factor such as sex, ethnicity, religion, age, or sexual orientation. Differences in salary based on skill level, achievement, or years of service are acceptable.

Questions to Consider Before Reading On

1. Have you used any of the theories discussed in this section to address ethical issues in your practice?

2. Which ethical theory or theories seem most relevant in Jonathan's situation with Mrs. Jackson and the surgeon?

Six Tenets for Decision Making

While principlism is the most often used theory in medical ethics, the system does not fully capture the nuances and ethics of care focus that are foundational to nursing. In addition to autonomy, beneficence, nonmaleficence, and justice, nurses have an ethical obligation of virtue and caring.

Virtue is the tenet that a nurse has an obligation to maintain her or his own integrity as well as the integrity of the profession. When considering a case or a decision through the lens of virtue, one should ask how the decision affects personal or professional integrity. How does the choice affect the virtues of nursing—honesty, transparency, standard of care and conduct? One should also consider how similar cases were handled in the past and whether that led to a good outcome.

Caring is the obligation to provide compassion and nurturing to all patients and peers. This tenet asks how a choice supports the patient, the patient's family, and their relationship. It asks if all perspectives have been considered from a cultural, social, religious, and familial point of view. Caring is not only toward the patient, but also toward the self and one's peers. Does an action compromise caring for oneself? For example, if a patient needs to be moved and there is no help around nor transfer equipment, the nurse is not obligated to put herself or himself at personal risk to move the patient improperly even if that would be more convenient. Caring also means supporting other nurses in their work, in mentoring, and in their desires to grow in the profession.

The other four tenets echo the four principles. As tenets they provide guiding questions to assist in moral deliberation. While autonomy is the notion of self-governance, knowing how to apply it to a particular case is facilitated by asking a few questions. For example, is the patient competent and capacitated to make decisions? If the patient is not competent and capacitated, then who makes the decisions? Does the patient or proxy decision maker understand the health condition? Is the patient or proxy capable of expressing the choice? And what are the patient's preferences?

Beneficence is the obligation to provide benefit. How can the nurse help the patient's physical and psychological well-being? How does an action (test, medication, or procedure) stand to improve a patient's condition? And perhaps the question that is often overlooked: In your professional opinion, what is best for the patient? The last question does not mean that you will direct care, or that the patient has to follow your recommendation (autonomy allows the patient to choose). This question acknowledges that as someone who has substantial education and experience in the practice of nursing, your professional opinion should be recognized.

Nonmaleficence holds that we should do no harm. Some methods of prevention are clear—be competent, work within your scope of practice, be aware of any limitations you may have. Some may not be so clear. What biases do you have? These could be biases about the role of the patient, or feelings about people of certain ages, sexes, genders, religions, ethnicities, socioeconomic statuses, sexual orientations, and more. Do you have a bias against people whose behaviors may have been a factor in the disease such as a smoker with lung cancer, an alcoholic with liver disease, or a sun tanner with melanoma? Once a bias is acknowledged, one should ask if that bias is affecting how a patient is treated. Nonmaleficence asks us to look at the negative side effects of a proposed course of action or with no action at all.

Justice is about the community perspective: Are there factors outside the patient–care provider relationship that impact the case? This might include finances, legal obligations, institutional policy, public health interests, and using scarce resources.

When making an ethical decision, going through the six tenets serves as a guide as to what questions you should ask about the ethical dilemma or issue. After working through the chart, you will find that one or two tenets are the crux of the ethical issue. Knowing that, you can use that tenet to solve the case.

For example, take the case of Mrs. Jackson and Nurse Jonathan. By completing the analysis, one sees that the patient's consent may not have been voluntary. Although giving the transfusion may save the patient's life, there is a risk to Mrs. Jackson's psychological and spiritual well-being as well as a threat to her relationships—receiving blood could lead to exile from her church and family. It also becomes clear that her health care surrogate—likely the husband—has not been asked about what her preferences would be. And to protect Jonathan's professional integrity, he has an ethical obligation to speak out. The issue here is autonomy and virtue: Was the patient's autonomy respected and is the nurse being asked to act in a manner that injures integrity?

The third component of Rest's model is moral motivation—making a choice because it is the moral one rather than the personal or convenient one. Using the analysis table, the tenets show that Jonathan should have spoken out at the time that he viewed problems with the consent process. That he did not is because he chose the course that was more convenient, avoided conflict, and prevented any personal consequences to his action. Although Jonathan did not report his concerns before surgery, he has a second chance to demonstrate moral motivation when the surgeon requests blood for the patient. The convenient choice here again is simply to follow the physician and give the blood. The moral choice, however, is something else. Jonathan could speak and say that since Mrs. Jackson changed her mind only under pressure, perhaps they should ask her proxy decision maker. If that is not possible because that individual is not available or time is too short, then if Jonathan feels consent was truly coerced and not what Mrs. Jackson wanted, he should refuse to give the blood (autonomy and virtue). However, if he thinks there is any chance that Mrs. Jackson truly wanted the blood, then he should err on the side of life (beneficence).

During a case such as this, there is not necessarily time to go through the full deliberation. But thinking about these issues beforehand can provide you with some guidelines and thought experiments to help you know what to do when faced with various real-life situations.

Caring and virtue ethics are central to nursing practice and exemplified in the Code of Ethics. They represent the focus of the nurse–patient relationship and the character of the nurse.

Questions to Consider Before Reading On

1. How could an understanding of caring/virtue ethics enhance Jonathan's moral motivation?

2. Recall a recent ethical issue in your practice. How could aspects of caring/virtue ethics be used to reflect on the issue?

ETHICS IS ACTION

Aristotle said that knowing the right thing to do was not enough; you have to actually do the right thing. How you approach the doing is a key detail. Aristotle felt that you had to volunteer to do the right thing; that you had to be deliberately aware that you were doing it; and that making good choices had to be a consistent and established part of your character (Aristotle, 1962). The notion of moral character is the fourth component of Rest's model, which he defines as "executing and implementing a play of action" (Rest et al., 1986, p. 15). A person must follow through with the moral choice, work around barriers, and demonstrate courage and strength to see that the moral choice happens.

For the purposes of the opening case, let us assume that Jonathan knows not giving the blood is the right thing to do because informed consent did not happen. Is Jonathan willing to say "no" to the surgeon, thus creating conflict? Would he accept possible consequences of being removed from the operating room at the surgeon's request or even being brought before a review panel or hearing? In other words, will he put his ethics into action and accept the consequences?

CONCLUSION

The ethical theories presented here provide you with perspectives and methods for identifying ethical dilemmas and issues, analyzing cases, determining the possible choices, and selecting a more right choice.

Ethics in terms of nursing is about what behaviors and attitudes a nurse ought to practice. In general, ethics is a process of moral deliberation. For the profession, such deliberation has led to the nursing Code of Ethics that dictates the virtues, values, skills, attitudes, and knowledge that a nurse should have. Morality is one's personal belief about what is right and wrong. An ethical dilemma is when there is a conflict in values. An ethical issue is when there is a question about what one ought to or ought not to do.

Nursing ethics is part of the modern movement of bioethics. Bioethics evolved out of rapid advances in health sciences technology, human research abuses, public engagement, and the Civil Rights movement. Concerns about nursing etiquette were espoused by Florence Nightingale and other early nurses. This notion of etiquette—acceptable courteous behaviors—became part of the Florence Nightingale Pledge in 1893. In 1950, The Code for Professional Nurses established the values, duties, and ideals of nursing.

Psychologist James Rest suggests that there are four steps to making an ethical decision—moral sensitivity, moral judgment, moral motivation, and moral character. Ethical theories can help one in analyzing cases to determine the "more right" choice. Nursing ethics are based in the ethics of care theory, which focuses on caring for and nurturing individuals as its highest good. Other theories believe the good action is one that follows rules (deontology) or provides the greatest outcome for the greatest number (utilitarianism). The principles of biomedical ethics are a set of four midlevel principles to guide one in ethical thought—autonomy, nonmaleficence, beneficence, and justice.

The six tenets of nursing ethics incorporate the four principles of autonomy, nonmaleficence, beneficence, and justice, but also add virtue and caring as reflective of the unique nature of the nursing profession and the relationships nurses have with their patients and society-at-large. An understanding of nursing ethics is essential in providing competent care and supporting the profession, nurse, patients, and society.

Question to Consider Before Reading On

Box 1.3 presents Quality and Safety Education for Nurses (QSEN) competencies relevant to the discussion in this chapter.

1. How might Jonathan have demonstrated these competencies in the situation with Mrs. Jackson and the surgeon?

Box 1.3

Ethical Terms, Theories, and Principles: Relevant QSEN Competencies

Acknowledge the tension that may exist between patient rights and the organizational responsibility for professional, ethical care. (Attitudes)

Communicate patient values, preferences, and expressed needs to other members of health care team. (Skills)

Describe strategies to empower patients or families in all aspects of the health care process. (Knowledge)

Elicit patient values, preferences, and expressed needs as part of clinical interview, implementation of care plan, and evaluation of care. (Skills)

Explore ethical and legal implications of patient-centered care. (Knowledge)

Respect patient preferences for degree of active engagement in care process. (Attitudes)

Value active partnership with patients or designated surrogates in planning, implementation, and evaluation of care. (Attitudes)

Source: Cronenwett et al. (2007), pp. 123–129.

Critical Thinking Questions and Activities

Eunice Rivers Laurie was a public health nurse who played a central role in the Tuskegee syphilis study. Considering the time frame of the study (1932–1972), read the following article by Susan Reverby (1999) and discuss Nurse Rivers's role in the study.

1. Discuss the ethical theories, tenets, and components of ethical decision making (Rest) that would have been applicable in Nurse Rivers's situation.

http://ftp.columbia.edu/itc/hs/pubhealth/p9740/readings/reverby.pdf

Read the following article by Epstein and Turner (2015) that addresses the value and history of the Code of Ethics.

1. Discuss the reasons for the major changes to the 2015 Code of Ethics and the implication for your current practice.

(continued)

Critical Thinking Questions and Activities *(continued)*

2. The 2015 Code "requires each nurse to demonstrate ethical competence in professional life" (ANA, 2015, p. vii). What does it mean to be ethically competent?

http://www.nursingworld.org/MainMenuCategories/ANAMarketplace/
ANAPeriodicals/OJIN/TableofContents/Vol-20-2015/No2-May-2015/
The-Nursing-Code-of-Ethics-Its-Value-Its-History.html

REFERENCES

American Nurses Association. (1926). A suggested code. *American Journal of Nursing, 26*(8), 599–601.

American Nurses Association. (2015). *Code of ethics for nurses with interpretive statements*. Silver Spring, MD: Nursesbooks.org. Retrieved from www.nursingworld.org/MainMenuCategories/EthicsStandards/CodeofEthicsforNurses/Code-of-Ethics-For-Nurses.html

Aristotle. (1962). *Nichomachean ethics* (M. Ostwald, Trans.). Englewood Cliffs, NJ: Library of Liberal Arts.

Beauchamp, T. L., & Childress, J. F. (2013). *Principles of biomedical ethics* (7th ed.). New York, NY: Oxford University Press.

Bentham, J. (2007). *An introduction to the principles of morals and legislation*. Mineola, NY: Dover Philosophical Classics.

Cronenwett, L., Sherwood, G., Barnsteiner J., Disch, J., Johnson, J., Mitchell, P., . . . Warren, J. (2007). Quality and safety education for nurses. *Nursing Outlook, 55*(3), 122–131.

Epstein, B., & Turner, M. (2015). The nursing code of ethics: Its value, its history. *The Online Journal of Issues in Nursing, 20*(2). Retrieved from http://www.nursingworld.org/MainMenuCategories/ANAMarketplace/ANAPeriodicals/OJIN/TableofContents/Vol-20-2015/No2-May-2015/The-Nursing-Code-of-Ethics-Its-Value-Its-History.html

Ethics. (2014). *Oxford English Dictionary* (3rd ed.). Retrieved from http://www.oed.com.ezproxy.depaul.edu/view/Entry/355823?redirectedFrom=ethics#eid

Gilligan, C. (1982). *In a different voice: Psychological theory and women's development*. Cambridge, MA: Harvard University Press.

Gretter, L. E. (1893). Florence Nightingale Pledge. Retrieved from http://nursingworld.org/FunctionalMenuCategories/AboutANA/WhereWeComeFrom/FlorenceNightingalePledge.aspx

Kant, I. (1995). *Foundations of the metaphysics of morals* (L. W. Beck, Trans., 2nd ed.). Upper Saddle River, NJ: Library of Liberal Arts.

Nightingale, F. (2010). In V. Skretkowicz (Ed.), *Notes on nursing & notes on nursing for the labouring classes*. New York, NY: Springer Publishing Company. Retrieved from http://www.springerpub.com/florence-nightingale-s-notes-on-nursing-and-notes-on-nursing-for-the-labouring-classes.html

Reich, W. T. (1995). Bioethics. In W. T. Reich (Ed.), *Encyclopedia of bioethics* (2nd ed.). New York, NY: Macmillan Publishing.

Rest, J. R., Bebeau, M., & Volker, J. (1986). An overview of the psychology of morality. In J. R. Rest (Ed.), *Moral development: Advances in research and theory* (pp. 1–27). New York, NY: Praeger.

Reverby, S. (1999). Rethinking the Tuskegee Syphilis Study. Retrieved from http://ftp.columbia.edu/itc/hs/pubhealth/p9740/readings/reverby.pdf

Developing Ethical Skills: A Framework

CATHERINE ROBICHAUX

Upon completion of this chapter, the reader will be able to:

- Describe the role of personal values clarification in ethical skills development
- Discuss how ethical sensitivity contributes to the interpretation of an ethical situation
- Distinguish ethical from nonethical situations
- Apply the components of an ethical decision-making model
- Explain strategies to maintain ethical motivation and overcome personal/professional barriers to implementing an ethical decision
- Discuss the purpose of reflection on and evaluation of an ethical decision

Nurses encounter ethical questions in their everyday clinical practice and often experience uncertainty about patient/family concerns related to informed consent, quality of life, surrogate decision making, and other issues. As members of an interdisciplinary health care team, nurses may also confront ethical situations in their professional relationships with peers. Increased challenges are posed when these issues occur in an environment with a deficient ethical climate that does not support the moral agency of the nurse. As a registered nurse, you may have had an ethics course or some content in your initial nursing preparatory program. However, you will find that more in-depth knowledge and skills will be very useful to assist you with effectively addressing the existing and potential ethical issues you face on a daily basis.

This chapter presents a framework for the development of ethical skills in nursing practice (Robichaux, 2012; Robinson et al., 2014): James Rest's four-component model (FCM; 1986). The FCM describes the deliberative thought processes that occur from recognition of situation with ethical content, as in the Case Scenario, to implementation of a justifiable action. The FCM integrates the cognitive and affective processes that form an understanding of ethical nursing practice: sensitivity, judgment, motivation, and action. As with attainment of clinical skills and expertise, ethical skills can be experientially learned and refined over time through role modeling and other strategies that are presented.

CASE SCENARIO

John received his BSN after serving in the army as a medic. He has worked in the critical care unit (CCU) of a 400-bed community hospital in the Southwest for several years and recently attained certification as a critical care nurse (CCRN). John has become very familiar with Mr. T and his family as the patient has been admitted to the CCU three times within the last 6 months for exacerbations of severe heart failure (HF). On this admission, Mr. T's condition deteriorated rapidly with episodes of hypotension and worsening renal function requiring use of inotropes, intubation, and dialysis.

Following 8 days of aggressive treatment, Mr. T is alert and showing signs of improvement and a decision is made to begin weaning him from the ventilator. After numerous unsuccessful weaning attempts over the next week, Mr. T is diagnosed with ventilator dependence and a decision is made to perform a tracheotomy. John has cared for Mr. T and his family during this hospitalization. He believes that Mr. T and his family do not fully understand various treatment options and possible implications despite discussing them in a family care conference.

VALUES AND ETHICAL SKILLS

Ethical behavior and action in nursing practice evolve from personal values that inform and direct our decisions in all aspects of our lives. An understanding of our values requires self-awareness and continual appraisal of our motivations in situations with ethical content. This understanding can be considered preliminary to the first component in developing ethical skills, ethical sensitivity.

"A value can be defined as a belief upon which one acts by preference" (Olpin & Hesson, 2016, p. 135). Values inform our actions and provide direction and meaning in life. Personal values are formed over time and can be influenced by family, culture, education, and the environment, among other factors. Certain values may be constant while others may change or evolve in response to experiences. Rokeach (2008) identified two types of values: instrumental and terminal. Instrumental values are personal characteristics that we possess or aspire to, such as being ambitious, caring, or intelligent. Terminal values are those that we consider most important or desirable and may include security, love, and independence. Instrumental values assist in attaining terminal values. As these core values become part of who we are, they may influence recognition of ethical situations and/or impact decision making in less than conscious ways.

Awareness of one's values is an important first step in developing ethical skills and competence. This recognition also enables us to identify and articulate these values when they are challenged in professional and/or organizational contexts. Approaches to value clarification can involve the use of real or hypothetical situations, group or individual work, self-analysis, or other methods. It is a continual, reflective process that promotes alignment of our thoughts with our actions, thus enhancing personal integrity (Burkhardt & Nathaniel, 2014).

Developing self-awareness includes being actively conscious of our thoughts and physical/emotional reactions and questioning, in a nonjudgmental manner, why we are feeling that way. This awareness may enable us to identify the underlying value that is reflected or challenged in a given situation. It may also assist in developing the ability to step back and listen to others' interpretations of the same situation. Listening to and discussing our reactions with others help us to articulate our own values and perhaps revise our perspectives (Olpin & Hesson, 2016).

Case Scenario (CONTINUED)

Returning to the Case Scenario, John considers why he thinks that Mr. T and his family are not fully informed of treatment alternatives. He believes Mr. T would not want to be placed in a facility for ventilator-dependent patients, a likely outcome that was presented briefly during the family conference. John also has difficulty imagining a life dependent on a machine. Although he understands the benefits of technology in achieving therapeutic outcomes, he does not think that will happen for Mr. T. who had told John that he does not want to be a burden for his family.

In exploring his reactions to the situation, John realizes that he highly values his ability to engage in and enjoy many different sports and be independent. He is very physically fit, similar to his father and brothers. John discusses his thoughts with Jackie who has been a nurse for over 10 years and was his preceptor. Jackie asks if Mr. T, who is Japanese American, and his family have discussed possible future outcomes. She also suggests that culturally they may have a more communal approach to making these decisions. John states, "Mrs. T is not well and her two daughters live out of town. She has said that she can't care for Mr. T at home and would not be able to visit him very often. I don't think he would want to live that way. No one has talked with the family enough about the possible need for long-term care."

As nurses increasingly work with both patients and providers from different cultural backgrounds, awareness of personal values and understanding those of others are essential to ethical practice. This understanding is also considered an essential Quality and Safety Education for Nurses (QSEN) competency for both undergraduate and graduate nurses, as presented in Table 2.1. Because values are learned within the context of a particular culture, a value such as respect for individual autonomy may not be shared in a culture that is relationship centered and prefers communal decision making. The provision of patient centered care that is culturally sensitive does not require the provider to ignore his/her values. It does, however, emphasize relationships and understanding of the cultural worldview of others rather than simply offering a choice to participate in clinical decisions about what treatments to forgo or accept. This cross-cultural reflection is especially important when exploring potential end-of-life care (Johnstone, 2012).

Question to Consider Before Reading On

You can begin to determine your personal values by answering general questions such as:

1. Where would I like to be in 5 to 10 years or what would I like someone to say about me in my eulogy?

ETHICAL SENSITIVITY

Ethical sensitivity involves the ability to interpret and identify with the reactions and feelings of others. This skill involves an awareness of how our actions or inactions in a given situation may affect others and, in so doing, assume a sense of responsibility or obligation. It can be said that all nursing actions and interactions are inherently ethical in nature as they are aimed at achieving good for patients, families, and all those who are recipients of care. Ethical sensitivity is also relevant in our relationships with peers and coworkers. As Benner (2003) has observed, "It is not an exaggeration to say that in every clinical encounter, there may ethical issues at the personal, provider, and social levels" (p. 375).

How do we distinguish between ethical situations or problems and those that are nonethical, what Burkhardt and Nathaniel (2014) refer to as "practical dilemmas" or "decisional conflicts"? Routine problems are generally those that focus on preference, expediency, and economy. They can usually be resolved with appropriate information and resources. In contrast, ethical problems are described by terms such as harm, benefit, right, wrong, and so on, and have elements of uncertainty, value, and conflict. A situation may have ethical content when an action freely performed or not performed has the potential to harm or cause considerably less benefit to others. Harms can include death, pain (physical, emotional, spiritual), loss of freedom, opportunity, or loss of dignity or self-esteem (Gert, 2005).

Table 2.1	

Developing Ethical Skills: Relevant QSEN Competencies

Integrate understanding of multiple dimensions of patient-centered care: patient/family/community preferences, values information, communication, and education. (Knowledge)

Elicit patient values, preferences, and expressed needs as part of clinical interview, implementation of care plan, and evaluation of care. (Skills)

Communicate patient values, preferences, and expressed needs to other members of health care team. (Skills)

Value seeing health care situations "through patients' eyes." (Attitudes)

Respect and encourage individual expression of patient values, preferences, and expressed needs. (Attitudes)

Willingly support patient-centered care for individuals and groups whose values differ from own. (Attitudes)

Describe basic principles of consensus building and conflict resolution. (Knowledge)

Participate in building consensus or resolving conflict in the context of patient care. (Skills)

Value continuous improvement of own communication and conflict resolution skills. (Attitudes)

Value the perspectives and expertise of all health team members. (Attitudes)

Respect the centrality of the patient/family as core member of any health care team. (Attitudes)

Act with integrity, consistency, and respect for differing views. (Skills)

Use effective practices to manage team conflict. (Skills)

Source: AACN (2012); Cronenwett et al. (2007).

Practical dilemmas or decisional conflicts may arise in situations in which moral claims compete with nonmoral claims that are characterized by self-interest or based on personal values (Burkhardt & Nathaniel, 2014). For example, in the Case Scenario, John may have been required to work overtime when caring for Mr. T during his initial admission crisis. John may have perceived a practical dilemma or a conflict of duties if he had promised his father that he would accompany him to a football game. This personal duty, however, does not have the same moral obligation as that of caring for Mr. T.

Sensitivity to situations that may contain ethical content can help nurses avoid erroneously identifying some issues as strictly clinical or administrative. As examples, nurse fatigue (ANA, 2014) and an inadequate number of registered nurses (Duffield et al., 2011) have been associated with a higher incidence of medication errors and increased patient mortality rates. In addition, fatigue impacts the health and safety of nurses resulting in a host of potential physical disorders and injury risk factors related to drowsy driving (ANA, 2014). Box 2.1 presents an application of Rest's FCM to a case of nurse fatigue.

Box 2.1

Application of the Four-Component Model to a Nurse Fatigue Case Scenario

Carmen and Charles have worked together on the pediatric oncology unit of a large, academic medical center for about 5 years. Recently, Charles has begun working the night shift, 7 p.m. to 7 a.m., so he can attend school during the day to finish his BSN. Carmen has received report from Charles and assumed care of his patients on the day shift on several occasions. In the past 2 weeks, Carmen notices that Charles appears very exhausted during morning report. She also found him dozing in the break room while his patient's infusion device was alarming and noticed several errors in his documentation. Today, Charles reported to Carmen that he rescheduled several medications for one patient because he had overlooked administering them at the proper time.

ETHICAL SENSITIVITY
Carmen thinks about the possible patient harm that could occur from Charles's fatigue but wonders if it might be temporary until he adjusts to the night shift. She is aware of her primary ethical obligation to the patients but also considers her professional relationship with Charles and the potential impact to his career if she reports the incidents. Carmen decides to first share her concerns with Charles who states: "Well, nothing really happened. I'll get used to the hours."

ETHICAL JUDGMENT
Carmen considers the components of the ethical decision-making framework. The questions assist her in recognizing her principal responsibility to protect the patients as presented in the Code of Ethics (2015), which is also consistent with maintaining her moral integrity. However, she also values her professional relationship with Charles and his usual consistent ability to provide excellent patient care. Carmen

(continued)

Box 2.1

Application of the Four-Component Model to a Nurse Fatigue Case Scenario *(continued)*

realizes that there is a conflict between the principles of beneficence (supporting Charles) and nonmaleficence (avoiding patient harm). She decides to talk with Charles once again before discussing the issue with the nurse manager.

ETHICAL MOTIVATION

In Carmen's second conversation with Charles about his fatigue and the potential for patient harm, he again states that he will get accustomed to the hours soon and she is not to worry. Carmen thinks about the next step and wonders if she will alienate Charles and the other nurses if she brings her concerns to the nurse manager. She does not want to jeopardize the cohesive nursing teamwork on the unit and is generally not a person who "speaks up" or "makes waves." Carmen discusses her hesitation with the nurse educator who agrees to go with her to speak with the nurse manager.

ETHICAL ACTION

After the nurse manager listens to Carmen's concerns, she and the nurse educator agree to speak with Charles about the possible consequences of his fatigue. They also know that the issue of nurse fatigue is not limited to Charles and there have been several "near misses" on the unit. The manager and nurse educator decide to present a class integrating the American Nurses Association (ANA) position statement on nurse fatigue (2014) and related evidence-based strategies designed to promote patient safety and the health of the nurse. One of these practices, creating a respite room where night nurses are encouraged to nap or rest, will be instituted immediately. The nurse manager will also work with Charles and other nurses to ensure that they do not work more than 12 hours a day or more than 40 hours in 7 days (Trossman, 2015).

Recognition of a situation with ethical content can be especially challenging in the present health care environment where the primary focus is often on efficiency and cost savings. Research suggests that professional socialization and organizational structures may impact nurses' and other providers' ability to be sensitive to the moral content of their practice. Insufficient or unsupportive coworkers and lack of time to provide adequate care may lead to perceptions of inadequacy and failed expectations resulting in erosion of ethical sensitivity and dulling of moral conscience (Gustafson, Eriksson, Strandberg, & Norberg, 2010).

Ethical sensitivity involves an understanding of alternate courses of action and how each might affect patients, family members, coworkers, administration, and others. This understanding may also avoid moral certainty, which can result in insensitivity to new information or alternative solutions. Moral certainty compels one to act on a chosen resolution to an uncomfortable situation but does not guarantee a positive outcome (Wurzbach, 2005). Respect for alternative perspectives, such as Jackie's and the surgeon's, is necessary if constructive dialogue is to occur and contribute to developing and sustaining a moral community. Gallagher and Tschudin (2010) describe a moral community as one in which values are made clear and shared, where these values direct ethical action, and where all feel safe to be heard.

Emotion and empathy are central in developing ethical sensitivity. To discriminate appropriately in an ethical situation, the nurse must be able to put himself or herself in the other's position as noted in the QSEN competency, "Value seeing health care situations 'through the patients' eyes'" (Table 2.1). Overidentification and the influence of personal motives must be avoided, however. This skill can be enhanced through self-knowledge, critical reflection, and awareness of individual values, biases, and assumptions.

Case Scenario (CONTINUED)

John thinks about his conversation with Jackie and her perspectives on the situation. He reflects on his motivation and still believes that Mr. T and his family do not fully understand treatment options and possible outcomes. John discusses his concerns with the surgeon performing the tracheotomy who states, "They seemed to understand everything during the care conference. I know the intensivist wants to move ahead with the trach quickly so the patient can be moved out of the ICU." John replies, "I don't think they completely understand the possibility that he will eventually be placed in a ventilator dependent facility or the chances that he may never be able to breath on his own. I understand the need to move the patient out of the ICU but the family requires more information like the option of terminal weaning." "You will have to speak to the intensivist about that," responds the surgeon, "I doubt that he will discuss that with the family."

Questions to Consider Before Reading On

1. Can you describe a situation in which you or a class peer/colleague "overidentified" with a patient and/or family member?

2. What skills may be needed to maintain ethical sensitivity while avoiding overidentification?

ETHICAL JUDGMENT

The second component of the Rest's framework, ethical judgment or decision making, has been widely studied in nursing and other disciplines (Page, 2012; Park, 2012). This deliberative process should reflect knowledge of ethical principles, theories, and professional codes. As with the decision-making model developed by Craig Klugman (see Table 2.2), used in this chapter and in several others in this text, most have elements that outline an approach to reaching a judgment through identifying and organizing facts so one can reflect on the issues. Use of a systematic and comprehensive process serves to improve the quality of ethical decisions (Grace, 2014).

Some decision-making models are linear while others revisit previous steps, as necessary with the overall goal of making a prudent choice, not achieving certainty. Most models integrate diverse ethical theories and approaches, as one alternative is not applicable for every ethical situation. Issues that arise during daily practice may not need in-depth consideration of all elements in a model. Others may be more complex such as in the Case Scenario and require careful evaluation (Robichaux, 2012).

The decision-making model can be applied at different stages in an ethical situation. It can be used by an individual nurse or the interdisciplinary team and patient/family to think through an ethical decision. In the Case Scenario, John may or may not be involved in the final decisions about Mr. T's treatment and placement. However, he can use the model to guide judgment regarding his concern about the patient's and family's lack of knowledge about treatment options and outcomes, as presented in Table 2.2.

The decision-making model presented in Table 2.2 contains specific questions to consider that relate to the four principles of bioethics: autonomy, beneficence, justice, and nonmaleficence. Those questions associated with virtue and care ethics acknowledge the moral integrity of the nurse and his or her caring relationship with the "other," in this case, the patient and his family. Every question in the model may not be relevant in every situation. In reality, there may never be enough information to ensure that a decision is perfect; however, it is possible to gain sufficient insight by considering the questions posed.

Questions to Consider Before Reading On

Recall an ethical situation that left you feeling concerned. Explore this situation with a class peer or colleague using the decision-making framework in Table 2.2.

1. What insights did you gain?

2. Would you or your class peer or colleague have done things the same or differently?

Table 2.2

Application of Ethical Decision-Making Model (developed by Craig Klugman)

VIRTUE	CARING
▪ Does the proposed action uphold the nurse's professional integrity? *Yes, by acting in accordance with professional value of advocacy.* ▪ Does the proposed action (and how it is discussed) uphold honesty and transparency? *Yes, by presenting action to all stakeholders.* ▪ Does the proposed action require any deviation from the nurses' standard of care? *No.* ▪ Does the proposed action coalesce with how the nurse has dealt with similar situations in the past? *Has not called for ethics consult before but discussed action with nurse mentor.*	▪ How does the proposed action support the care of the patient? *By ensuring that patient and family are aware of all options and potential outcomes.* ▪ How does the proposed action support the patient's relationships with family? With care providers? *All stakeholders will be involved in the ethics consultation.* ▪ What cultural/social/religious/and family issues need to be considered? *The family believes in communal decision making and respect for elders.* ▪ Have all necessary perspectives been considered? *Yes, and will be discussed during the ethics consult.*
AUTONOMY	**BENEFICENCE**
▪ Is the patient competent and capacitated to make decisions? *Yes.* ▪ Is the patient capable of expressing a choice? *Yes.* ▪ Who is the decision maker? *The patient and his family.* ▪ Does the patient understand his or her condition? *Yes, to a certain extent but perhaps not entirely.* ▪ What are the patient's preferences? *A purpose of the consult is to clarify the patient's preferences.*	▪ How can you the nurse help the patient's physical and psychological health? *I believe the ethics consult will help clarify options/outcomes for the patient/family.* ▪ How does the proposed treatment, test, or action benefit the patient? *As mentioned previously, hopefully, it will help them make better informed choices.* ▪ What are the likely positive outcomes of your actions? *The patient/family will have better understanding as will the care providers.* ▪ In your professional opinion, what is best for the patient? *What is best is what the patient/family wants, but they should know all the options.*

(continued)

Table 2.2

Application of Ethical Decision-Making Model Application of Ethical Decision-Making Model (developed by Craig Klugman) *(continued)*

NONMALEFICENCE	JUSTICE
■ What are your biases? *I would not want to be dependent on a machine and live in a long-term care facility. I think that the patient/ family should have all the information unless they say otherwise.* ■ What can be done to protect the patient? *If the patient/ family have already made up their minds, we should not try to impose our opinions* ■ Would the proposed action cause harm or make the patient worse? *I have talked with the patient/family about the purpose of the ethics consult and they have agreed.* ■ What negative outcomes are possible with and without the proposed action? *The patient has the tracheotomy without being aware of alternatives and possible outcomes. The patient is informed of alternatives and outcomes and chooses the tracheotomy or no intervention.*	■ What scarce resources are involved in patient care? *The patient has been in the ICU for 2 weeks. He has end-stage HF and is ventilator dependent. There is a possibility that he will be transferred to an LTC facility.* • If applicable, should these scarce resources be used on this patient? *This may be discussed during the consult.* ■ What is the patient's financial/insurance situation? *The patient does not have long-term care insurance.* ■ What are the larger social concerns? • Legal obligations • Institutional policy • Public health interests *Not noted at this point.*

HF, heart failure; ICU, intensive care unit; LTC, long-term care.

ETHICAL MOTIVATION

It can be said that all nurses want to be ethical and live in a manner consistent with their moral values. Although they may recognize an ethical issue and, like John, identify a justifiable course of action, they may encounter personal or professional barriers that impede their motivation to act. As the third element in the FCM, ethical motivation is the bridge between ethical judgment and action. Competing personal values such as protecting one's position or reputation can understandably obstruct action as can lack of ethical sensitivity or knowledge regarding professional obligations. For example, since John has been a nurse for only 2 years, he may be reluctant to speak out believing it may harm his relationship with other nurses and the physicians. He also realizes that very few nurses in the unit have called for an ethics consult. John may question his judgment about the situation or capacity to participate in the consultation process. In addition, he may believe that calling for an ethics consultation will jeopardize his relationship with and ability to care for Mr. T and his family (Gaudine, Lamb, LeFort, & Thorne, 2011; Pavlish, Brown-Saltzman, Jakel, & Fine, 2013).

"Persevering to do the right thing" in an ethical situation (Grace, Robinson, Jurchak, Zollfrank, & Lee, 2014, p.14) can also be affected by institutional barriers. There may be lack of supervisory support, fear of reprisal, or limited access to ethics resources. Poor collaboration with physicians in such ethically difficult situations may also silence nurses' moral voices (Pavlish et al., 2013). These obstacles may characterize a unit or organizational ethical climate that does not promote patient/family advocacy and nurse moral agency. The moral distress that can result from these perceived personal and institutional barriers may be overcome by developing moral courage, also discussed in Chapter 4.

Although not addressed by Rest (1986) in the original FCM framework, he and others (Bebeau, Rest, & Narvaez, 2009; Chambers, 2010) explored moral courage in discussions of personal characteristics that influence motivation and action. Individuals with moral courage have developed the skills of effective engagement and the "willingness to speak out and do what is right in the face of forces that would lead a person to act in some other way" (Lachman, 2007, p.131). Lachman (2007, 2009, 2010a, 2010b; Lachman, Murray, Iseminger, & Ganske, 2012) has written extensively about moral courage in nursing and links it to virtue ethics, which emphasizes the role of character in ethical situations. Hawkins and Morse (2014) describe moral courage in nursing practice as "risk taking actions, despite fear for self and others with the intent to ensure safe patient care," which can be "learned, practiced, and mentored" (p. 268). Nurses may develop moral courage by consistently practicing in an ethically courageous manner similar to developing expertise in clinical skills through constant application.

Many ethical situations are difficult and, despite excellent motivation, are emotionally and cognitively overwhelming. It may be challenging to remember what actions to take when encountering a situation that requires moral courage. Lachman et al. (2007, 2012) have developed a useful mnemonic (CODE; Box 2.2) that reminds nurses of their ethical obligations and actions as detailed in the Code of Ethics (2015). The CODE strategy helps recall these actions and includes ways to overcome fear and reluctance to speak up including reflection, reframing, and assertiveness skills.

The **C (courage)** in the CODE mnemonic refers to evaluating the necessity for moral courage in a situation. This step involves careful consideration of the relevant information to determine the need for further evaluation and possible intervention. The **O (obligations to honor)** in the mnemonic reminds the nurse to reflect on his or her obligations as contained in the Code of Ethics (2015). John may refer to Provision 1.4, The Right to Self Determination, which states:

> Patients have the moral and legal right . . . to be given accurate, complete, and understandable information in a manner that facilitates an informed decision . . . Nurses preserve, protect, and support those rights by assessing the patient's understanding of the information presented and explaining the implications of all potential decisions. (p. 2)

Time for reflection also avoids reaction and action based on unexamined moral certainty and allows a "time out" for thinking about those values and ethical principles that may be at risk for compromise. For example, John considers the surgeon and intensivist's differences of opinion regarding Mr. T's understanding of the situation. John does not want to engage in judgmental communication with other providers and reflects on the ethical principle(s) involved. If Mr. T and his family are not fully informed and knowledgeable about possible treatment alternatives and future outcomes, they cannot make fully autonomous choices. Although some information was provided during the family conference, John believes Mr. T and his family did not have adequate time to think about or discuss their values and preferences. The physicians may believe that avoiding additional discussion is in the patient's "best interest," a form of benevolence. They may also be concerned about justice issues related to continued use of scarce resources in the ICU. In shared decision making, a component of family-centered care, "clinicians and patients share the best available evidence when faced with the task of making decisions, and . . . patients are supported to consider options, to achieve informed preferences" (Elwyn et al., 2012, p. 1361). This approach is also supported by the Institute of Medicine (IOM; Alston et al., 2014).

Box 2.2

CODE: Components of Moral Courage

C Courage: Determine if moral courage is needed to address the situation.

O Obligations to honor: Take a time-out to reflect on your ethical obligations and determine what moral values or ethical principles are at risk in the situation.

D Danger management: Use cognitive approaches to handle your fear and risk aversion.

E Expression: Express your beliefs and take action through assertiveness.

Adapted from Lachman et al. (2012). Used with permission.

The **D (danger management)** in the CODE mnemonic represents danger management and addresses developing cognitive strategies and approaches to overcoming risk aversion such as cognitive reframing and self-soothing. Cognitive reframing involves learning how to substitute negative thought processes with positive self-talk. Moral courage can be facilitated by responding to the worry associated with the potential negative consequences of an interpersonal interaction with positive thoughts. Asking ourselves the "what if" question, that is, what if the horrible event or terrible reaction does really happen? What would be our response? This strategy allows us to consider ways to address the overwhelming situation and appreciate our ability to plan for and control the event to a certain extent. For example, John thinks, "What if the surgeon and intensivist are angry about my requesting an ethics consult and this affects our professional relationship?" To cognitively reframe these negative thoughts, he considers the tactics he learned and used in the military to deal with angry individuals and how they could be employed in the "what if" situation (Lachman et al., 2012).

In self-soothing, another danger-management strategy, the nurse can use various approaches to quiet or calm himself or herself when anticipating negative or fearful circumstances. In self-soothing, the nurse may find a middle ground between being detached and removed or experiencing an emotional crisis or upheaval. These methods generally involve physical techniques that activate different body senses. Spending time in a peaceful setting, taking a brief walk, listening to music, or even looking out the window can serve to self-sooth and build moral courage. Additional strategies include venting to a friend and journaling (Lachman, 2010a).

Case Scenario (CONTINUED)

John talks with Jackie and another nurse, Anita, about his decision to request an ethics consult. Anita has experience with submitting a request and Jackie has participated in an ethics consultation for one of her patients. He discusses his reservations about offending the surgeon and intensivist and thinks about his ability to participate in the consultation process. Anita and Jackie state that although "the physicians might not be happy," it seems to be "the right thing to do." They agree to help him with the consult request submission and review what might occur during the actual process.

Questions to Consider Before Reading On

1. Have you or a class peer/colleague experienced barriers that influenced your motivation after reaching an ethical decision?

2. How could the strategies presented previously assist you to maintain moral motivation in the future?

ETHICAL ACTION

Ethical action includes determining the best way to implement a chosen decision and having the ability and confidence to see it through to completion. This component requires consideration of possible resistance or objections that may occur and competencies associated with **E (expression)** in the CODE mnemonic: assertiveness and negotiation skills (Lachman et al., 2012). In using a systematic decision-making process, John can clearly explain and justify his decision to others employing effective communication and assertion techniques.

Most nurses receive education on using therapeutic communication with patients and families in their initial nursing programs. Additional skills are required, however, in situations of potential conflict and disagreement with patients/families and team members. Many new graduates and experienced nurses have been described as lacking conflict resolution skills in addition to assertiveness and confidence in times of distress or disagreement (Theisen & Sandau, 2011). The detrimental effects of conflict avoidance, overall poor communication among the health care team, impact on patient safety, and nurse turnover are well documented (Mahon & Nicotera, 2011; Sayre, McNeese-Smith, Leach, & Philips, 2012; Twibell et al., 2012). Effective communication and conflict engagement skills are also considered essential QSEN competencies for both undergraduate and graduate nurses (Table 2.1). As a result, various programs and approaches for strengthening communication skills have been developed. Among these are crucial conversations (Patterson, Grenny, McMillan, & Switzler, 2012), elements of TeamSTEPPS (AHRQ, 2016; Harvey, Echols, Clark, & Lee, 2014), and others also discussed in Chapter 4.

A crucial conversation may be necessary when an issue involves three components: differing opinions, high stakes, and strong emotions. While such conversations may revolve around ethical issues, others may not. The crucial conversation process involves observing our own behavior and asking if this approach will obtain the conclusion we desire in the situation. Avoiding blaming and using cognitive reframing as discussed previously may enable us to stop negative thought processes and "master our stories" (Patterson et al., 2012). For example, if John is hesitant to call for an ethics consult because he fears the potential anger of the intensivist, he is telling himself a story in which he has been hurt or injured. To master this emotion of fear, he can choose to tell himself a useful story that leads to constructive dialogue. Patterson et al. (2012) state that among other elements, a useful story turns "villains into humans" and "the helpless into the able" (p. 123). This approach may assist in separating the known facts (the intensivist is caring but can be very abrupt) from your story (he will object to the consult and be angry). Components of a structured crucial conversation are presented in Box 2.3.

CASE SCENARIO (*CONTINUED*)

With Anita and Jackie's assistance, and after discussing it with Mr. T and his family, John decides to request an ethics consultation. Although he does not have to inform the intensivist of his intended action, John decides to do so. He recalls several steps outlined for engaging in crucial conversations and approaches Dr. V in the breakroom after morning rounds. "Dr. V, I have cared for Mr. T and his family for some time during this admission and in the past. I also participated in his care conference and don't believe that he has had enough time or information to consider his preferences. I think an ethics consult is needed to further discuss treatment options and possible outcomes with Mr. T and his family who agree to participate. I know that we all want what is best for him and to provide quality, ethical care. I value your opinions and experience and hope that you will share them now and during the consultation." Dr. V appears somewhat upset and states, "I disagree about the need for a consult because it will delay an intervention that the patient requires and prolong his stay in the ICU. However, I will listen to their recommendations and thank you for informing me, John."

Box 2.3

Crucial Conversation Components

1. Start with heart—Before you begin, consider the following:
- What is your desired outcome for this conversation? Are your goals clear?
- What is at stake for you, other individuals, and relationships?
- How can you avoid looking for ways to win, appease, or punish?

2. Learn to look
- The goal is to maintain free-flowing dialogue.
- Are you becoming defensive? Is the other person becoming angry?

3. Make it safe
- State your mutual purpose/shared goal.
- Establish respect—tell the other person that you value his or her perspective and experience.
- Avoid ambiguity.

4. Master your story
- Control your emotions with positive thoughts.
- Explain how and why you have come to your conclusions.
- Ask yourself if you have contributed to the issue.

(continued)

Box 2.3

Crucial Conversation Components *(continued)*

5. State your path and explore the paths of others
- Share facts and perspectives and ask others to do the same.
- Look for areas of agreement.
- Be sincere and ask questions.

6. Move to action
- Decide together how to make decisions about the issue being discussed.
- Document the decisions and follow-up.

Questions to Consider Before Reading On

1. Can you identify a colleague who has good communication and conflict management skills?

2. What strategies does he or she use with patients/family members and coworkers?

ETHICAL OUTCOME AND EVALUATION

CASE SCENARIO *(CONTINUED)*

After speaking with John about his concerns regarding Mr. T and his family, the ethicist holds a bedside conference. With the intensivist, surgeon, and rehabilitation physician, the ethicist clarifies Mr. T's present condition, all treatment options and potential outcomes, including a tracheotomy, terminal weaning, and/or placement in a rehabilitation unit. Mr. T and his family are asked to think about what he values and considers quality of life in regard to the choices. He is told that although stable at present, his HF is end-stage and long-term placement in a rehabilitation unit is most likely. The rehabilitation physician informs Mr. T that this unit provides specialized multidisciplinary teams and a specific program to restore functional independence. He also states that they have achieved moderate success with aggressive weaning protocols. Following further discussion with his family, Mr. T decides to have the tracheotomy and be placed in the rehabilitation unit for 1 month after which he and his family will reconsider his choices.

Box 2.4

Ethical Evaluation: Debriefing Questions

Was the outcome anticipated or unexpected?

Did additional, new information provided affect the outcome?

Do similar issues keep reoccurring and further education or policy change is needed?

Could you have done things differently or what would you have liked to understand better?

What insights would you share with others?

Adapted from Grace (2014) and Robichaux (2012).

An often-neglected aspect of ethical decision making is processing or evaluating the event after the fact. This step may be crucial to nurses' development of confidence in their ethical skills. Self-reflection and reflection with others allow for sharing of insights and perspectives. Some possible questions to consider during this "debriefing" are presented in Box 2.4.

CASE SCENARIO *(CONTINUED)*

After the ethics consultation, John, Jackie, and Anita review and reflect on the process and outcome. John acknowledges his satisfaction with the consultation method and expresses appreciation of the values and perspectives of all those involved in the process a QSEN competency (Table 2.1). He expresses surprise, however, with Mr. T's choices. Jackie believes that the discussion of Mr. T's stable HF status and relationship to potential successful weaning in the rehabilitation unit impacted his decision. She asserts that having a follow-up consultation after 1 month to reevaluate the decision will be beneficial. Anita states that being more proactive regarding early ethics consultation may benefit patients, family members, and caregivers.

As nurses spend the most time with patients, they are often the first to realize an impending ethical situation and can intervene before it develops into a crisis. Having their moral voices heard in such circumstances is vital to interdisciplinary collaboration, ethical dialogue, and quality patient care (Pavlish, Brown-Saltzman, Jakel, & Fine, 2014).

STRATEGIES TO DEVELOP ETHICAL SKILLS

As Grace (2014) observes: "Gaining confidence in one's moral decision making is admittedly a slow process" (p. 78). This confidence is not bolstered by the pervasive belief that ethics in health care is always about difficult dilemmas that can be understood and solved only by specially trained individuals. The majority of ethical issues are the result of "lack of focus on either the goals or recipient of care" (Grace, 2014, p.79). Again, as nurses spend the most time with patients and family members, they tend to have the most comprehensive understanding of their (patients/families) narratives. Nurses' ability to engage in ethical deliberation, articulate these narratives, and initiate actions toward problem resolution is facilitated through ethical skill development.

While certain ethical skills such as sensitivity may be inherent, they cannot be developed or sustained in a moral vacuum. Health care facilities can contribute to administrative systems that either facilitate or undermine nurses' moral competency or agency. Nursing units can also be thought of as individual moral communities in which all should feel safe to be heard. At the individual level, recognizing that additional ethics education may be needed and taking advantage of courses offered by professional organizations such as ANA and American Association of Critical Care Nursing (AACN) may enhance ethical skills. Reading and discussing articles related to ethics in nursing practice, similar to a journal club, is another strategy. Forming a nursing ethics group or committee and conducting interdisciplinary or nursing ethics rounds may provide opportunities to identify and clarify issues with ethical or nonethical content. Although nurses may be members of an institutional bioethics committee, a nursing ethics group or committee provides a safe forum for expressions of perspectives and concerns unique to nurses. In addition, a bioethics committee may focus primarily on clinical ethics issues and not address organizational ethics topics such as bullying and incompetence (Bean, 2011).

Several health care institutions have developed ethics education programs for staff nurses and may serve as potential resources for ethics skills development (Grace et al., 2014; Sauerland, Marotta, Peinemann, Berndt, & Robichaux, 2015; Wocial, Hancock, Bledsoe, Chamness, & Helft, 2010). As an example, Robinson et al. (2014) created the Clinical Ethics Residency for Nurses (CERN) at two large, Northeast medical centers and their affiliates. This program incorporates specific ethics content and experiential learning in conjunction with participants' clinical experiences to enable them to effectively address existing and potential ethical issues. Content is based on Rest's FCM (1986), Doris's (2010) discussion of moral psychology, the Code of Ethics (2015), and the American Society for Bioethics and Humanities (2009) ethics competencies. Various learning strategies are utilized including online and classroom presentations/discussions, role play, high fidelity simulation, and clinical mentorship with ethics faculty. Evaluation of this comprehensive intervention indicates that participants' ability to effectively prevent or intervene in ethical situations has increased while their moral distress has diminished.

Creating comprehensive ethics education programs for practicing nurses may not be feasible for every institution as it generally requires financial support and dedicated faculty. However, recognizing that enhancement of ethical skills is needed may begin with one motivated individual nurse. This was the case at the author's affiliated hospital where the nurse educator in the perioperative unit became concerned about ethically challenging situations in that area and throughout the facility. She questioned her ability to do the ethically right thing for patients and their families and wondered if other nurses shared her concerns. Upon questioning, many of the nurses appeared to lack knowledge about what constituted an ethical situation or, if recognized, where to seek resources. These discussions also suggested that nurses were experiencing moral distress. After presenting these anecdotal findings to the Magnet® project director, the nurse educator collaborated with a faculty member (Catherine Robichaux [CR]) to obtain research-based results regarding registered nurses' levels of moral distress and their perceptions of the ethical climate (Sauerland et al., 2014, 2015).

The findings from the moral distress/ethical climate study were presented to the hospital chief nursing officer (CNO), nursing directors, and members of administration. As a result, and in conjunction with recommendations by Magnet consultants, a nursing ethics council (NEC) and unit-based ethics steward program were developed. The council meets monthly and has representatives from various units in addition to members from other disciplines such as child life and physical therapy. Meeting agendas may include identified ethics educational topics presented by members or invited speakers and/or open discussion of members' concerns. For example, responses to the two open-ended questions in the study described many instances of bullying and lateral violence. Consequently, one NEC meeting discussed relevant provisions and interpretive statements from the Code of Ethics (Interpretive statements 1.5 and 6.3, ANA, 2015) that specifically address these issues. As avoidance is the most common conflict resolution approach used by many nurses in such damaging interactions, conflict engagement strategies and skills were presented and practiced. These skills and strategies were further reinforced at a follow-up conference. Reluctance to use formal avenues to report bullying/lateral violence behaviors because of fear of retaliation or the belief that "nothing will be done" was addressed by having a representative from the risk department address the NEC. Nurses were also informed of the process involved in requesting and participating in an ethics consultation that is also available as a podcast on the hospital intranet.

NEC meetings serve as a safe place for participants to share their stories and those of patients and families and to gain support to face ethical challenges. This sharing of narratives is believed to enhance ethics knowledge and contribute to the development of resilience and a moral community (Austin, 2012; Lawrence & Maitlis, 2012). These strategies could be adapted for use in individual units or the overall facility in which nurses are employed.

CONCLUSION

This chapter presented a four-component framework for developing ethical skills in nursing practice: sensitivity, judgment, motivation, and action. Analyzing and clarifying personal values were identified as a preliminary step to exploring and refining ethical sensitivity, the ability to identify and distinguish situations with ethical content from those that are practical or decisional in nature. Application of an ethical judgment or decision-making model was discussed in addition to strategies to maintain motivation through moral courage. Approaches to overcoming barriers to implementation of a chosen ethical action were presented. Practical methods to develop ethical skills such as nursing ethics groups, ethics rounds, and journal clubs were identified.

Critical Thinking Questions and Exercises

1. Using the following websites, describe your personal values and how they may or may not have affected your interpretation of a recent ethical situation.

http://hrweb.mit.edu/system/files/Value%20Clarification%20Exercise.pdf
http://cbwc.ca/wp-content/uploads/2012/05/Values-Clarification.pdf

2. Explore the ethical decision making frameworks in the links provided. Discuss the similarities and differences with the framework provided in this chapter.

http://depts.washington.edu/bioethx/tools/4boxes.html
https://www.scu.edu/ethics/ethics-resources/ethical-decision-making/
a-framework-for-ethical-decision-making/

3. Using the websites provided as follows, that of another professional nursing organization, library, or the references from this chapter, choose a relevant ethics article, source, or online CE offering to discuss with nursing peers.

http://www.nursingworld.org/MainMenuCategories/EthicsStandards/Resources
http://www.bioethicsinstitute.org/nursing-ethics-summit-report/resources

REFERENCES

Agency for Healthcare Research and Quality. (2016). TeamSTEPPS: Strategies and tools to enhance performance and patient safety. Rockville, MD. Retrieved from http://www.ahrq.gov/professionals/education/curriculum-tools/teamstepps/index.html

Alston, C., Berger, Z., Brownlee, S., Elway, G., Fowler, F., Hall, L., . . . Henderson, D. (2014). Shared decision making strategies for best care: Patient decision aids. Discussion Paper, Institute of Medicine, Washington, DC. Retrieved from https://www.mainequalitycounts.org/image_upload/SDM%20Strategies%20for%20Best%20Care_Alston%20et%20al_IOM_Sept%202014.pdf

American Association of Colleges of Nursing (AACN). (2012). *Graduate level QSEN competencies: Knowledge, skills, and attitudes.* Washington, DC: Author.

American Nurses Association. (2014). Addressing nurse fatigue to promote safety and health: Joint responsibilities of registered nurses and employers to reduce stress. Retrieved from http://www.nursingworld.org/MainMenuCategories/Policy-Advocacy/Positions-and-Resolutions/ANAPositionStatements/Position-Statements-Alphabetically/Addressing-Nurse-Fatigue-to-Promote-Safety-and-Health.html

American Nurses Association. (2015). *Code of ethics for nurses with interpretive statements.* Silver Spring, MD: Author.

American Society for Bioethics and Humanities. (2009). *Improving competencies in clinical ethics.* Glenview, IL: Author.

Austin, W. (2012). Moral distress and the contemporary plight of health professionals. *HEC Forum*, *24*(1), 27–38.

Bean, S. (2011). Navigating the murky intersection between clinical and organizational ethics: A hybrid case taxonomy. *Bioethics*, *25*(6), 320–325.

Bebeau, M., Rest, J., & Narvaez, D. (1999). Beyond the promise: A perspective on research in moral education. *Educational Research*, *28*(4), 18–26.

Benner, P. (2003). Enhancing patient advocacy and social ethics. *American Journal of Critical Care*, *12*(4), 375–375.

Burkhardt, M., & Nathaniel, A. (2014). Values clarification. In M. Burkhardt & A. Nathaniel (Eds.), *Ethics and issues in contemporary nursing* (pp. 92–106). Stamford, CT: Cengage Learning.

Chambers, D. (2010). Developing a self-scoring comprehensive instrument to measure Rest's four-component model of moral behavior: The moral skills inventory. *Journal of Dental Education*, *75*(1), 23–35.

Cronenwett, L., Sherwood, G., Barnsteiner, J., Disch, J., Johnson, J., Mitchell, P., . . . Warren, J. (2007). Quality and safety education for nurses. *Nursing Outlook*, *55*(3), 122–131.

Doris, J. (2010). *The moral psychology handbook.* New York, NY: Oxford University Press.

Duffield, C., Diers, D., O'Brien-Pallas, L., Aisbett, C., Roche, M., King, M., & Aisbett, K. (2011). *Applied Nursing Research*, *24*(4), 244–255.

Elwyn, G., Frosch, D., Thomson, R., Joseph-Williams, N., Lloyd, A., Kinnersely, P., . . . Barry, M. (2012). Shared decision-making: A model for clinical practice. *Journal of General Internal Medicine*, *27*(10), 161–1367.

Gallagher, A., & Tschudin, V. (2010). Educating for ethical leadership. *Nursing Education Today*, *30*(3), 224–227.

Gaudine, A., Lamb, M., LeFort, S., & Thorne, L. (2011). Barriers and facilitators to consulting hospital ethics committees. *Nursing Ethics*, *18*(6), 767–780. doi: 10.1177/0969733011403808. Epub 2011 Jun 6.

Gert, B. (2005). *Morality: Its nature and justification.* New York, NY: Oxford University Press.

Grace, P. (2014). *Nursing ethics and professional responsibility in advanced practice.* Burlington, MA: Jones & Bartlett.

Grace, P., Robinson, E., Jurchak, M., Zollfrank, A., & Lee, S. (2014). Clinical ethics residency for nurses: An education model to decrease moral distress and strengthen nurse retention in acute care. *Journal of Nursing Administration*, *44*(12), 640–646.

Gustafson, G., Eriksson, S., Strandberg, G., & Norberg, A. (2010). Burnout and perceptions of conscience among health care personnel: A pilot study. *Nursing Ethics*, *17*(1), 23–28.

Harvey, E., Echols, S., Clark, R., & Lee, E. (2014). Comparison of two TeamSTEPPS training methods on nurse failure to rescue. *Clinical Simulation in Nursing, 10*(2), e57–e64. doi: http://dx.doi.org/10.1016/j.ecns.2013.08.006

Hawkins, S., & Morse, J. (2014). The praxis of courage as a foundation for care. *Journal of Nursing Scholarship, 46*(4), 263–270.

Hendricks, J., & Cope, V. (2013). Generation differences: What nurse managers need to know. *Journal of Advanced Nursing, 69*(3), 717–725.

Johnstone, M. J. (2012). Bioethics, cultural differences and the problem of moral disagreement in end of life care: A terror management theory. *Journal of Medicine and Philosophy, 37*, 181–200.

Lachman, V. (2007). Moral courage in action: Case studies. *MEDSURG Nursing, 16*(4), 275–277.

Lachman, V. (2010a). Strategies necessary for moral courage. *The Online Journal of Issues in Nursing, 15*(3), Manuscript 3. Retrieved from http://www.nursingworld.org/MainMenuCategories/Ethics Standards/Courage-and-Distress/Strategies-and-Moral-Courage.html

Lachman, V. (2010b). Do not resuscitate orders: Nurse's role requires moral courage. *MedSURG Nursing, 19*(4), 249–251.

Lachman, V., Murray, J., Iseminger, K., & Ganske, K. (2012). Doing the right thing: Pathways to moral courage. *American Nurse Today, 7*(5), 24–29. Retrieved from https://americannursetoday.com/doing-the-right-thing-pathways-to-moral-courage/

Lawrence, T., & Maitlis, S. (2012). Care and possibility: Enacting an ethic of care through narrative practice. *Academy of Management Review, 37*(4), 641–663.

Mahon, M., & Nicotera, A. (2011). Nursing and conflict communication: Avoidance as preferred strategy. *Nursing Administration Quarterly, 35*(2), 152–163.

Olpin, M., & Hesson, M. (2016). The importance of values. In M. Olin & M. Hesson (Eds.), *Stress management for life: A research-based experiential approach* (pp. 134–149). Belmont, CA: Thomson Higher Education.

Page, K. (2012). The four principles: Can they be measured and do they predict ethical decision making? *BMC Medical Ethics, 13*(10), 1–8. Retrieved from http://www.ncbi.nlm.nih.gov/pmc/articles/PMC3528420/pdf/1472-6939-13-10.pdf

Park, E. (2012). An integrated ethical decision-making model for nurses. *Nursing Ethics, 19*(1), 139–159.

Patterson, K., Grenny, J., McMillan, R., & Switzler, A. (2012). Crucial conversations: Tools for talking when the stakes are high. New York, NY: McGraw-Hill.

Pavlish, C., Brown-Saltzman, K., Jakel, P., & Fine, A. (2014). The nature of ethical conflicts and the meaning of moral community in oncology practice. *Oncology Nursing Forum, 41*(2), 130–140.

Pavlish, C., Hellyer, J., Brown-Saltzman, K., Miers, A., Squire, K. (2013). Barriers to innovation: Nurses' risk appraisal in using an ethics screening and early intervention tool. *Advances in Nursing Science, 36*(4), 304–319.

Rest, J. (1986). *Moral development: Advances in research and theory.* New York, NY: Praeger.

Robichaux, C. (2012). Developing ethical skills: From sensitivity to action. *Critical Care Nurse, 32*(2), 65–72.

Robinson, E., Lee, S., Zollfrank, A., Jurchak, M., Frost, D., & Grace, P. (2014). Enhancing moral agency: Clinical ethics residency for nurses. *Hastings Center Report, 44*(5), 12–20.

Rokeach, M. (2008). *Understanding human values.* New York, NY: Simon & Schuster.

Sauerland, J., Marotta, K., Peinemann, M., Berndt, A., & Robichaux, C. (2014). Assessing and addressing moral distress and ethical climate: Part 1. *Dimensions of Critical Care Nursing, 33*(4), 234–245.

Sauerland, J., Marotta, K., Peinemann, M., Berndt, A., & Robichaux, C. (2015). Assessing and addressing moral distress and ethical climate, part II: Neonatal and Pediatric Perspectives. *Dimensions in Critical Care Nursing, 34*(1), 33–46.

Sayre, S., McNeese-Smith, D., Leach, L., & Philips, L. (2012). An educational intervention to increase "speaking up" behaviors in nurses and improve patient safety. *Journal of Nursing Care Quality, 27*(2), 154–160.

Sherman, R. (2013, July 14). How to have that crucial conversation. (Web log comment). Retrieved from http:/www.emergingrnleader.com/crucial-conversation

Theisen, J., & Sandau, K. (2013). Competency of new graduate nurses: A review of their weaknesses and strategies for success. *The Journal of Continuing Education in Nursing, 44*(9), 406–414.

Trossman, S. (2015, January/February). More than just tired. *The American Nurse, 1,* 6. Retrieved from http://www.theamericannurse.org/index.php/2015/03/01/more-than-just-tired/

Twibell, R., St. Pierre, J., Johnson, D., Barton, D., Davis, C., Kidd, M., & Rook, G. (2012). Tripping over the welcome mat: Why new nurses don't stay and what the evidence says we can do about it. *American Nurse Today, 7*(6). Retrieved from https://americannursetoday.com/tripping-over-the -welcome-mat-why-new-nurses-dont-stay-and-what-the-evidence-says-we-can-do-about-it/

Wocial, L., Hancock, M., Bledsoe, P., Chamness, A. & Helft, P. (2010). An evaluation of unit-based ethics conversations. *JONA's Healthcare Law, Ethics, and Regulation, 12*(2), 48–54.

Wurzbach, M. (2005). Nursing ethics and Hagar the Horrible. *Reflections on Nursing Leadership, 31*(3). Retrieved from http://www.reflectionsonnursingleadership.org/Pages/Vol31_3_Wurzbach.aspx

Skills and Resources for Ethical Decision Making

3

Using Ethical Decision Making and Communication Skills to Minimize Conflict

DOUGLAS HOUGHTON

LEARNING OBJECTIVES AND OUTCOMES

Upon completion of this chapter, the reader will be able to:

- Understand the types of health care decisions faced by patients/families
- Describe several types of advance care planning and documentation
- Understand the role of the surrogate decision maker in health care settings
- Describe the role of cultural background on the communication and decision-making processes
- Describe important components of the communication process between the health care team and patients/surrogates
- Understand the role of the nurse in the communication and decision-making processes in health care situations
- Describe key elements of the goals-of-care conference
- Discuss strategies to minimize conflict in the health care decision-making process

DECISION MAKING AND HEALTH CARE

As RNs, we know that health care consumers (i.e., our patients) often face some of the most challenging decision situations imaginable. These decisions are challenging due to the often serious consequences of these decisions; it is not an exaggeration to state that life or death may be in the balance. These decisions may be made for oneself or for loved ones while serving as their surrogate, and may need to be made based on information given by a health care provider (HCP) they do not know well, if at all. The health issues at stake and prognoses given may be difficult to understand clearly for decision makers without health care experience. Additionally, in the inpatient environment these critical decisions are frequently made at a time of emotional distress, exhaustion, uncertainty, and fear. Communication between the patient/family and health care team may be limited or nonexistent, misunderstood, or fail to address prognosis and meaningful goals of care. Consequently, conflict is a common occurrence between involved parties in health care decisions (Kayser, 2014). This conflict may arise between HCPs and families, HCPs and patients, patients and families, or within families themselves. Fortunately, knowledge of available evidence from pertinent research, strong communication skills, and a sound ethical decision-making framework can minimize such conflict. RNs need a strong set of communication and conflict resolution skills and an understanding of the multiple factors that may influence the health care decision-making process, so that they may provide expert guidance to support patients and families during this often-complex process. These skills are an essential Quality and Safety Education for Nurses (QSEN) competency.

CASE SCENARIO

AJ is a 22-year-old male, whose family has recently located to south Florida from Colombia. AJ has had a high-speed motorcycle crash and sustained life-threatening injuries, including multiple rib fractures, a pelvic fracture, and a severe traumatic brain injury (TBI). He had difficulty breathing at the scene and was endotracheally intubated by paramedics en route, but only after much difficulty during which he experienced a 5-minute hypoxic period. He arrived at the trauma center with a Glasgow Coma Score (GCS) of 3. He is admitted to the intensive care unit with respiratory distress, anemia related to bleeding from his pelvic fracture, and altered mental status from his TBI. His primary nurse is Kevin, a Caucasian male from upstate New York. Kevin has 10 years of experience as an RN in critical care, and 5 years in his current position. Kevin is keenly aware of the long and complicated hospital course that AJ will likely experience.

Importance and Types of Decisions in Health Care

Most everyday treatment decisions in health care in the United States are made collaboratively between mentally competent patients and providers. Whether or not to start a new medication for a chronic illness, undergo recommended routine screening exams, and how to execute a plan to quit smoking are common scenarios in routine outpatient care which elicit minimal drama and contain little or no ethical content. However, health care decisions become much more complicated in the acute care or inpatient setting. These decisions may involve life and death, comfort or pain, and may require patients, families, and providers to make end-of-life care decisions they are not prepared to face. There is often little or no relationship between the patient and these HCPs, and there is the added stress of an acute illness and hospitalization. The illness or injury leading to the hospitalization may have been unexpected, or it may be an exacerbation of a chronic health condition. Guiding patients and decision makers through end-of-life care choices poses a particularly significant and complex problem often faced by nurses. In spite of significant national efforts by the health care community to improve end-of-life care, a recent study showed that patient/surrogate reports of pain, depression, confusion, and other symptoms actually increased during the time period from 1998 to 2010 (Singer et al., 2015).

Unfortunately, many older persons and even those with chronic illnesses fail to clarify the kind of care they would prefer in the event they become unable to decide for themselves. Only about one quarter of the U.S. adult population has some type of advance directive describing what kind of care they would like at the end of life. This number approaches 50% in senior populations, but this leaves a vast number of Americans without clearly described wishes should a health crisis arise (Institute of Medicine, 2014). These numbers demonstrate that a great deal of ambiguity often exists for those left to decide among care options for incapacitated loved ones. The advance care planning process can eliminate or ease the concerns of health care surrogates and HCPs and help ensure that care provided is consistent with patient values and wishes. Nurses can play a key role in educating the public and their own patients about available options, and encouraging them to complete some type of advance directive. See Box 3.1 for a description of advance care planning options.

Questions to Consider Before Reading On

1. Do *you* have an advance directive stating the kind of care you would prefer? How about your loved ones?

2. How would you assist a patient/family in understanding the advance care planning options presented in Box 3.1?

Influencing Factors in Health Care Decision Making

Many factors influence the decision-making process, including personal values and culture (of both the provider and the patient/family), level of education, religion, prognostic (un)certainty, and patient/family trust in the HCP (Institute of Medicine, 2014; Philipsen, Murray, Wood, Bell-Hawkins, & Setlow, 2013). The influence of culture is pervasive, and providers must

Box 3.1

Advance Care Planning Options

Definition of advance care planning: A process of *ongoing discussions* regarding one's wishes for future medical care, particularly end-of-life care. Participants may include individual patients, families or support systems, HCPs, and legal representatives.

Advance directives: Patient-initiated documents that describe future care wishes or name a health care surrogate should the patient be incapacitated. These include:

Living will: a document describing care preferences should the patient be medically determined to be in terminal condition.

Durable power of attorney for health care: written legal designation of a person named by the patient to make health care decisions for the patient should he or she be incapacitated.

Medical orders: Order sets created and signed with a physician or other HCP governing emergency, inpatient, and/or end-of-life care for a seriously ill person. These may include:

Physician orders for life-sustaining treatment (POLST): medical orders covering a range of care topics common in serious or terminal illness, to designed to cross-care settings. Appropriate for frail or terminally ill persons, binding in many states (www.polst.org).

Do-not-resuscitate, allow natural death, do-not-hospitalize, do-not-intubate: medical orders written to apply in a given health care setting governing end-of-life care.

Adapted from Institute of Medicine (2014).

often listen diligently in order to hear and understand cultural nuances in communication and decision-making styles (Pascual & Marks, 2014). Race and religion have been demonstrated to have a significant effect on illness perception by patients and families, which may result in a situational "perception gap" between patient/families and providers (Ford, Zapka, Gebregziabher, Yang, Sterba, 2010). Cultural background has been found to influence end-of-life care costs, with Black and Hispanic groups choosing more aggressive support and costly care near the end of life (Hanchate, Kronman, Young-Xu, Ash, Emanuel, 2009; Institute of Medicine, 2014; Johnson et al., 2010). Level of religiosity has also been identified as a predictor of more aggressive life support choices (Pew Research Center, 2013; Phelps et al., 2009). Caution must be used when applying such research data to individual situations, since wide variations exist within cultural groups. Nurses must also be aware of the effect of their own cultural background on their values, decision styles, and communication styles. This is particularly relevant in the United States, a country with significant cultural diversity. Some groups may reflect blending of cultural norms through assimilation ("hyphenated" groups, such as African American, Irish American, Italian American), while others remain largely true to their culture of origin (Purnell, 2012).

Communication Styles

Communication is an essential part of the decision-making process. It is vital that necessary information such as prognosis is communicated from the health care team to the patient/surrogate, and equally important that the patient/surrogate communicate patient preferences, values, and questions to the team. Culture influences how we prefer to receive and transmit information to others, and significant conflict can result if communication (HCP–patient–surrogate) is not effective. Awareness of our own communication style and how it may differ from that of the patient/surrogate is key to providing culturally sensitive and high-quality health care in a multicultural society such as the United States (Purnell, 2012). In U.S. and Western European cultures (predominantly individualistic cultures), communication styles are more direct, with eye contact being common and a sign of attention. In collectivistic cultures such as Japan, India, and many Latin cultures, communication may be less direct and contain significant nonverbal cues (Giri, 2006). Nurses providing care to persons of cultures other than their own are encouraged to become familiar with cultural variances, particularly with regard to health beliefs, end-of-life beliefs and practices, and communication styles.

Decision-Making Styles

As with communication style, culture also has a profound influence on how patients/surrogates make decisions. Collectivist-oriented cultures place more value on the social impact of situations, and may undertake the decision process as a family group instead of as individual members making autonomous decisions. Family conferences may include a large number of participants, which may be intimidating for some clinicians. The patient/surrogate may consult clergy members to participate and offer opinions in the decision-making process.

In contrast, predominantly individualist cultures like the United States emphasize personal responsibility for decision making, and for the consequences of the decision process. Gathering information through asking questions and an active, assertive decision process and conflict resolution style is the norm. Individual patients/surrogates who are not accustomed to the predominantly direct, decisive communication and decision-making style of U.S. HCPs may find it difficult to communicate health care preferences and decisions in this fashion (Guess, 2004; Purnell, 2012; Ting-Toomey & Chung, 2011).

Questions to Consider Before Reading On

1. Have you or a peer experienced a patient/family care situation in which culture (either your own or that of the patient/family) may have influenced the communication/decision-making process?

2. How could cultural awareness and competence improve this process in the future?

CASE SCENARIO (CONTINUED)

AJ's family arrives at the trauma center. They are brought to the intensive care unit to see AJ for the first time. His family consists of his mother, 52, his father, 54, two younger sisters ages 12 and 14, and an uncle (his father's brother). They speak only Spanish, as they have been in the country for only 6 months. AJ's parents do not allow his sisters to see him, as they are afraid they may be overwhelmed and faint. His father, mother, and uncle proceed to the bedside. They are shocked by the sight of AJ, whose body is swollen and has multiple severe skin abrasions and lacerations.

AJ's family is greeted by Kevin, his nurse. Kevin speaks some Spanish and he is able to communicate basic information to the family. AJ's mother is very emotional, crying, and unable to focus well on what Kevin is telling them. Kevin, knowing that many health care decisions will need to be made for AJ, calls both AJ's primary physician, Dr. B, and the unit social worker in order to arrange an informational meeting and to complete paperwork to designate AJ's mother or father to serve as his health care surrogate (or proxy) while he is incapacitated. Kevin also calls for professional interpreter assistance, knowing that the family speaks little English.

The Role of the Surrogate in Decision Making

In Western society, the ethical principle of autonomy has come to dominate the health care decision-making process. The right of the patients to decide for themselves is supported by significant medical-legal precedent cases, which include support for decisions made by health care surrogates on behalf of incapacitated patients, in accordance with state laws (Wolf, Berlinger, & Jennings, 2015). Recent data show that more than 40% of older hospitalized patients are unable to make their own informed choices about health care options due to acute or chronic illness–related reasons and require involvement of a surrogate; 23% were completely reliant upon a surrogate decision maker (Torke et al., 2014). As described previously, many people fail to actively participate in the advance care planning process, leaving surrogate decision makers without clear guidance as to what type or level of care the individual would prefer in a health care situation, should they be unable to decide for themselves.

Conversely, the events leading to a health care crisis may have been unantici-pated, as in the case of a young trauma victim who had been previously in good health. Nurses in an inpatient environment will frequently be working with and supporting surrogate decision makers, which serves to protect the patient's autonomy.

From an ethical perspective, the surrogate has a duty to act in accordance with the patient's preferences and values, if such had been expressed verbally or in writing. The primary ethical principle guiding decision making is auton-omy, although the principles of caring and beneficence are also applicable to the surrogate decision-making process. Many health care surrogates struggle in their role due to multiple emotional and cognitive factors, leading to pro-found distress. Surrogates who have no prior experience in the role, as well as those who had not engaged in prior discussions with the patient about their treatment preferences, have reported increased stress and decreased confidence in their ability to act for the patient (Majesko, Hong, Weissfeld, & White, 2012). Nurses can improve and support the decision-making process of sur-rogates by educating them on their role, emphasizing that all decisions made should reflect the *patients'* wishes and values and how they would likely decide for themselves if they were able to do so (the legal concept of "substituted judgment"). Should surrogates have no direct knowledge of patients or their values prior to their incapacity, the standard for decision making is "best inter-est," which requires that surrogates decide (in *their* judgment) what decision or course of treatment would be in the best interest of patients. This triad (HCP–surrogate–patient) complicates the decision-making process, in addi-tion to the fact that patients who require surrogates are sicker, have more in-hospital transfers, and more often die when compared to patients who do not require surrogates (Torke et al., 2014).

Questions to Consider Before Reading On

1. Who would serve as AJ's surrogate decision maker if his parents were unavailable?

2. As the nurse caring for AJ, how should Kevin assist this surrogate to understand his or her role?

The Role of the Health Care Provider in Decision Making

HCPs, most commonly physicians, are the primary source of medical infor-mation regarding patient condition and prognosis for recovery. This role may also be filled or supplemented by a nurse practitioner or physician assistant. The communication of this information in a respectful, complete, and under-standable manner is essential to an ethical decision-making process reflecting virtue, caring, and beneficence. Establishing a trusting relationship and mak-ing time to elicit patient values are critical, especially in situations where end-of-life choices are needed (Cook & Rocker, 2014; Kayser, 2014). An important nursing role is to ensure that the communication process is taking place, identify any anticipated problems, and help clarify care options with patients, families, and surrogates.

Provider decision-making behaviors can be described in four common roles:

- Informative (HCP provides information only, no guidance.)

- Facilitative (HCP provides information, elicits patient preferences, and guides the surrogate in his or her decision-making process to apply these preferences.)

- Collaborative (HCP provides information, elicits patient preferences, provides surrogate guidance, and makes a recommendation.) This may also be described as a shared decision-making model, which is most often recommended by professional guidelines, societies, and available evidence.

- Directive, or paternal (HCP makes a decision without patient/surrogate consultation.) This is less often recommended but may be appropriate for some situations such as emergencies or routine medical care (Cook & Rocker, 2014; Manara, 2015; Uy, White, Mohan, Arnold, & Barnato, 2013).

A recent U.S. study of physicians' decision-making roles in a simulated intensive care unit scenario identified 1% as informative, 49% were facilitative, 37% were collaborative, and 12% used a directive role (Uy, White, Mohan, Arnold, & Barnato, 2013). Another large survey of critical care physicians found that the vast majority of critical care physicians feel comfortable making life support recommendations (92%) and believe it is appropriate for them to do so (93%); however, only 22% reported always doing so (Brush, Rasinski, Hall, & Alexander, 2012). Debate continues in medical literature regarding the role of the physician and his or her responsibility to make treatment recommendations to patients/surrogates (Hutchinson, 2015; Veatch, 2015), although a shared decision-making model is recommended by the Society for Critical Care Medicine and the American Association of Critical Care Nurses, among others. A recent joint policy statement from multiple medical and nursing organizations explicitly states that "it is ethically untenable to give complete authority for treatment decisions to either patient/surrogates or individual clinicians. Instead, clinicians and patient/surrogates should work collaboratively to make treatment decisions" (Bosslet, 2015).

An important part of the role of nurses in patient/family discussions is to identify their own values and biases, and make every attempt to distance their own views from the expressed wishes of the patient, should there be any. The acknowledgment and setting aside of one's own biases and values reflect an understanding of the ethical concept of nonmaleficence. Cultural and personal values may conflict with those of the patient/surrogate, leading to moral distress on the part of the nurse and other providers when they are asked to provide care they believe is inappropriate, burdensome, or nonbeneficial to the patient (Keyser, 2014; Pascual & Marks, 2014).

CASE SCENARIO *(CONTINUED)*

Kevin, Dr. B, the social worker, an interpreter, and AJ's mother, father, and uncle meet in the unit conference room. Dr. B, through the interpreter, describes AJ's prognosis, multiple injuries, and what needs to be done at present. The prognosis for functional recovery is very poor, because of anoxic brain damage from the prolonged period when AJ was not able to breathe well. His other injuries are severe but likely survivable in a young healthy person. His pelvic fracture would need surgical repair, but because of AJ's poor neurological prognosis, Dr. B recommends not doing the surgery. He explains that this is because AJ will not walk due to his brain damage and the surgery would be extensive and has risks. AJ's family appears overwhelmed and tearful, and his mother is repeating prayers aloud in Spanish through her tears. Kevin provides emotional support. Dr. B, knowing that the family will need time to process the prognosis, says he must leave but schedules another meeting in 2 days. The family asks if they may bring other family members to the next meeting, and the team agrees to the request.

Question to Consider Before Reading On

1. Have you or a peer experienced a patient/family care situation in which you disagreed with a treatment decision because you believed it to be inappropriate, burdensome, or nonbeneficial? What was the outcome? What were your feelings?

The Role of the Nurse in the Decision-Making Process

The nurse plays a vital role in the health care decision-making process, since he or she is often the most visible and present member of the health care team, especially in the inpatient environment. Families often ask the nurse for his or her opinion when weighing care decisions, and informal, honest dialogue about the patient situation may help patients/surrogates clarify priorities and goals of care. Through application of the ethical concepts of virtue, caring, and beneficence, the RN can play a valuable role in helping patients/surrogates to understand their choices and the ramifications of various options. The nurse can also support the patient/surrogate emotionally, advocate for them, and help them formulate questions and understand the choices they are facing. This is especially important when the patient/surrogate is of a different cultural background than the primary HCP responsible for the patient's care. These actions are supported by the American Nurses Association's (ANA) Code of Ethics (2015), Provision One, which states, "The nurse practices with compassion and respect for the inherent dignity, worth, and unique attributes of every person" (p. 1).

Guides to Inform Ethical Decision Making

James Rest's four-component model (FCM; 1986), described in Chapter 2, and the framework for ethical decision making utilized in this book offer assistance to nurses seeking to provide guidance through the decision-making process for patients/surrogates and families. See Tables 3.1 and 3.2 for application of these models to the Case Scenario presented here.

Table 3.1

Application of Rest's Four-Component Model to AJ's Case Scenario

COMPONENT	NURSING CONSIDERATIONS AND ACTIONS
Ethical sensitivity	Kevin knows that AJ's family's culture is different from his own. This awareness allows him to set aside his own values and guide the family through the decision-making process using their values and cultural norms, such as a family (collective) group decision-making process.
Ethical judgment	Kevin is aware that the family's inability to speak English impairs communication vital to the decision-making process. He knows this type of decision will be difficult for AJ's family. He is aware that holding a conference with a large family group may be more difficult for Dr. B.
Ethical motivation	Kevin is motivated to assist the family in the decision process, in his nursing role as patient advocate. He does so knowing that the interpreter and multiple family members may make Dr. B uncomfortable.
Ethical action	Kevin acted on his understanding of the family communication challenges. He secured interpreter services, and facilitated the presence of multiple family members and their clergyman in the care conference.

Source: Rest (1986).

Table 3.2

Framework for Ethical Decision Making: Application to AJ's Case Scenario

VIRTUE	CARING
Does the proposed action uphold the nurses' professional integrity? *Yes, Kevin acts as family advocate.* Does the proposed action (and how it is discussed) uphold honesty and transparency? *Yes, through obtaining an interpreter and ensuring family understanding.* Does the proposed action require any deviation from the nurses' standard of care? *No.* Does the proposed action coalesce with how the nurse has dealt with similar situations in the past? *Yes, Kevin has had similar experiences with different cultural groups and has learned from them.*	How does the proposed action support the care of the patient? *Ensuring effective communication is vital to care-related decision making.* How does the proposed action support the patient's relationships with family? With care providers? *AJ's family relationships are supported through Kevin's actions, and family / provider trust is improved.* What cultural/social/religious/family issues need to be considered? *Kevin knows that in many Latino cultures, a collective or group (family) decision-making process is common. He also understands the importance of encouraging the family to bring a religious representative for support.*
AUTONOMY	**BENEFICENCE**
Is the patient competent and capacitated to make decisions? *No.* Is the patient capable of expressing and choosing? *No.* Who is the decision maker? *Kevin has facilitated the process of AJ's father becoming his legal surrogate for decision making.* Does the patient understand his/her condition? *No, but Kevin acts to ensure that AJ's family understands on AJ's behalf.*	How can you the nurse help the patient's physical and psychological health? *In this case, Kevin's responsibility as a nurse is to provide family-centered care as well as provision of skilled intensive care nursing.* How does the proposed treatment, test, or action benefit the patient? *Through facilitation of effective communication, AJ's family is assisted in making care decisions on his behalf.* What are the likely positive outcomes of the nurses' actions? *The family may experience sadness and grief, but they will likely feel trust in AJ's health care team.*

(continued)

Table 3.2

Framework for Ethical Decision Making: Application to AJ's Case Scenario *(continued)*

AUTONOMY	BENEFICENCE
What are the patient's preferences? *Unfortunately these are not known in this case.*	In your professional opinion, what is best for the patient? *In this case, Kevin feels that it may be best to allow a peaceful death for AJ, knowing the long course of suffering ahead for both the patient and family. However, Kevin also knows that other values may lead to other choices and he must respect their choice.*
NONMALEFICENCE	**JUSTICE**
What are your biases? *In this case, Kevin is aware of his bias toward not prolonging life support in the face of a grim prognosis.* What can be done to protect the patient? *Most important here is to ensure that AJ's family truly understands the care choices available and their implications.* Would the proposed action cause harm or make the patient worse? *While the nurse may have conflicting feelings about what is ethically right in this case (i.e., potential future patient/ family suffering), most important is supporting the patient physically while supporting his family through the decision-making process.* What negative outcomes are possible with and without the proposed action? *Through facilitating effective communication and family education, Kevin minimizes the possibility of them struggling to understand their options and make a choice. If he did not do so, their decision would not be truly informed.*	What scarce resources are involved in patient care? *Although the choice of long-term care for AJ will use expensive resources, no resources in question are particularly scarce.* What is the patient's financial/insurance situation? *This is not addressed in the present Case Scenario, but this could be an important factor in other scenarios.* What are the larger social concerns? *Discussions of the high cost of health care in the United States are applicable here, although caution is warranted in applying societal issues to individual cases.* Legal concerns? *None.* Institutional policy? *None relevant.* Public health interests? *Again, the U.S. citizenry must engage in national conversations about appropriate use of limited health care dollars. However, this should not be applied to this individual case.*

Note: See Table 2.2 for a further description of Klugman's decision-making model.

MINIMIZING CONFLICT IN THE DECISION-MAKING PROCESS

Health care has improved dramatically during the past several decades, enabling many people to live longer and healthier lives. However, this improvement has come at a cost. Our ability to keep many critical and terminally ill persons alive indefinitely through the use of aggressive and invasive care has caused countless ethical dilemmas (Institute of Medicine, 2014; Rothman, 2014). These dilemmas are problematic because making ethical decisions in these situations is incredibly complex and fraught with individual value and cultural judgments. Values held by nurses and other health care team members may conflict with the values of their patients/families. These situations often lead to moral distress on the part of health care team members who may find themselves providing care that they view as burdensome, futile, or a waste of resources (ethical concepts of nonmaleficence and justice). In addition, patients/surrogates/families often find themselves facing health care decisions with an unclear understanding of the situation and potential future consequences of these decisions. The nurse and the multidisciplinary team have a professional responsibility (ethical concepts of caring, virtue, and benevolence) to assist and guide decision makers through a difficult, confusing, and emotionally stressful time.

Questions to Consider Before Reading On

1. It is not uncommon for family members to ask nurses, "What would you do?" in situations such as Kevin's. How would you answer this question?

2. What direction does the Code of Ethics provide for such a situation?

Establish Prognosis as Soon as Possible

At present, the vast majority of deaths in the intensive care unit occur after some type of limiting or withdrawing of aggressive life support therapies (Morgan, Varas, Pedroza, & Almoosa, 2013). The identification and management of persons who will not benefit from further aggressive interventions are extremely difficult and subjective. Few evidence-based tools have proven useful in prognosticating in complex patient care scenarios, leaving the establishment of prognosis in the hands of providers with varying degrees of skill, knowledge, and experience. Even in the most experienced hands, prognosis is often uncertain, which thwarts the ability of the patient/surrogate/HCP to make informed, ethical decisions. Often, the level of aggressiveness of life support interventions is based on unit/setting cultural norms and physicians' practice styles (Hart et al., 2015). Even when the prognosis is clear to the health care team, we may fail to recognize that the patient/surrogate/family does not have the same understanding or perception of the clinical picture (Brown, 2014). This misunderstanding may be a result of an inadequate communication process, health care team avoidance of prognosis discussions, lack of patient/family readiness to hear and accept a poor prognosis, or language and other cultural barriers (Brown, 2014; Chiarchiaro, Buddadhumaruk, Arnold, White, 2015; Pascual & Marks, 2015). It is recommended that the health care team discuss prognosis regularly and attempt to reach consensus among team members while making patient care rounds, to ensure that team members are prepared to discuss this prognosis with family from a unified position and that patients/surrogates/families do not receive conflicting messages from team members. Patient/surrogate/family education may also be useful in improving understanding of prognosis and life support measures and is an important role for nurses in acute care settings. A recent study found that an educational video presentation regarding cardiopulmonary resuscitation (CPR) options improved patient and surrogate knowledge about CPR; however, this did not result in a change in documented resuscitation preferences (Wilson et al, 2015).

Establish Goals of Care as Early as Possible

Early HCP/patient/surrogate discussions to elicit patient values (if known), discuss prognosis, and establish goals of care are interventions well supported by professional guidelines from multiple Western medicine associations (Cook & Rocker, 2014; Truog et al., 2008; You, Fowler, Heyland, & CARENET, 2014). Despite this, these crucial conversations do not happen effectively for many critical or terminally ill persons. Many barriers to communication between the health care team and patients/families/surrogates exist, including provider avoidance or discomfort with the topic, lack of time, provider lack of end-of-life and communication training, and perceived lack of patient/family readiness to accept a poor prognosis (Durall, Zurakowski, & Wolfe, 2012; Iglesias, Pascual, & de Bengoa Vallejo, 2013). Recent research shows that goals of care and patient values are not addressed in a large number of patient/surrogate/HCP meetings (Scheunemann, Cunningham, Arnold, Buddadhumaruk, & White, 2015; You et al., 2014), demonstrating significant opportunity for improvement. If the patient prognosis is not yet clear, a trial of aggressive therapy may be warranted with curative therapy as the stated goal of care. Often, such trials of aggressive therapy may yield poor results (i.e., failure to improve patient health status) and therefore goals of care may need to be readdressed. This is a common scenario in the intensive care unit and may occur as a sudden shift from curative to palliative care, or in a step-wise fashion, first shifting to a practice of "no escalation of care" (continuation of current therapy, but no additional interventions/therapies). Morgan and colleagues (2013) found this goal of care shift preceded death in 30% of decedent patients in a large academic medical center. It is important that the primary HCP, usually the physician, consider the patient's likely long-term functional prognosis when discussing care goals with patients/surrogates. Turnbull and colleagues (2014), in a large survey of intensivists, showed that these professionals were 49% more likely to discuss withdrawal of aggressive support when they were asked to record the patient's likely 3-month functional prognosis. Nurses need to be involved in discussions of prognosis, in order to be able to clarify and discuss any patient/family/surrogate questions.

The previous data demonstrate the importance of goals of care discussions, occurring on a regular basis during the illness or hospitalization. An obvious reason that these discussions may not occur as often as they should is that HCPs do not relish being the bearer of bad news, and may dislike or feel uncomfortable relaying a poor prognosis to a patient/family and/or surrogate decision maker. The bedside nurse may play an important role in advocating for the patient and ensuring that regular goals of care discussions occur, with an honest and open communication process. This role is supported by the ethical concepts of virtue, caring, and beneficence. The ANA Code of Ethics for Nurses (2015) provides further ethical support for this nursing role in Provision Two: "The nurses' primary commitment is to the patient, whether an individual, family, group, community, or population" (p. 5). Interpretive statement 2.1 (Primacy of the Patient's Interests) of this provision describes the role of the nurse as patient advocate, ensuring that honest, open discussions about treatment options occur, as well as nursing duty to help resolve situations where the HCP treatment regimen may be in conflict with the values or desires of the patient. Key elements of goals of care conferences for seriously ill patients are described in Box 3.2.

Box 3.2

Key Elements of Goals of Care Conferences for Seriously Ill Patients

- Ask about prior patient discussions or documentation regarding the use of life-sustaining treatment.
- Offer to meet to discuss goals of care.
- Provide information about advance care planning to review prior to health care team discussion.
- Upon meeting, disclose prognosis.
- Ask about patients' values and what is important to them.
- Provide information about outcomes, potential benefits, and risks of life-sustaining treatment.
- Provide information about outcomes, potential benefits, and risks of comfort measures.
- Prompt for questions about goals of care and plan of treatment.
- Provide time for patient/family to express fears and/or concerns.

(continued)

Box 3.2

Key Elements of Goals of Care Conferences for Seriously Ill Patients *(continued)*

- Ask about care preferences in case of life-threatening illness (such as cardiac arrest—allow natural death [AND] or do-not-resuscitate [DNR]).
- Provide documents necessary to record patient wishes (such as POLST—physician orders for life sustaining treatment).

Adapted from You et al. (2014).

Questions to Consider Before Reading On

1. Using the elements provided in Box 3.2, what should be addressed in the goals of care conference for AJ?

2. What information should be provided? What questions asked?

Case Scenario *(continued)*

Two days later, the group meets again to discuss AJ's condition, prognosis, and goals of care. Five additional family members are present; several cousins, two aunts, and the family's clergyman, a Catholic priest. Kevin has facilitated the logistics of this meeting in spite of being quite busy caring for AJ and another patient, because he knows how important the meeting will be to ensure that goals of care are clarified for his patient AJ. AJ's father has been appointed his health care surrogate.

Further diagnostic testing has confirmed that AJ has significant anoxic brain damage, and his prognosis for neurological recovery is nil. As the interpreter relays this message from Dr. B to the family group, many break out in tears and exclamations. AJ's mother repeats, "No, no, no, it is not true" in Spanish while wringing her hands over and over. AJ's father appears stoic but grim faced. Dr. B offers two alternative plans of care: the first would be to perform a tracheostomy and gastrostomy, and seek placement for AJ in a long-term care facility; the second would be to choose comfort measures only and withdraw his ventilator support, artificial hydration and nutrition, allowing a natural death to occur. AJ's father becomes incensed when he hears that option suggested, and he loudly tells Dr. B that he will not give up on his son (in Spanish). He leaves the room and storms down the hall. Other family members are tearful and sob, holding each other for support. Kevin and the priest provide as much support as possible. Dr. B suggests that they meet again in 24 hours so that they may consider what they have heard.

EFFECTIVE COMMUNICATION STRATEGIES

Making informed decisions (autonomy) requires information, and communicating information effectively requires patience, self-awareness, and skill. Information regarding patient prognosis and available care options must be communicated from the lead HCP/physician to the patient/family/surrogate, and information regarding patient values, questions, and goals of care must in turn be communicated from the patient/surrogate to the lead HCP/physician. Communication styles vary significantly among cultural groups and it is essential that nurses are keenly aware and sensitive to these variations. Native language and patient/family understanding of the health care team's language is vital, and a professional interpreter should be used, not a family member. Even with a professional interpreter, care conferences using interpretation have been found to contain fewer elements of shared decision making and greater imbalance of physician/family speech (Van Cleave et al., 2014).

Significant opportunity for improvement exists in this vital communication and goal-setting process, as described in the Establish Goals of Care As Early As Possible section. In addition, a majority of family members consistently overestimate the patient's prognosis for recovery after receiving prognostic information from the ICU team, which may adversely affect the decision-making process and lead to undue suffering for patients with a poor prognosis (Chiarchiaro et al., 2015). These data reveal that a significant communication gap frequently exists and likely contributes to team–patient/family conflict. This disconnect may jeopardize the honoring of patient preferences when they are known, due to a surrogate's lack of understanding or acceptance of a poor patient prognosis. Thoughtful and consistent attention to the communication process and knowledge of available evidence-based strategies to improve HCP/patient/surrogate communication can decrease or eliminate much conflict and drama. Both the quality and the quantity of patient/family/team meetings are important, and regular, structured meetings providing written information to educate decision makers have been proven helpful in improvement of communication (Harvey, 2014; Scheunemann, McDevitt, Carson, & Hanson, 2011). Communication training for the multidisciplinary health care team has also demonstrated improved communication as a result and is recommended, in addition to consideration of early ethics and/or palliative care consultation if appropriate. These interventions improve family emotional outcomes and reduce ICU length of stay and treatment intensity (Scheunemann et al., 2011; Shaw, Davidson, Smilde, Sondoozi, & Agan, 2014). Effective communication with families may also be improved through attention to some key points, which are described in Box 3.3. Related evidence-based practice findings on family support are described in Box 3.4.

Box 3.3

Effective Communication Strategies in the Health Care Environment

GENERAL STRATEGIES

1. Identify the patient/family-preferred communication style (individual, small group, or family unit).

2. Choose a time and place for the meeting that allows for unhurried, uninterrupted conversation.

3. Clarify patient/family/surrogate understanding of situation.

4. Assess the patient/family/surrogate readiness to hear information about prognosis.

5. Transmit information clearly (avoid jargon, assess understanding of medical terms).

6. Establish/reiterate common goals of care.

VALUE mnemonic*

  V = Value comments made by the family
  A = Acknowledge family emotions
  L = Listen
  U = Understand the patient as a person
  E = Elicit family questions

*Developed by U. Washington End-of-life Care Research Program; Lautrette et al. (2007).

Box 3.4

Evidence-Based Practice—Family Support

IMPROVE FAMILY SATISFACTION AND INCREASE DECISION-MAKING PARTICIPATION

Problem: Families of patients in this surgical intensive care unit were not satisfied with their level of participation in the decision-making process. There was also a family perception of a lack of multidisciplinary teamwork.

Intervention: The researchers developed an algorithm to bundles of communication interventions at specific points in the patient ICU

(continued)

Box 3.4	

Evidence-Based Practice—Family Support *(continued)*

stay: at 24, 72, and 96 hours after unit admission. These bundles contained clinical triggers to expedite multidisciplinary care meetings as indicated by the patient condition, as well as specific family educational interventions (both written and verbal).

Results: Pre- and postintervention scores were compared for family participation in decision making (45% pre, 68% post) and perception of how well the health care team worked together (64% pre, 83% post).

Conclusions: Use of a structured family communication algorithm improved family satisfaction with decision making and perception of health care team functionality. Although specific to this unit, similar algorithms to improve family communication may provide similar positive outcomes.

Source: Huffines et al. (2013).

Questions to Consider Before Reading On

1. Have you or a peer participated in a discussion or family conference in which communication and understanding were less than optimal? Describe the problems.

2. How could the strategies and evidence provided in Boxes 3.3 and 3.4 improve future discussions/conferences?

SOURCES OF CONFLICT IN HEALTH CARE DECISION MAKING

Despite our best efforts, conflict is nearly inevitable when dealing with health situations that may be uncertain, unwelcome, unanticipated, and laden with personal preferences and value judgments. The emotional nature of health situations also contributes to a stressful decision-making process for all concerned, especially when the illness is sudden and life-threatening. When the values of the nurse (or other health care team member) are different from those of the patient/family, the nurse may experience moral distress from having to provide treatments with care team disagreement about prognosis and the viability of various treatment options.

- Patient/family misunderstanding of the situation or prognosis

- Lack of communication

- Feeling that moving to comfort measures is a sign of "giving up" or failure

- Team loss of focus from macro- to micro-level (i.e., focus on small irrelevant gains and missing the "big picture")

- Patient/family feelings of powerlessness

- Mistrust of the health care team

It may be useful to distinguish between ethical conflicts and decisional conflicts, as this may help the nurse frame the issue and act accordingly with decreased moral distress.

Ethical Conflict

A situation may be determined to contain ethical content when "an action performed or not performed has the potential to harm or benefit others" (Robichaux, 2012, p. 69). This harm in a health situation may include death, pain, disability, further injury, and emotional or spiritual suffering. Based on this definition, the vast majority of end-of-life care situations contain significant ethical content, making this a particularly complex decision-making arena. Patients/families as well as HCPs may experience ethical conflict, or an ethical dilemma, when ethical principles collide. As an example, a nurse caring for a seriously ill patient (unable to make his or her own decisions) knows that further aggressive treatment will only prolong suffering for the person. However, the decision maker for the patient chooses aggressive care instead of comfort care because the patient had "always been a fighter." The nurse experiences ethical conflict between the principles of caring, beneficence, and nonmaleficence (knowing that further aggressive care will lead to prolonged suffering, and the nurse's desire to do good for the patient) versus a desire to respect the autonomy of the patient/surrogate to make his or her own decisions. Provision 1.4 of the Code of Ethics for Nurses (ANA, 2015), the right to self-determination, helps clarify that in this example the primacy of the patient's right to self-determination (through the surrogate) and the ethical principle of autonomy overshadows the nurse's feelings of "doing wrong" for the patient. This example can also serve to demonstrate how this nurse may experience moral distress as a result of the situation.

Decisional Conflict

Decisional conflict may be defined as a situation in which differing values or preferences are the cause of the conflict. In this type of situation, the choices made and actions taken (or not taken) do not harm others (Robichaux, 2012). Often the consequences of various courses of action in health situations are uncertain, complicating our ability to choose or make recommendations effectively. Decisional conflicts may exist within or between persons involved, often resulting from uncertainty about what choice is best for them, given the circumstances. This kind of conflict may often arise within families making choices for a family member, and also within health care teams where differing opinions may exist about the viability of various treatment options.

CASE SCENARIO (CONTINUED)

Twenty-four hours later, most of the group members meet again. Kevin and AJ's night nurse Maria have spent significant efforts answering the family's questions and educating them on the choices they face, trying consciously not to project their own values and opinions on the family. AJ's father has regained his composure and he appears tense but not visibly angry. The mother relays to Kevin that the family has discussed the two alternative plans of care and has decided as a group that the family cannot give up on AJ. They will consent to a tracheostomy and gastrostomy for long-term care, and express hope that divine intervention will allow AJ to recover. Kevin and Dr. B personally disagree with the decision as they would not want that for themselves knowing the grim future for AJ and his family, but they support the family in their decision and do not voice their opinions, knowing that different values guide AJ's family's decision.

Resolving Conflict Effectively

Conflict exists in epidemic proportions in health care situations, especially those in the acute and critical care environment where patient/family stress, surrogate decision making, and emotional exhaustion are common (Institute of Medicine, 2014; Kayser, 2014; Long & Curtis, 2013). Practicing nurses are likely to be drawn into these conflicts, and Provision 2.1 of the Code of Ethics, Primacy of the Patients' Interests (ANA, 2015) clarifies the role of the nurse in supporting the patients in resolving conflicts and assisting them in understanding all available treatment options. As the profession consistently rated as the most trusted (Gallup, 2014), nurses are strongly positioned to resolve conflicts effectively.

Recent data also reveal a significant disconnect in perceived conflict between physicians and patients/families. Either the physician or the surrogate identified conflict in 63% of cases in a four-ICU study, but the agreement between physicians and surrogates regarding the presence of conflict was poor, revealing a "perception gap" between the health care team and the surrogate (Schuster, Hong, Arnold, & White, 2013). Conflict contributes to adverse patient outcomes, and resolution of conflict between the health care team and patient/surrogates is a critical step toward improving care, especially end-of-life care. This conflict also contributes to burnout (and/or moral distress), anxiety, mistrust, and patient/family dissatisfaction (Institute of Medicine, 2014). A consensus working definition of conflict in critical care is "a dispute, disagreement, or difference of opinion related to the management of a patient in the ICU involving more than one individual and requiring some decision or action" (Fassier & Azoulay, 2010). These situations may arise in any clinical area, but are more common in the inpatient environment. In general, these conflicts arise in situations of inadequate or ineffective communication, or situations in which the patient/family has a poor opinion of the physician or health care team. Therefore, improving communication as described earlier is likely the most effective way to minimize conflict in health care situations. Valuable assistance may be received in conflict resolution via pastoral care, ethics, and/or palliative care consultations. However, in most cases, nursing intervention and patient advocacy to improve, clarify, or augment the communication process will be the most important conflict resolution tool.

Question to Consider Before Reading On

1. Do you think Kevin and Dr. B may experience moral distress in this case, since they did not agree personally with the choice that AJ's family made? If so, how could they deal with those feelings? What resources should be available?

CONCLUSION

Making decisions in health care settings is challenging for patients, surrogates, nurses, and other members of the multidisciplinary health care team. Advance care planning is essential for any persons with significant health challenges or advanced age, and is recommended for all adults. These important health decisions and the ways in which they are made are strongly influenced by one's cultural background, previous health care experiences, trust in the health care team, and the effectiveness of the communication process between all parties involved. Nurses play an important role in this decision-making process through patient advocacy, ensuring the integrity and effectiveness of the communication process, helping clarify the prognosis and its meaning to individual patient/family groups, and guiding decision makers through the decision process using a sound ethical framework. Ethical decision-making frameworks such as the FCM and the ethical framework described in this text can help guide nurses through the decision-making process by prompting thoughtful questions. Familiarity with the concepts they contain may help nurses minimize personal moral distress while advocating effectively for patients.

Critical Thinking Questions and Activities

1. In the case of AJ, what actions did the nurse take to uphold AJ's autonomy?

2. What other actions could Nurse Kevin have taken to uphold the ethical principle of beneficence?

3. Is it ethical to bring a discussion of the patient financial/insurance status into the care conference discussions between the multidisciplinary team and the family? Explain.

4. "The global migration of populations presents nurses with the challenge of delivering care to unprecedented numbers of patients with health care beliefs and practices that may differ from their own" (Douglas et al., 2014, p.109). Read the guidelines for implementing culturally competent nursing care in the following link. Discuss how these guidelines were illustrated in the chapter Case Scenario and how they may be implemented in your current practice.

http://www.tcns.org/files/Standards_of_Practice_for_Cult_Comp_Nsg_care
-2011_Update_FINAL_printed_copy_2_.pdf

REFERENCES

American Nurses Association. (2015). *Code of ethics for nurses with interpretive statements*. Silver Spring, MD: Nursebooks.org.

Bosslet, G. T., Pope, T. M., Rubenfeld, G. D., Lo, B., Truog, R. D., Rushton, C. H., . . . White, D. B. on behalf of The American Thoracic Society ad hoc Committee on Futile and Potentially Inappropriate Care. (2015). An official ATS/AACN/ACCP/ESICM/SCCM Policy Statement: Responding to requests for potentially inappropriate treatments in intensive care units. *American Journal of Respiratory and Critical Care Medicine, 191*(11), 1318–1330.

Brown, T. (2014). Lost in clinical translation. *New York Times* Opinion Pages. Retrieved from http://opinionator.blogs.nytimes.com/2014/02/08/lost-in-clinical-translation/?_r=0

Brush, D. R., Rasinski, K. A., Hall, J. B., & Alexander, G. C. (2012). Recommendations to limit life support: A national survey of critical care physicians. *American Journal of Respiratory and Critical Care Medicine, 186*(7), 633–639.

Chiarchiaro, J., Buddadhumaruk, P., Arnold, R. M., & White, D. B. (2015). Quality of communication in the ICU and surrogate's understanding of prognosis. *Critical Care Medicine, 43*(3), 542–548.

Cook, D., & Rocker, G. (2014). Dying with dignity in the intensive care unit. *The New England Journal of Medicine, 370*(26), 2506–2514.

Douglas, M., Rosenkoetter, M., Pacquiao, D., Callista, L., Hattar-Pollara, M., Lauderdale, J., . . . Purnell, L. (2014). Guidelines for implementing culturally competent nursing care. *Journal of Transcultural Nursing, 25*(2), 109–121.

Durall, A., Zurakowski, D., & Wolfe, J. (2012). Barriers to conducting advance care discussions for children with life-threatening conditions. *Pediatrics, 129*(4), e975–e982.

Fassier, T., & Azoulay, E. (2010). Conflicts and communication gaps in the intensive care unit. *Current Opinion in Critical Care, 16*(6), 654–665. doi:10.1097/MCC.0b013e32834044f0

Ford, D., Zapka, J., Gebregziabher, M., Yang, C., & Sterba, K. (2010). Factors associated with illness perception among critically ill patients and surrogates. *Chest, 138*(1), 59–67.

Gallup. (2014). Honesty/ethics in professions. Retrieved from http://www.gallup.com/poll/1654/honesty-ethics-professions.aspx

Giri, V. N. (2006). Culture and communication style. *The Review of Communication, 6*(1–2), 124–130.

Guess, C. (2004). Decision making in individualistic and collectivistic cultures. *Online Readings in psychology and culture, 4*(1). Retrieved from http://scholarworks.gvsu.edu/cgi/viewcontent.cgi?article=1032&context=orpc

Hanchate, A., Kronman, A. C., Young-Xu, Y., Ash, A. S., & Emanuel, E. (2009). Racial and ethnic differences in end-of-life costs. *Archives of Internal Medicine, 169*(5), 493–501.

Hart, J. L., Harhay, M. O., Gabler, N. B., Ratcliffe, S. J., Quill, C. M., & Halpern, S. D. (2015). Variability among U.S. intensive care units in managing the care of patients admitted with pre-existing limits on life-sustaining therapies. *JAMA Internal Medicine, 175*(6), 1019–1026.

Harvey, M. (2014). Tapping a vital resource: Increasing the yield of family care conferences. *Critical Care Medicine, 42*(2), 450–451.

Huffines, M., Johnson, K. L., Smitz Naranjo, L. L., Lissauer, M. E., Fishel, M. A., D'AngeloHowes, S. M., . . . Smith, R. (2013). Improving family satisfaction and participation in decision making in an intensive care unit. *Critical Care Nursing, 33*(5), 56–69.

Hutchinson, P. J. (2015). Do physicians have a responsibility to provide recommendations regarding goals of care to surrogates of dying patients in the ICU? Yes. *Chest, 147*(6), 1453–1455.

Iglesias, M. E., Pascual, C., & de Bengoa Vallejo, R. B. (2013). Obstacles and helpful behaviors in providing end-of-life care to dying patients in intensive care units. *Dimensions of Critical Care Nursing, 32*(2), 99–106.

Institute of Medicine. (2014). *Dying in America: Improving quality and honoring individual preferences near the end of life.* Washington, DC: National Academies Press.

Johnson, R. W., Newby, K. L., Granger, C. B., Cook, W. A., Peterson, E. D., Echols, M., . . . Granger, B. B. (2010). Differences in level of care at the end of life according to race. *American Journal of Critical Care, 19*(4); 335–344.

Kayser, J. B. (2014). Ethics, communication and the ICU: Charting a course for resolving conflict. *Critical Connections, 13*(4), 1,9.

Lautrette, A., Darmon, M., Megarbene, B., Joly, L. M., Chevret, S., Adrie, C., . . . Azoulay, E. (2007). A communication strategy and brochure for relatives of patients dying in the ICU. *The New England Journal of Medicine, 356*(5), 469–478.

Long, A. C., & Curtis, J. R. (2013). The epidemic of physician–family conflict in the ICU and what we should do about it. *Critical Care Medicine, 42*(2), 461–462.

Majesko, A., Hong, S. Y., Weissfeld, L., & White, D. B. (2012). Identifying family members who may struggle in the role of surrogate decision maker. *Critical Care Medicine, 40*(8), 2281–2286.

Manara, A. (2015). Bespoke end-of-life decision making in ICU: Has the tailor got the right measurement? *Critical Care Medicine, 43*(4), 909–10.

Morgan, C. K., Varas, G. M., Pedroza, C., & Almoosa, K. F. (2013). Defining the practice of "No escalation of care" in the ICU. *Critical Care Medicine, 42*(2), 357–361.

Pascual, J. L., & Marks, J. A. (2014). Key to cultural awareness and ethical decision-making in the ICU: Effective communication. *Critical Connections, 13*(4), 8.

Pew Research Center. (2013). Views on end-of-life medical treatments. Retrieved from http://www.pewforum.org/2013/11/21/views-on-end-of-life-medical-treatments

Phelps, A. C., Maciejewski, P. K., Nilsson, M., Balboni, T. A., Wright, A. A., Paulk, M. E., . . . Prigerson, H. G. (2009). Religious coping and use of intensive life-prolonging care near death in patients with advanced cancer. *JAMA, 301*(11), 1140–1147.

Philipsen, N., Murray, T., Wood, C., Bell-Hawkins, A., & Setlow, P. (2013). Surrogate decision-making: How to promote best outcomes in difficult times. *Journal of Nursing Practice, 9*(9), 581–587.

Purnell, L. (2012). *Transcultural health care: A culturally competent approach* (4th ed.). Philadelphia, PA: F. A. Davis.

Rest, J. (1986). *Moral development: Advances in research and theory*. New York, NY: Praeger.

Robichaux, C. (2012). Developing ethical skills: From sensitivity to action. *Critical Care Nursing, 32*(2), 65–72.

Rothman, D. J. (2014). Where we die. *The New England Journal of Medicine, 370*(26), 2457–2460.

Shaw, D. J., Davidson, J. E., Smilde, R. I., Sondoozi, T., & Agan, D. (2014). Multidisciplinary team training to enhance family communication in the ICU. *Critical Care Medicine, 42*(2), 265–271.

Schuster, R. A., Hong, S. Y., Arnold, R. M., & White, D. B. (2013). Investigating conflict in ICUs: Is the clinicians' perspective enough? *Critical Care Medicine, 42*(2), 328–335.

Scheunemann, L. P., Cunningham, T. V., Arnold, R. M., Buddadhumaruk, P., & White, D. (2015). How clinicians discuss critically ill patients' preferences and values with surrogates: An empirical analysis. *Critical Care Medicine, 43*(4), 757–764.

Scheunemann, L. P., McDevitt, M., Carson, S. S., & Hanson, L. C. (2011). Randomized, controlled trials to improve communication in intensive care. *Chest, 139*(3), 543–554.

Singer, A. E., Meeker, D., Teno, J. M., Lynn, J., Lunney, J. R., & Lorenz, K. A. (2015). Symptom trends in the last year of life from 1998–2010. *Annals of Internal Medicine, 162*(3), 175–183.

Ting-Toomey, S., & Chung, L. C. (2011). *Understanding intercultural communication* (2nd ed.). New York, NY: Oxford University Press.

Torke, A. M., Sachs, G. A., Helft, P. R., Kianna Montz, M. A., Hui, S. L., Slaven, J. E., & Callahan, C. M. (2014). Scope and outcomes of surrogate decision making among hospitalized older adults. *JAMA Internal Medicine, 174*(3), 370–377.

Truog, R. D., Campbell, M. L., Curtis, J. R., Haas, C. E., Luce, J. M., . . . American Academy of Critical Care Medicine. (2008). Recommendations for end-of-life care in the intensive care unit: A consensus statement by the American College (corrected) of Critical Care Medicine. *Critical Care Medicine, 36*(3), 953–963.

Uy, J., White, D. B., Mohan, D., Arnold, R. M., & Barnato, A. E. (2015). Physician's decision-making roles for an acutely unstable and terminally ill patient. *Critical Care Medicine, 41*(6), 1511–1517.

Van Cleave, A. C., Roosen-Runge, M. U., Miller, A. B., Milner, L. C., Karkazis, K. A., & Magnus, D. C. (2014). Quality of communication in interpreted versus noninterpreted PICU family meetings. *Critical Care Medicine, 42*(6), 1507–1517.

Veatch, R. M. (2015). Do physicians have a responsibility to provide recommendations regarding goals of care to surrogates of dying patients in the ICU? No. *Chest, 147*(6), 1455–1457.

Wilson, M. E., Krupa, A., Hinds, R. F., Litel, J. M., Swetz, K. M., Akhoundi, A., . . . Kashani, K. (2015). A video to improve patient and surrogate understanding of cardiopulmonary resuscitation choices in the ICU: A randomized controlled trial. *Critical Care Medicine, 43*(3); 621–629.

Wolf, S. M., Berlinger, N., & Jennings, M. A. (2015). Forty years of work on end-of-life care: From patients' rights to systemic reform. *The New Englang Journal of Medicine, 372*(7), 678–682.

You, J. J., Fowler, R. A., & Heyland, D. K., Canadian researchers at the End of Life Network (CARENET). (2014). Just ask: Discussing goals of care with patients in hospital with serious illness. *Canadian Medical Association Journal, 186*(6), 425–432.

You, J. J., Dodek, P., Lamontagne, F., Downar, J., Sinuff, T., Jiang, X., . . . Heyland, D. K. for the ACCEPT Study Team and the Canadian Researchers at the End of Life Network (CARENET). (2014). What really matters in end-of-life discussions? Perspectives of patients in hospital with serious illness and their families. *Canadian Medical Association Journal, 186*(18), E679–E687.

Recognizing and Addressing Moral Distress in Nursing Practice: Personal, Professional, and Organizational Factors

CATHERINE ROBICHAUX

LEARNING OBJECTIVES AND OUTCOMES

Upon completion of this chapter, the reader will be able to:

- Identify and discuss four responses to ethical situations: moral uncertainty, moral dilemma, moral distress, and moral residue
- Describe personal, professional, and organizational causes of moral distress
- Analyze current interventions and strategies to address moral distress at the personal, professional, and organizational levels

In a 2009 investigation, 71.6% of nurses and physicians from 24 countries reported experiencing an ethical conflict the week before completing the study survey (Azoulay et al., 2009). Current sources of ethical conflict reflect advances in technology, consumers' expectations of medical care, differing values/goals, poor communication, disruptive provider behaviors, and a business-focused model of health care, among others (Pavlish, Hellyer, et al., 2015). As a nurse, you may encounter such conflicts on a daily basis and believe you know what kind of ethical action is needed, but are unable to act on that knowledge. This inaction may result in feelings of moral distress.

CASE SCENARIO

Marcia taught high school math for several years and then received her BSN 2 years ago at the age of 42. Recently, Marcia enrolled in the master in science nurse educator program at a smaller university. This semester, she is taking the clinical practicum course in which she and a faculty preceptor, Ann, have a group of eight senior associate degree students in a 40-bed medical–surgical unit. One of the students, Jackie, has been having difficulty in both the clinical and didactic components of the course and is often late in the morning and for clinical conferences. Marcia has recently observed Jackie conducting a very superficial physical assessment and documenting inaccurate findings in the patient's electronic record. When she attempts to discuss this situation with her, Jackie states, "You have no authority over me; you're just a student, too!" Although Ann, the faculty preceptor, had Jackie repeat the physical assessment and correct her charting, Jackie continues to take shortcuts and narrowly avoids making a medication error on the following clinical day. Marcia decides to discuss her concerns regarding Jackie's competence and professionalism with Ann, who says "I agree, but she has been passed along by the other faculty and is about to graduate. The former dean didn't want to lose any more students from the program and I'm not sure about the new dean. In addition, Jackie works nights right now and is the main provider for her three kids. She really needs a better job, like nursing." Marcia considers Ann's comments and thinks, "Well, I am just a student in this program and I don't want to get in an argument with the dean or ruin Jackie's chance for a career, but what if she continues to be unsafe?"

Marcia is both a student and a practicing nurse who has a primary professional obligation to protect patients; however, she does not want to harm her own career by potentially angering the dean of the school in which she is a student. Marcia is also concerned that the university faculty "passed along" Jackie and believes it should have been their responsibility to take action sooner in the program. She does not want to jeopardize Jackie's future and ability to care for her family, but is aware of Provision 3 of the Code of Ethics: "The nurse promotes, advocates for, and protects the rights, health, and safety of the patient" (ANA, 2015a, p. 9). In addition, Statement 3.3 mandates: "Nurse educators, whether in academics or direct care settings, must ensure that basic competence and commitment to professional standards exist prior to entry into practice" (p. 11). As the practicum continues, Jackie's clinical skills and didactic performance remain marginal and Marcia begins to have headaches and bouts of sleeplessness. Marcia is experiencing moral distress, described as the psychological, emotional, and physiological suffering that nurses and other health professionals endure when they act in ways that are inconsistent with deeply held ethical values, principles, or commitments (McCarthy & Gastmans, 2015). Another definition proposes that moral distress is "mental anguish as a result of being conscious of a morally appropriate action, which despite every effort cannot be performed owing to organizational or other constraints" (Schluter, Winch, Holzhauser, & Henderson, 2008, p. 306).

Despite its apparent prevalence across nursing specialties and among all health care disciplines, both nationally and internationally, moral distress remains a contested concept. For some, the notion of moral distress remains ambiguous and they maintain that further examination will not contribute to quality deliberation or ethical nursing practice (Johnstone & Hutchinson, 2015; Pauly, Varcoe, & Storch, 2012). Others propose that inattention to moral distress among nurses and other providers will continue to result in burnout and/or leaving the profession (Whitehead, Herbertson, Hamric, Epstein, & Fisher, 2015). To bridge this gap, Peter (2015) suggests that our understanding of moral distress has expanded and may serve as a window through which nurses and others can describe the nuances of their ethical experiences. She proposes that perhaps "we have asked too much of this concept [moral distress] by attempting to articulate more about the nature of nurses' ethical lives than it can reliably hold" (p. 3). Although recognition of moral distress is essential, developing and implementing interventions to reduce its impact is critical. Thus, the purpose of this chapter is to describe the origins of moral distress, its contributing factors, and potential interventions designed to mitigate its deleterious effects on ethical nursing practice.

RESPONSES TO ETHICAL SITUATIONS

Question to Consider Before Reading On

1. How would you describe Marcia's initial responses in this situation?

As initially described by philosopher Andrew Jameton in his book, *Nursing Practice: The Ethical Issues* (1984), and experienced by Marcia in the Case Scenario, moral distress can occur when a nurse or other provider believes he or she knows what ethical action is needed but is unable to act on that knowledge. Recall that in Chapters 1 and 2 we discussed Rest's four-component model (FCM, 1986) for developing ethical skills or competence in nursing practice: sensitivity, judgment, motivation, and action. Moral distress inhibits or impedes motivation, resulting in inaction. This response to an ethical situation differs from other reactions described by Jameton (1984) and Rushton & Kurtz (2015), moral/ethical uncertainty, dilemmas, and conflicts, presented in Box 4.1.

CASE SCENARIO *(CONTINUED)*

If Marcia were unsure whether the situation with Jackie constituted an ethical issue or did not understand which ethical principles or provisions/statements from the Code of Ethics were relevant, she would be experiencing moral uncertainty. *This uncertainty may be the result of lack of sensitivity or ethics*

(continued)

CASE SCENARIO (CONTINUED)

education and there may be no resolution of the issue. However, Marcia may still experience emotional or physical symptoms that suggest something is "not quite right" and continue with ethical deliberation and action as presented in the FCM.

Box 4.1

Responses to Ethical Situations

Moral uncertainty—uncertainty about which ethical principles and/or provisions from the Code of Ethics apply in an ethical situation.

Moral dilemma—two ethically viable principles or goals are in opposition to each other in an ethical situation and only one may be chosen.

Moral conflict—stakeholders in an ethical situation have opposing views about how it should be resolved.

Moral distress—a nurse or other provider believes he or she knows what ethical action is needed but is unable to act on that knowledge.

Moral residue—painful feelings that remain after experiencing morally distressing situations.

Sources: Jameton (1984); Rushton and Kurtz (2015).

As discussed in Chapter 1, an *ethical* or *moral dilemma* occurs when there are two competing principles or values that are in opposition to one another. While each option may be ethically viable, only one may be chosen and the nurse may feel that he or she is compromising one value for another. Nursing care situations in which patient autonomy may be compromised to maintain safety and prevent harm are examples of possible ethical dilemmas. Differing values or goals of the organization may also conflict with those of the nurse or other provider. In the Case Scenario, Marcia may feel that her core values of protecting patients and maintaining professional standards conflict with the educational institution's goal of retaining students.

Providers and others involved in an ethical dilemma may have opposing views about how the situation should be resolved, resulting in *moral conflict*. As Rushton and Kurtz (2015) observe, conflicts generally arise over disagreements about the goals of care or perceived treatment outcomes. They describe resuscitation status as a decision that may result in conflict among or within health care team members and the patient/family. The decision to resuscitate extremely premature infants provides an example of this potential moral conflict (Molloy, Evans, & Coughlin, 2015). Those involved in the decision may have differing opinions regarding whether the benefits of resuscitation outweigh the risks of possible long-term health issues and compromised quality of life for the infants and families. The intensely emotional nature of such conflicts makes reasoning very difficult. In the communication process necessary to address these ethical conflicts, it is critical that those involved are not required to abandon their core values or professional integrity.

Questions to Consider Before Reading On

1. How would you define moral distress?

2. Do you believe you have experienced moral distress?

3. How did you learn to deal with it in your initial nursing program or in continuing education since you graduated?

DEFINING MORAL DISTRESS

In describing the origins of the concept of moral distress, Jameton (2013) discusses the introduction of bioethics courses in medical school curricula in the 1970s and 1980s. Faculty teaching these courses recognized that nurses and nursing students were very interested in the study of ethics and, consequently, the courses were offered campus wide. Although often labeled "medical ethics," many more nurses enrolled in these courses than students in other health care professions. While faculty had previously taught major ethical theories and representative dilemmas that highlighted the central role of the physician, the predominance of nurses in the classroom shifted that focus. As a result, Jameton notes, Davis and Aroskar published one of the first modern nursing ethics books in 1978, *Ethical Dilemmas and Nursing Practice.*

Jameton (2013) observes that nurses in the ethics courses discussed concerns that were practical and relational in nature. As the time period (1970s–1980s) coincided with a beginning interest in feminism and feminist ethics, these concerns also included issues of powerlessness, inequality, and bureaucratic constraints on ethical nursing practice. Although many students had several years of clinical experience, Jameton states "they expressed little confidence in their own views" on ethical issues and expected to "receive little support from physicians or nursing administrators" (p. 298). The concept of moral distress then appeared to represent a more comprehensive depiction of nurses' moral problems and challenges.

While the original definition of moral distress is credited to Jameton (1984), both he and Fowler (2015) maintain that Kramer's 1974 work on reality shock in nursing predates his identification of the phenomenon. Kramer's seminal research explored the transition of recently graduated nurses into the workforce and "the discrepancy and shock like reactions that follow"

(p. 19) when they realized that their professional values and identity were not congruent with or supported by the immediate practice environment and/or employing organization. Given the increasing complexity of the current health care environment, many contend that this reality shock continues and is perhaps even more serious today (Dyess & Sherman, 2010; Kramer, Brewer, & Maguire, 2013). This experience of reality shock is reflected in Jameton's definition of moral distress, "one knows the right thing to do but institutional constraints make it nearly impossible to pursue the right course of action" (p. 6). As Epstein and Delgado (2009) observe, with moral distress, the appropriate or right action has been identified and discussion of the precipitating ethical situation is less critical. Rather, addressing moral distress requires consideration of both personal and professional factors and identification of organizational constraints.

CAUSES OF MORAL DISTRESS

Personal and Professional Factors

While Jameton's original definition of moral distress focused on organizational constraints on moral action, others propose that personal factors also hinder ethical practice (Epstein & Hamric, 2009; Rushton & Kurtz, 2015; Webster & Bayliss, 2000). In addition to those personal characteristics and internal constraints discussed in Chapter 2, such as individual values, protecting one's position, or lack of ethical sensitivity, these authors include perceived powerlessness, past experiences, and emotional stability.

Perceived Powerlessness

The often hierarchal nature of the health care system contributes to power differentials based on whose work may be considered more important (Pavlish, Brown-Saltzman, et al., 2015). As a result, nurses may feel that they have little influence on directing patient care or on decision making in general. Implementing the decisions of others while lacking authority and experiencing increased responsibility may contribute to moral distress. In the Case Scenario, Marcia may feel powerless as she is "just a student" and has to adhere to the decisions of the dean and faculty while feeling responsible for the impact of Jackie's incompetence on present and future patient care.

Past Experiences

In studies exploring moral distress in nursing, several researchers found that those who had been in practice for a longer period experienced more moral distress than those newer to the profession (Epstein & Delgado, 2010; Sauerland, Marotta, Peinemann, Berndt, & Robichaux, 2014; Sauerland, Marotta, Peinemann, Berndt, & Robichaux, 2015). As those past experiences causing moral distress may recur, nurses can have a "here we go again" response associated with dread, helplessness, and disengagement. These recurrent ethical situations may or may not be resolved and the painful feelings linger, resulting in *moral residue*. As defined by Webster and Bayliss (2000), moral residue is "that which each of us carries with us from those times in our lives when in the face of moral distress we have seriously compromised ourselves or allowed ourselves to be compromised" (p. 208). Frequent situations associated with moral distress and residue include providing aggressive, prolonged futile care, working with incompetent clinicians, and conflicts with other health care providers (Hamric, Borchers, & Epstein, 2012; Sauerland et al., 2014, 2015; Whitehead et al., 2015).

While nurses and other providers who have been practicing longer may have higher levels of moral distress, those newer to the profession may also be susceptible to its damaging effects. Indeed, the resulting "reality shock" and moral distress experienced by novice nurses have been identified among undergraduate nursing students who report witnessing poor nursing practice and experiencing bullying from preceptors (Grady, 2014; Sasso et al., 2015; Yoes, 2012). Students and recent graduates may not have sufficient experience and coping skills to address such morally distressing situations and/or may not be aware of existing resources to assist them.

CASE SCENARIO (*CONTINUED*)

Returning to the Case Scenario, Marcia continues to think about her preceptor Ann's comments regarding the former dean's goal of retaining students in the associate degree nursing (ADN) program. Marcia realizes that she is unfamiliar with the academic role of the nursing instructor; however, she is aware of the impact that "passing along" unprepared students has on faculty and the reputation of a school. Having taught high school for several years, Marcia recalls students who should not have progressed from the previous year into her class. These students continued to struggle and Marcia believed that the school was doing them a disservice. At that time, she spoke with the principal about her concerns and the potential repercussions for the school if the students could not pass state-mandated examinations. Her experience and maturity enabled Marcia to discuss the issue in a calm manner and the principal listened to her concerns and agreed to address the issue. After reflecting on this experience, Marcia talks with Ann, and they decide to make an appointment to speak with the dean of the nursing school.

Emotional Stability

Rushton and Kurtz (2015) state that a nurse's ability to remain mentally and emotionally stable in morally distressing situations may also be a factor in his or her experience of moral distress. Feeling helpless or unable to act in these circumstances can initiate stress responses such as "fight (anger), flight (abandonment), or freeze (numbing)" (p. 13). The fact that nurses are expected to be stoic and endure without overt reaction may add to these overwhelming stress responses. The experience of emergency department (ED) nurses working in resuscitation rooms provides a graphic example of struggling to maintain emotional control in these situations.

Houghtaling (2012) describes the moral suffering of nurses in the ED, who often witness unnecessary suffering and must perform painful procedures while "literally holding themselves together": "When seconds are all these nurses have, there is no time to premeditate or look inward; they must perform—whether or not they agree with the care practices that are carried out in the situation immediately unfolding around them" (p. 235). The stress and pressure to endure in such scenarios may cause the nurse to vent his or her frustration on another staff member and/or experience moral distress and moral residue. Houghtaling suggests that when nurses learn to recognize highly volatile and morally, ethically charged dilemmas, they may become more effective in finding skills within themselves to maintain a sense of well-being and balance. Strategies to increase resilience and mental/emotional stability when experiencing moral distress are discussed in the section on addressing moral distress.

Organizational Factors

Question to Consider Before Reading On

1. How would you describe the ethical climate in the organization in which you currently work or have worked in the past?

Ethical climate is described as the organizational conditions and practices in which problems with ethical implications are identified, discussed, and decided (Olson, 1998). As discussed in Chapter 2, moral distress can be exacerbated in organizations with a deficient ethical climate. Fear of reprisal for actions and/or limited access to ethics resources when dealing with ethical situations can result in moral distress. Additional institutional factors include lack of ethical, supervisory support, inadequate and/or incompetent staff, excessive workloads, and bullying, lateral violence, incivility, and workplace violence (Hamric, 2014; Whitehead et al., 2015). These organizational influences may create sources of moral distress and inhibit its resolution. Several of these factors are discussed in more detail as follows.

Lack of Ethical, Supervisory Support

Question to Consider Before Reading On

1. What level of ethical, supervisory support have you received where you are currently employed or have been employed in the past?

Effective, supportive leadership is essential to ethical nursing practice and is associated with a healthy work environment, improved patient safety and satisfaction, and decreased nurse turnover (Laschinger & Smith, 2013; Zook,

2014). Lack of such leadership can contribute to or directly cause moral distress (De Veer, Francke, Struijs, & Willems, 2013; Galletta, Portoghese, Battistelli, & Leiter, 2013). As noted previously, if the nurse feels that he or she will not be supported when speaking up in an ethical situation, patient safety may be compromised and nurse moral integrity impaired.

While supportive, ethical leadership has been examined extensively in the business literature, it has received far less attention in nursing (Makaroff, Storch, Pauly, & Newton, 2014; Storch, Makaroff, Pauly, & Newton, 2013). Although leadership theories discussed in nursing contain moral components and behaviors, ethical leaders focus *explicitly* on ethical obligations and guidelines and hold others accountable to do the same. Thus, their potential impact goes beyond simply increasing sensitivity to ethical issues and standards. Peers and employees trust ethical leaders and display more positive attitudes and greater job performance because of this heightened trust. In addition, these nurse leaders may influence the ethical conduct of others by modeling critical thinking and action regarding situations with ethical content (Zheng et al., 2015). The importance of ethical, supervisory support and leadership to ethical nursing practice is discussed more fully in Chapter 10.

CASE SCENARIO *(CONTINUED)*

Returning to the Case Scenario, Marcia and Ann arrive for their appointment with the dean of the nursing school and are escorted into her office. Marcia describes their concerns regarding Jackie's clinical competence and lack of attention to constructive feedback from both her and Ann. Marcia shares her distress regarding possibly jeopardizing Jackie's future but believes it is a professional, ethical responsibility to share their assessment. Dr. B, the dean, thanks Marcia and Ann for coming forward with their honest appraisal. She continues by adding that nurses in all roles, including education, administration, and research, share the primary, ethical commitment of providing high-quality care to the patient. Dr. B then refers to interpretive statement 7.3 in the Code of Ethics (2015a), "Academic educators must also seek to ensure that all their graduates possess the knowledge, skills, and moral dispositions that are essential to nursing" (p. 28). Dr. B. states that she, Marcia, and Ann will meet with Jackie to discuss her continued progression in the program. She also notes that, as contained in the undergraduate student handbook, students who have a documented pattern of unsafe or unprofessional clinical performance and have not improved following remediation may not be permitted to repeat the course. After leaving the dean's office, Ann thanks Marcia for arranging the appointment and states, "I feel more supported now in making these difficult decisions about students."

Inadequate and/or Incompetent Staff

Questions to Consider Before Reading On

1. Have you ever worked with incompetent staff?

2. What was the outcome?

3. Use the Box 4.2 to assess any personal, professional, or organizational factors that are present where you are employed that may lead to moral distress.

Several studies that have used the original Moral Distress Scale (MDS; Corley, Elswick, Gorman, & Clor, 2001) or the revised version (MDS-R; Hamric et al., 2012) or a qualitative, open-ended survey reported that nurses and other providers identified working with inadequate and/or incompetent staff as both highly distressing and occurring frequently (Sauerland et al., 2014, 2015; Wilson, Goettemoeller, Bevan, & McCord, 2013). In addition, research participants described providers who offered less than optimal treatment that did not meet the standard of care, witnessing poor patient care because of inadequate staff communication. Despite the prodigious amount of research documenting the direct relationship between inadequate registered nurse staffing and poor patient outcomes and increased mortality, this issue remains an ongoing concern (Dent, 2015; Needleman, 2015; West et al., 2014). As discussed in Chapter 10, the American Nurses Association (2012) and several specialty organizations (Thompson & Davidson, 2014) have proposed guidelines and strategies for adequate and competent nurse staffing. In addition, federal legislation regarding safe nurse staffing is presently under review in the U.S. Senate (Registered Nurse Safe Staffing Act of 2015).

Continued work is needed to develop an optimal staffing model that integrates site specific variables such as acuity, provider preparation, and the relational work of nursing, among other factors (Malloch, 2015; Needleman, 2015). As Malloch observes, much of the work of nursing is relational and therefore difficult to measure and integrate in a staffing model. In addition, nursing requires critical thinking, the synthesis of disparate data items, teamwork coordination around episodes of patient care, and ensuring safe navigation through the health care system. This complexity requires not only innovative measures, but new classifications of the work of nursing (Archibald, Caine, & Scott, 2014). Meanwhile, nurses may remain caught between their obligations to care for a potentially unsafe number of patients and maintaining their professional and ethical integrity. The Code of Ethics (2015a) is explicit in identifying the frontline nurse and nurse administrator's responsibility to take action in situations of incompetent or unsafe care (Box 4.2). Developing and contributing to moral environments that support and encourage such action is essential to ethical practice.

Box 4.2

Recognizing and Addressing Moral Distress in Nursing Practice: Personal, Professional, and Organizational Factors

Relevant Provisions and Selected Statements from the Code of Ethics (2015a)

PROVISION 1
INTERPRETIVE STATEMENT 1.5
RELATIONSHIP WITH COLLEAGUES AND OTHERS

Respect for persons extends to all individuals with whom the nurse interacts. Nurses maintain professional, respectful, and caring relationships with colleagues and are committed to fair treatment, transparency, integrity preserving compromise, and the best resolution of conflicts. The nurse creates an ethical environment and culture of civility and kindness, treating colleagues, coworkers, employees, students, and others with dignity and respect. This standard of conduct includes an affirmative duty to act to prevent harm. Disregard for the effects of one's actions on others, bullying, harassment, intimidation, threats, and violence are always morally unacceptable behaviors.

PROVISION 3
INTERPRETIVE STATEMENT 3.5
PROTECTION OF PATIENT HEALTH AND SAFETY BY ACTING ON
    QUESTIONABLE PRACTICE

Nurses must be alert to and must take appropriate action in all instances of incompetent, unethical, illegal, or impaired practice or actions that place the rights or best interests of the patient in jeopardy.

PROVISION 4
INTERPRETIVE STATEMENT 4.4
ASSIGNMENT AND DELEGATION OF NURSING ACTIVITIES OR TASKS

Nurses in management and administration have a particular responsibility to provide a safe environment that supports and facilitates appropriate assignment and delegation. This includes orientation, skill development; licensure, certification, continuing education, competency verification; adequate and flexible staffing; and policies that protect both the patient and the nurse from inappropriate assignment or delegation of nursing responsibilities, activities, or tasks.

(continued)

Box 4.2

Recognizing and Addressing Moral Distress in Nursing Practice: Personal, Professional, and Organizational Factors *(continued)*

PROVISION 5

INTERPRETIVE STATEMENT 5.2

PROMOTION OF PERSONAL HEALTH, SAFETY, AND WELL-BEING

Fatigue and compassion fatigue affect a nurse's professional performance and personal life. To mitigate these effects, nurses should eat a healthy diet, exercise, get sufficient rest, maintain family and personal relationships, engage in adequate leisure and recreational activities, and attend to spiritual or religious needs.

INTERPRETIVE STATEMENT 5.4

PRESERVATION OF INTEGRITY

When the integrity of the nurse is compromised by patterns of institutional behavior or professional practice, thereby eroding the ethical environment and resulting in moral distress, nurses have an obligation to express their concern or conscientious objection individually or collectively to the appropriate authority or committee. Nurse administrators must respond to concerns and work to resolve them in a way that preserves the integrity of the nurses. They must seek to change enduring activities or expectations in the practice setting that are morally objectionable.

PROVISION 6

INTERPRETIVE STATEMENT 6.2

THE ENVIRONMENT AND ETHICAL OBLIGATION

Nurses in all roles must create a culture of excellence and maintain practice environments that support nurses and others in the fulfillment of their ethical obligations.

Many factors contribute to a practice environment that can either present barriers or foster ethical practice and professional fulfillment.

Source: ANA (2015a).

Bullying, Lateral Violence, Incivility, and Workplace Violence

Question to Consider Before Reading On

1. What types of bullying, lateral violence, incivility, and/or violence have you witnessed or experienced in your work place?

Rushton and Kurtz (2015) suggest that nurses' support or lack of support for one another can affect the level of moral distress in the health care environment.

The complexity of patient care demands that all health care professionals work together collaboratively as a team; however, that is often not the reality. The old adage of "nurses eat their young" still exists and, sadly, remains quite robust. Indeed, the health care professions have one of the highest levels of bullying in the workplace (Farouque & Burgio, 2013) and with incivility, and lateral violence behaviors, contribute to and result in moral distress. It is difficult to find a recent professional journal in any health care discipline that does not contain an article on these and other disruptive behaviors, their effects on the quality of patient care, and the morale of providers (Fink-Samnick, 2015; Trossman, 2015; Van Norman, 2015).

The terms *bullying*, *lateral* or *horizontal violence*, and *incivility* are often used interchangeably. Although there are commonalities among these behaviors, there are also differences. Bullying is repeated, long-term, health-harming mistreatment of one or more persons by one or more perpetrators and is marked by behavior that is threatening, humiliating, or intimidating. Bullying can be a reflection of the hierarchal system in health care and other organizations in which those who occupy higher levels or are more experienced bully individuals who are new and/or at lower levels. Recent graduates continue to be victims of bullying despite overwhelming evidence that these behaviors contribute to moral distress, turnover, and leaving the profession. In addition, as seen in Box 4.2, bullying and other destructive conduct are a direct violation of the Code of Ethics and countermand Quality and Safety Education for Nurses (QSEN) competencies associated with teamwork and collaboration (Box 4.3).

Lateral or horizontal violence is described as "Unkind, discourteous, antagonistic interactions between nurses who work at comparable organizational levels and commonly characterized as divisive backbiting and infighting" (Alspach, 2007, p. 13). While behaviors associated with lateral violence, such as sarcastic comments and withholding support, are similar to those used in bullying, the perpetrator and victim are at comparable levels in the organization or unit.

The prevalence of bullying and lateral violence behaviors in nursing has been attributed to prior victimization and oppressed group theory, among other reasons. Being the recipient of such destructive conduct may cause the nurse to retaliate in kind with a peer or other employee, thus continuing the cycle of victimization and moral distress. Oppressed group theory proposes that people who are victims of a situation of dominance turn on each other rather than confront the system, which oppresses them both. If the nurse in these situations is unable to speak up because of fear of retribution and is forced to work under such duress, he or she may experience moral distress. Dellasaga and Volpe (2013) note that those who repeatedly witness bullying and lateral violence may also experience moral distress if they are reluctant to intervene for fear of becoming a victim themselves.

Disrespectful and uncivil interactions in health care not only contribute to an unethical, morally distressing environment but also jeopardize patient safety. For example, a new graduate makes a medication error because he or

Box 4.3

Recognizing and Addressing Moral Distress in Nursing Practice: Relevant QSEN Competencies

Teamwork and Collaboration

Definition: Function effectively within nursing and interprofessional teams, fostering open communication, mutual respect, and shared decision making to achieve quality patient care.

Act with integrity, consistency, and respect for differing views. (Skills)

Appreciate importance of intra- and interprofessional collaboration. (Attitudes)

Value the perspectives and expertise of all health team members. (Attitudes)

Initiate actions to resolve conflict. (Skills)

Source: AACN (2012); Cronenwett et al. (2007).

she did not want to clarify the dosage with his or her preceptor for fear of being ridiculed again. Dr. R. continually berates and intimidates the perioperative staff, "fostering an atmosphere in which medical errors become more likely and interpersonal interactions erode the primary goal of putting the patients' welfare foremost" (Van Norman, 2015, p. 215). Studies have reported startling statistics indicating a direct relationship between these egregious behaviors, adverse events, and staff turnover. In Rosenstein's (2010) survey of over 4,500 respondents (nurses, physicians, pharmacists, and administrators) from more than 100 hospitals, 67% identified a strong relationship with adverse event occurrence, while 27% felt that the behaviors contributed to patient mortality. Rawson, Thompson, Sostre, and Deitte (2013) estimated that in a 400-bed hospital, the combined costs of disruptive physician behaviors resulting in staff turnover, medication errors, and procedural errors exceeded $1 million annually. According to a recent national survey (Nursing Solutions Incorporated, 2016), the average cost of turnover for a bedside registered nurse ranges from $37,700 to $58,400, resulting in the average hospital losing $5.2 million to $8.1 million.

The National Institute for Occupational Safety and Health (NIOSH) defines workplace violence as those physically and psychologically damaging actions that occur in the workplace or while on duty (2002). Although often discussed in the same context as bullying, lateral violence, and incivility, workplace violence includes actions perpetrated by patients and/or family members. The findings of an American Nurses Association (ANA) survey of 3,765 registered nurses and nursing students demonstrate evidence of the prevalence of these behaviors committed by those to whom we provide care.

Forty-three percent of the respondents reported having been verbally and/or physically threatened while 24% had been physically assaulted by a patient or family member of a patient in the previous 12 months (ANA, 2014). That these behaviors are considered endemic in certain settings such as EDs and psychiatric units suggests "that workplace violence is a culturally accepted and expected part of one's occupation" (ANA, 2015b).

There has been a great deal of research on moral distress across health care disciplines (Whitehead et al., 2015). It has been identified as a reality of nursing practice that is not going away (Rushton & Kurtz, 2015). Development of evidence-informed interventions to address its often deleterious effects, however, remains ongoing. Although nurses and other providers may be familiar with the feelings associated with moral distress, they may not be aware of the term itself. Consequently, recognition and labeling of the experience is an initial first step toward implementing any intervention. As one nurse shared in a recent study, "When I first joined the NEC (Nursing Ethics Council), I had no idea how to define moral distress. Now, I am more vigilant about situations that can cause moral distress, seek to address those situations early, and try to act as a resource for my peers." (Sauerland et al., 2015). The NEC mentioned by this nurse is part of a multilayered approach initially discussed in Chapter 2. In conjunction with developing ethical skills, this approach also has relevance in addressing moral distress. The personal and professional causes of moral distress were identified in addition to organizational sources. The following section will discuss building competencies at each level to address moral distress.

Personal and Professional Competencies

Ethics Education

Questions to Consider Before Reading On

1. What types of formal or continuing education have you had in ethics?

2. What resources do you have to turn to when you experience moral distress?

The necessity of ethics education for nurses is well documented and has been shown to influence moral confidence and action (Grady, 2014; Laabs, 2015; Witt, 2011) and decrease moral distress (Robinson et al., 2014). The inclusion of a specific course on ethics in undergraduate or master's programs, however, does not universally exist (Bartlett, 2013). While some programs do have identified ethics courses, others "integrate" content across curricula which, as Rushton observes, "means that it can be pretty invisible" (as quoted in Der Bedrosian, 2015). In addition, current didactic approaches to teaching ethics content may not prepare students to recognize day-to-day ethical issues and engage in problem solving. Krautscheid and Brown (2014) reported that

senior baccalaureate students were unable to recall or apply principles presented in an ethics course to a simulated medication safety scenario. Rushton
(as quoted in Der Bedrosian, 2015) states that nurses' potential, inadequate
ethics preparation is exacerbated by a lack of continuing education opportunities in ethics. As a result, nurses may be challenged to "demonstrate ethical
competence in professional life" (p. viii) as directed in the Code of Ethics
(ANA, 2015a).

It may not be necessary to have extensive knowledge regarding ethical
terms, theories, and principles. However, nurses should have an adequate
understanding of these components to be able to identify and engage in situations with ethical content from the day-to-day issues or "microethics" to those
more complicated. Frequently, nurses believe they have this understanding
when in actuality they are referring to their morality (i.e., they are good people
who were raised well, have values, and can therefore make appropriate ethical
decisions). While an understanding of personal values is essential, it is not sufficient for ethical practice. Although the terms "ethical" and "moral" are often
used interchangeably in this book, Klugman notes an important distinction
between ethics and morality, stating that the latter is sometimes "irrational
and illogical" (Chapter 1). Chapter 1 also provides an overview of ethics terms,
theories, and principles needed to initiate and participate in ethical discussions, including those causing moral distress.

Recognizing that additional education in ethics and moral distress may
be beneficial, the individual nurse can take advantage of material offered by
professional organizations such as the ANA. Resources available on the ANA
website "Ethics" tab include several articles on moral distress and moral
courage in addition to position statements on end of life and other ethical
issues of concern to nurses (2016a). The American Association of Critical
Care Nurses (AACN) identifies addressing moral distress as a strategic initiative in creating a healthy workplace environment. The organization has
issued a position statement on moral distress (AACN, 2012) and developed
a handbook, *The 4 A's to Rise Above Moral Distress: Ask, Affirm, Assess, and Act*
(2004). The three-part Moral Distress Education Project at the University
of Kentucky (2015) is a free, multimedia CE program that provides an overview of the root causes of moral distress and presents strategies to prevent
its recurrence.

Reading and discussing articles related to ethics such as those contained
in the references in this book is another approach to enhancing ethical skills
and competence. As mentioned earlier, forming a nursing ethics group or
committee and conducting interdisciplinary or nursing ethics rounds may
provide opportunities to identify and clarify issues with ethical or nonethical
content. The author participates in a NEC at University Health System in San
Antonio, Texas. The council, which meets monthly, serves as a supportive
environment for discussion of ethical issues pertinent to nurses and provides
opportunities for ethics education.

Effective Communication and Conflict Engagement Competencies

Questions to Consider Before Reading On

1. How do you usually respond when faced with moral distress or conflict?

2. Does this work for you?

3. How would you improve theses skills?

Baccalaureate essential VI states that the nursing program prepares the graduate to "Incorporate effective communication techniques, including negotiation and conflict resolution to produce positive professional working relationships" (AACN, 2008, p. 23). These skills are also considered essential QSEN competencies, as presented in Chapter 2. Despite these mandates, new graduates and experienced nurses continue to be described as lacking assertive communication skills and using avoidance when confronted by conflict (Pavlish, Brown-Saltzman, et al., 2015; Theisen & Sandau, 2011). We continue to hear about the detrimental effects of conflict avoidance and overall poor communication among health care team members and the impact on patient safety and mortality (Okuyama, Wagner, & Bijnen, 2014; Sayre, Mc Neese-Smith, & Leach, 2012). More than 15 years after the Institute of Medicine (IOM) report, *To Err is Human: Building a Safer Health System* (1999), and the follow-up report, *Crossing the Quality Chasm* (2001), and following national ongoing initiatives from The Joint Commission (2015) and the Institute for Healthcare Improvement (2013a, 2013b), little progress has been reported in improving quality and safety (Dolansky & Moore, 2013; Rainer, 2015).

As a result of this lack of improvement, several programs have been developed to strengthen communication and conflict resolution skills and perhaps decrease the incidence of moral distress among health care providers. Crucial conversations training (Patterson, Grenny, Mc Millan, & Switzler, 2011), discussed in Chapter 2, has been shown to specifically increase perioperative nurses' ability to address physicians' disruptive behaviors (Saxton, 2012). The program has been implemented successfully in several health care organizations including Spectrum Health in West Michigan and Maimonides Medical Center in Brooklyn, New York. Results indicated that, after crucial conversations training, nurses and staff members addressed issues and concerns with one another instead of relying on managers and there was a 39% improvement in confronting violations of respect (VitalSmarts, 2015). Additional communication and conflict engagement skills include elements of TeamSTEPPS (AHRQ, 2016; Harvey et al., 2013) and cognitive rehearsal (Griffin, 2004; Griffin & Clark, 2014). These skills are based on scripting and require actual practice, as with developing any technical competency. Ideally, they should be practiced in a group setting using role play but can also be applied by the individual nurse.

Cognitive rehearsal is an evidence-based strategy used in behavioral health that involves memorization, learned, although not by rote, of a thought or an expression "designed to help an individual cue a certain behavior or express a desire to others" (Glod, 1998, pp. 58–59, as quoted in Griffin & Clark, 2014, p. 540). This strategy can take several forms and be used to address common, uncivil behaviors and/or patient safety and conflict situations. Table 4.1 lists several common uncivil behaviors and associated cognitive rehearsal responses. Being able to recall these responses may allow the nurse to address the behavior or situation in the moment rather than experiencing anger and/or regret later for not speaking up.

The "CUS" technique and "DESC" scripting methods associated with TeamSTEPPS (AHRQ, 2016) are variants of the cognitive rehearsal strategy. CUS, an acronym for **c**oncerned, **u**ncomfortable, and **s**afety, is an assertive communication technique used when a patient safety issue or change in status is identified and can also be used to address uncivil behaviors. For example, the CUS technique can be applied in the following way: "Dr. Smith, I am concerned about Mr. Brown's rapid increase in heart rate. I am uncomfortable with his change in status. I don't think this it is safe for him to be unmonitored." Similarly, a nurse may respond to a bullying or lateral violence

Table 4.1

Uncivil Behaviors and Cognitive Rehearsal Responses

Nonverbal behaviors (sighing, eye rolling, etc.)	"I sense from your expression that there is something you wish to say to me. Please speak directly to me."
Spreading rumors, gossiping, sabotaging	"I don't feel right talking about him/her/situation when I wasn't there. I suggest you speak directly to them."
Using silent treatment or withholding information	"I understand that there was more information about this patient/situation. Please share all relevant information as safe patient care depends on collaboration."
Sarcastic comments, yelling, demeaning remarks	"I do not appreciate your comments/yelling as it is unprofessional behavior. If there is something you wish to discuss with me, we can do so privately."
Distracting, disruptive behaviors, inattention during handovers/meetings	"Can I speak with you about your conduct in handovers/meetings? It is distracting and may jeopardize patient care/effective communication."

Sources: ANA (2012); Griffin (2004); Griffin and Clark (2014).

experience by saying, "I am concerned about your uncivil tone. I am uncomfortable and stressed by this unprofessional situation which makes it difficult to work together and provide safe patient care."

The DESC communication model is used in TeamSTEPPS and described as "carefronting" by Briles (2007). The DESC acronym refers to **d**escribe the behavior/situation, **e**xplain the effect of the behavior/situation, **s**tate the desired change or outcome, and **c**onsequences, or what will happen if the behavior/situation continues. It is an assertive but caring technique based on work by Augsberger (1973), a family therapist, and adapted to nursing by Kupperschmidt (1994, 2006, 2008). Carefronting is similar to having a crucial conversation in that it involves holding someone accountable by confronting them in situations involving disrespect and/or those jeopardizing patient safety. Nurses have reported experiencing moral distress and remorse when they are unable to speak up and get others to listen to them or respect their opinions (Maxfield, Greeny, Lavandero, & Groah, 2011; Maxfield, Lyndon, Kennedy, O'Keefe, & Zlatnik, 2013). The goal of all these techniques is to develop an ethical environment based on mutual respect in which providers can work together to provide safe patient care. Kupperschmidt (2008) notes that carefronting is honest, courageous communication that requires courage (Chapter 2) and rigor. She states that rigor "means having the discipline to plan for effective carefronting: to make optimal use of resources, to say what one will do, and to do what one says. We cultivate rigor, and thus courage, by putting personal convenience in perspective, letting logic prevail, and ensuring that we are not blaming and shaming" (p. 15). Box 4.4 provides an example of a carefronting DESC script.

Rainer (2015) reminds us that providers from different cultures, including nurses, may have additional challenges employing effective communication and conflict engagement skills. While some difficulties are related to language barriers, others reflect differences in values associated with perceptions of patient autonomy, decision making, and workplace hierarchy. In a qualitative study exploring the ability to speak up and be heard, Garon (2012) reported that nurses who self-identified as Asian or Hispanic (n = 15) described endeavoring to emulate the assertive behavior of peer role models. The support of nurse managers in establishing an open, ethical environment that encouraged nurses to voice their concerns was also recognized as essential to speaking up by these participants.

Self-Care Competencies

Questions to Consider Before Reading On

1. What are your attitudes or feelings when you experience an ethical concern or conflict?

2. How would you describe your current level of moral courage?

Authors and researchers observe that moral distress in health care is not likely to go away and is "becoming part of our new normal" (Lavandero, as quoted in

---

Box 4.4

Application of a Carefronting DESC Script

Dr. C is a senior resident in the PICU and has had a good working relationship with the nurses. Recently, the unit has expanded to accommodate transplant patients and more nurses were hired. You are one of several newly hired nurses who feel intimidated by Dr. C as she is often rude and unhelpful. She is also slow to respond to pages and insists that only certain, "more experienced" nurses care for "her" patients.

Today, Dr. C has loudly complained about your assessment skills in front of others:

Describe the behavior/situation:
Dr. C, this morning you shouted at me in the nurses' station in front of others. This is not the first time you have spoken to me in that manner. (Stay silent)

Explain how the situation/behavior makes you feel and your concerns:
I feel angry and humiliated because it seems like you are trying to make me appear incompetent.

Suggest alternatives and seek agreement:
In the future, I would like you to talk to me personally if you have questions about my patient assessments as we are both here to provide safe patient care. Please do not raise your voice to me again. Are you committed to doing this? (Stay silent)

Consequences should be stated in terms of impact on goals/patient safety:
If you continue with this behavior, which I have documented, I will report it to (manager, supervisor, director) as it is bullying, against hospital policy, and affects my ability to provide safe care.

Sources: Kupperschmidt (1994, 2006, 2008).

Wood, 2014). Others note that experiences of moral distress can have a positive effect by increasing awareness of personal and institutional obstacles to ethical practice. This awareness can initiate a learning process that may contribute to a proactive approach as demonstrated by one nurse in a recent study who wrote, "I do more good by staying and correcting these distressing situations than I would if I left because they bothered me so!" (Sauerland et al., 2014, p. 242). A positive and proactive attitude may be enhanced by developing self-care competencies that address cognitive, somatic, and affective dimensions. These self-care competencies may also mitigate the physical and psychological symptoms associated with moral distress including headache, insomnia, and depression (Rushton, Kasniak, & Halifax et al., 2013; Sauerland et al., 2014, 2015).

Although Provision 5 of the Code of Ethics states, "The nurse owes the same duties to self as to others including the responsibility to promote health and safety" (ANA, 2015a, p. 19), self-care education is rarely addressed in nursing or medical school curricula (Sanchez-Reilly et al., 2013). Indeed, as Blum (2014) observes, nurses express reluctance to take the time for self-care or have difficulty finding relevant activities that are easily adapted to their lives. A comprehensive review of the numerous self-care activities available is beyond the scope of this chapter. As Sanchez and colleagues note, however, self-care activities include a spectrum of knowledge, skills, and attitudes that contribute to personal resilience, defined as the ability to adapt coping strategies to minimize distress or the capacity to keep functioning in the face of stress, trauma, adversity, or tragedy (Rushton, Batcheller, Schroeder, & Donohue, 2015; Sullivan et al., 2012).

A fundamental, personal self-care strategy includes maintaining a healthy lifestyle by ensuring adequate nutrition, sleep, and exercise. In addition, time for vacations, family, and hobbies contributes to overall resilience. The Wellness Wheel, such as that used by the Vanderbilt University Wellness Center (2016), is an instrument that addresses eight dimensions of wellness (Figure 4.1). The Vanderbilt website link to each dimension of the wheel provides a definition and associated attributes in addition to suggested resources and articles. Consideration of each dimension may encourage reflection on current life balance and self-care activities. The American Nurses Association HealthyNurse initiative (2016b) offers a healthy nurse toolkit that provides information on nurse fatigue and preventing back injuries, among other issues. ANA has also collaborated with Pfizer to develop The HealthyNurse Health Risk Appraisal survey. This instrument provides real-time data on individual health, safety, and wellness, both personally and professionally. Upon completion of the survey, a nurse can compare his or her results to national averages and ideal standards and access resources individualized to his or her responses. The American Holistic Nurses Association (2015) also has extensive resources on stress management modalities including mindfulness meditation, journaling, and cognitive restructuring.

Lachman (as quoted in Jones, 2015) observes that moral courage (Chapter 2) is a means to overcome fear through practical action. Similarly, developing resilience to deal with ethical challenges may require a change in how nurses think about their roles and responsibilities, for example:

- Accepting change as a part of living

- Keeping things in perspective

- Avoiding seeing crises as insurmountable problems

- Looking for opportunities for self-discovery

- Maintaining a hopeful outlook

- Getting needed social support (Jones, 2015, p. 16)

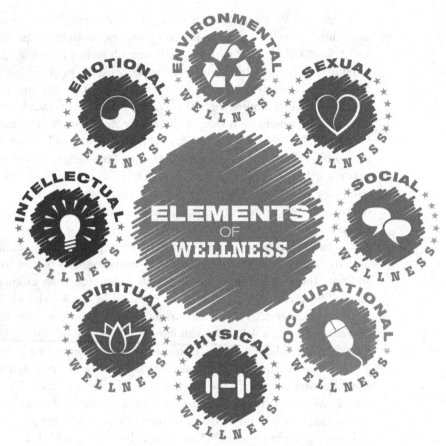

Figure 4.1 Wellness wheel—elements of wellness.
Source: Vanderbilt University Wellness Center. Used with permission.

Use of the tools and resources included in this section may enhance self-care competencies, increase resilience, and reduce the incidence of overall stress and moral distress.

Organizational Competencies

Supportive, Ethical Leadership

 Question to Consider Before Reading On

1. How do your leaders provide you support in ethical situations in your work place?

Lack of supportive, ethical leadership is identified as contributing to a deficient ethical climate and subsequent moral distress among health care providers (Galletta et al., 2013; Makaroff et al., 2014). In contrast, the presence of ethical leaders who serve as mentors and role models for nurses enhances the moral community and may mitigate the causes and effects of moral distress (Edmonson, 2015). Chapter 8 discusses the components and behaviors of the ethical leader in more detail and recognizes that he or she can serve in an informal or formal leadership capacity. For example, the majority of members of the NEC at University Health System in San Antonio, Texas, are staff nurses. These informal nurse leaders provide ethics resources to their peers and may assist them in identifying, articulating, and addressing ethical conflicts and instances of moral distress (Sauerland et al., 2015).

As indicated in the Code of Ethics (Box 4.3), formal nurse leaders and administrators have a particular obligation to recognize and respond to issues that erode the ethical environment and contribute to moral distress among nurses. These leaders can preserve the moral integrity of nurses by developing and implementing policies and protocols that address identified concerns such as provider incompetence or incivility, unsafe staffing, and disruptive patient/family behavior, among others. They can also ensure that nurses are aware of and have access to ethics resources, continuing ethics education, and consultation services. In addition, they can support and respect those nurses who choose to exercise conscientious objection and serve as a representative voice in forums with other providers and health care administrators (Rushton & Kurtz, 2015).

To assist nurse leaders in being proactive about moral distress in clinical practice, Pavlish et al. (2016) developed the SUPPORT model. This model "provides strategies for nurse leaders to simultaneously develop nurses' ethical skills and team based dialogue while also creating policies shaped by standards of healthy work environments and the American Nurses Association Code of Ethics" (p. 319).

Organizational Policies and Support Services

Organizational policies and programs that address specific causes of health provider moral distress such as disruptive patient/family behavior, provider incivility/bullying, and workplace violence are becoming more prevalent. Nurses should be familiar with and use those available at their facilities. If they are not available, nurses can work with other leaders to develop these resources and policies using examples provided in this chapter and in Box 4.5. One resource is The Safe at Hopkins (2015) program at Johns Hopkins University in Baltimore, Maryland. As with many institutions, Johns Hopkins has adopted a policy that calls for "zero tolerance of violent behavior, threats, bullying, intimidation, and any behavior of concern that contributes to an abusive environment" (2014, p. 2). The Safe at Hopkins program website provides online tools and resources to recognize and act upon behaviors of concern including a training module (2015). Another example with extensive resources and information is the stopbullyingtoolkit (2015) created by members of the Robert Wood Johnson Foundation Executive Nurse Fellows program.

Moral distress can occur when patient safety and patient/family satisfaction are given priority over the nurse's safety and moral integrity (Lipscomb & London, 2015). Noting that the "nursing profession will no longer tolerate violence of any kind from any source" (p. 1), the ANA (2015b) has issued a

Box 4.5

Moral Distress Resources

POSITION STATEMENTS/DOCUMENTS

American Association of Critical Care Nurses. (2004). *The 4 A's to rise above moral distress: Ask, affirm, assess, act.* Retrieved from http://www.aacn.org/wd/practice/docs/moral_distress.pdf

American Association of Critical Care Nurses. (2008). AACN position statement: Moral distress. Retrieved from http://www.aacn.org.WD/Practice/Docs/Moral_Distress.pdf

American Nurses Association. (2015a). *Code of ethics for nurses with interpretive statements.* Silver Spring, MD: ANA. Retrieved from http://www.nursingworld.org/MainMenuCategories/EthicsStandards/CodeofEthicsforNurses/Code-of-Ethics-For-Nurses.html

American Nurses Association. (2015b). Position statement on incivility, bullying, and workplace violence. Silver Spring, MD: ANA. Retrieved from http://www.nursingworld.org/DocumentVault/Position-Statements/Practicc/Position-Statement-on-Incivility-Bullying-and-Workplace-Violence.pdf

American Nurses Association. (2016a). Moral courage/distress. Retrieved from http://www.nursingworld.org/MainMenuCategories/EthicsStandards/Courage-and-Distress

American Nurses Association. (2016c). Incivility, bullying, and workplace violence. Retrieved from http://www.nursingworld.org/MainMenuCategories/WorkplaceSafety/Healthy-Nurse/bullyingworkplaceviolence

McPhaul, K., London, M., & Lipscomb, J. (2013). A framework for translating workplace violence intervention research into evidence-based programs. *The Online Journal of Issues in Nursing, 18*(1), Manuscript 4. Retrieved from http://www.nursingworld.org/MainMenuCategories/ANAMarketplace/ANAPeriodicals/OJIN/TableofContents/Vol-18-2013/No1-Jan-2013/A-Framework-for-Evidence-Based-Programs.html

WEBSITES, WEBINARS, VIDEOS, TOOLKITS

Agency for Healthcare Research and Quality. (2015). Successful outcome using TeamSTEPPS techniques. Retrieved from https://m.youtube.com/watch?v=yWd56QVL1VQ; https://m.youtube.com/watch?v=VX1kHduTHng; https://m.youtube.com/watch?v=ny1kr93_sKk

American Holistic Nurses Association. (2015). Holistic stress management for nurses. Retrieved from http://www.ahna.org/Resources/Stress-Management/Managing-Stress

(continued)

Box 4.5

Moral Distress Resources *(continued)*

Emergency Nurses Association. (2010). Workplace Violence Toolkit. Retrieved from https://www.ena.org/practice-research/Practice/ToolKits/ViolenceToolKit/Documents/toolkitpg1.htm

Johns Hopkins University Health System. (2015). Safe at Hopkins. Retrieved from http://www.safeathopkins.org

Institute for Healthcare Improvement. (2015). Web-based training: On demand: Improving skills to empower frontline nurses. Retrieved from http://www.ihi.org/education/WebTraining/OnDemand/NurseQI/Pages/default.aspx

National Institute for Occupational Health and Safety. (2014). Workplace violence prevention for nurses. Retrieved from http://www.cdc.gov/niosh/topics/violence/training_nurses.html

Robert Wood Johnson Foundation. (2015). PACERS: Civility Toolkit: Resources to empower healthcare leaders to identify, intervene, and prevent workplace bullying. Retrieved from http://stopbullyingtoolkit.org

University of Kentucky College of Medicine. (2015). The Moral Distress Education Project. Retrieved from http://www.cecentral.com/moraldistress

Vanderbilt University Wellness Center. (2016). Retrieved from http://www.vanderbilt.edu/recreationandwellnesscenter/wellness

position statement on incivility, bullying, and workplace violence. This statement contains recommendations and resources for individual nurses and employers related to preventing and mitigating these damaging behaviors. An example resource is the NIOSH (2014) free online course entitled Workplace Violence Prevention for Nurses. The Emergency Nurses Association has also developed a Workplace Violence Toolkit (2010) to assist leaders at various levels in an institution to create a customized violence prevention plan. Mc Phaul, London, and Lipscomb (2013) have also created a research- and regulatory-based framework for establishing a comprehensive workplace violence prevention program.

In the Case Scenario presented in this chapter, the ADN student Jackie demonstrated uncivil behavior toward Marcia, the MSN student who attempted to speak with her about her inaccurate charting by stating, *"You have no authority over me; you're just a student too!"* Clark, Barbosa-Leiker, Gill, and Nguyen (2015) observe that bullying and general incivility, whether instigated or experienced by students or faculty, is also a serious issue in nursing education. Clark has conducted extensive research on incivility in academic and work environments. She has developed a number of assessment tools, interventions, and programs that can be adapted by students, practicing nurses, and formal leaders. For example, Clark's civility curriculum includes signing a civility pledge, establishing classroom and clinical behavioral norms, and participating in communication and conflict negotiation simulations among other strategies (as quoted in Nikitas, 2014). The Clark Workplace Civility Index (CVI, 2013) is a tool for self-reflection that allows an individual nurse or other health care team member to assess his or her own civility level (Figure 4.2).

To complete the index, consider the 20 statements listed below. Read each statement carefully. Using a scale of 1–5; (5) always, (4) usually, (3) sometimes, (2) rarely, (1) never, select the response that most accurately represents the frequency of each behavior by asking yourself . . .

How often do I . . .

	Always (5)	Usually (4)	Sometimes (3)	Rarely (2)	Never (1)
1. Assume goodwill and think the best of others	○	○	○	○	○
2. Include and welcome new and current colleagues	○	○	○	○	○
3. Communicate respectfully (by e-mail, telephone, face-to-face) and really listen	○	○	○	○	○
4. Avoid gossip and spreading rumors	○	○	○	○	○
5. Keep confidences and respect others' privacy	○	○	○	○	○
6. Encourage, support, and mentor others	○	○	○	○	○
7. Avoid abusing my position or authority	○	○	○	○	○
8. Use respectful language (no racial, ethnic, sexual, age, or religiously biased terms)	○	○	○	○	○
9. Attend meetings, arrive on time, participate, volunteer, and do my share	○	○	○	○	○

Figure 4.2 Clark workplace civility index.
Source: Clark (2013). Used with permission. (The Clark Workplace Civility Index used herein is the copyrighted property of Dr. Cynthia Clark. The material should not be reproduced in any form without Dr. Clark's expressed written permission.)

	Always (5)	Usually (4)	Sometimes (3)	Rarely (2)	Never (1)
10. Avoid distracting others (misusing media, side conversations) during meetings	○	○	○	○	○
11. Avoid taking credit for someone else's ideas/work/contributions	○	○	○	○	○
12. Acknowledge others and praise their ideas/work/contributions	○	○	○	○	○
13. Take personal responsibility and accountability for my actions	○	○	○	○	○
14. Speak directly to the person with whom I have an issue	○	○	○	○	○
15. Share pertinent or important information with others	○	○	○	○	○
16. Uphold the vision, mission, and values of my organization	○	○	○	○	○
17. Seek and encourage constructive feedback from others	○	○	○	○	○
18. Demonstrate approachability, flexibility, and openness to other points of view	○	○	○	○	○
19. Bring my 'A' Game and a strong work ethic to my workplace	○	○	○	○	○
20. Apologize and mean it when the situation calls for it	○	○	○	○	○
Subtotal					
Add the scores for each column; Enter your TOTAL score in the column to the right					

Scoring the Clark Workplace Civility Index

90–100:	Very civil	60–69:	Barely civil
80–89:	Moderately civil	50–59:	Uncivil
70–79:	Mildly civil	Less than 50:	Very uncivil

Figure 4.2 (*continued*)

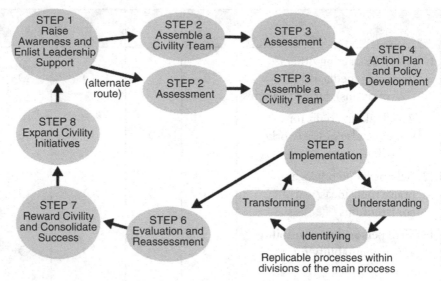

Figure 4.3 Pathway for fostering organizational civility.

The CVI is designed to raise individual awareness and recognize civility strengths and areas for improvement (Clark, 2013).

To create and sustain civility at the organizational level, Clark (2013) has developed an eight-step framework, the Pathway for Fostering Organizational Civility (PFOC, Figure 4.3). As can be seen, this is a cyclical process designed to engage nursing and other leaders at various levels in the organization with the goal of promoting "collegiality, teamwork, and collaboration—and ultimately a culture of civility" (p. 182). As Clark observes, this process is based on the premise that simply raising awareness is insufficient; rather a sustained and dedicated commitment coupled with adequate resources is needed for transformational change. In addition, pre- and postorganizational evaluations are required. These assessments are done to identify areas needing improvement and those with clear policies and procedures for addressing incivility and rewarding civil, collegial behaviors (as cited in Nikitas, 2014).

Questions to Consider Before Reading On

1. Do you feel there is a need for improvement in your workplace civility?

2. How do you think that could be accomplished?

This chapter has emphasized the need to have organizational support services such as ethics consultation, education, and employee assistance programs for those experiencing moral distress. Chaplaincy departments and ethics consultation services may also provide individual assistance or unit-based debriefings when moral distress is affecting health care team members. Epstein and Hamric (2009) observe, however, that traditional ethics consultation for moral dilemmas or conflicts may overlook the presence of moral distress, which may be the underlying reason for calling the consult. They instituted a Moral Distress Consult Service (MDCS) at the University of Virginia Health System that seeks to address the three levels of moral distress concerns or causes: the patient/family, the unit/team, and the organization. The consultants endeavor to find a time where all members of the team can meet, talk about the issue, and try to identify the "right" thing to do and barriers preventing them from doing so. The team then works together to identify and prioritize strategies to get around the barriers that may be at one or more of the three levels. Dr. Epstein states that team members have to realize that they are not weak or unusual in their experiences of moral distress and what they see as the right action might have several different avenues. She observes that "the key is addressing it [moral distress] somehow," whether it be through a formal consult or unit-based discussions (E. Epstein, personal communication, July 9, 2015). Jeanie Sauerland, the assistant director of nursing ethics at University Health System in San Antonio, Texas, and an ethics consultant, provides an example of a unit-based discussion/consultation for moral distress in Box 4.6.

Box 4.6

Moral Distress—Unit-Based Discussion/Consultation

BACKGROUND

The consult was initiated by a staff nurse and the unit nurse manager in response to a patient/family situation resulting in moral distress among the health care team members. The patient, Mr. S, had been hospitalized for many weeks, was experiencing organ failure, and was in great pain. On several occasions, he had requested that interventions be stopped and providers were willing to honor his wishes. The patient's wife, however, objected to withdrawing care and instituting a do not resuscitate (DNR) order. Mrs. S would speak with her husband, resulting in his autonomous decision to continue aggressive care. Nurses who cared for Mr. S believed that they were contributing to his pain and suffering by continuing to provide nontherapeutic interventions. In addition, the providers were angry with Mrs. S whom they saw as prolonging the dying process.

DISCUSSION/CONSULTATION

Ms. Sauerland and the nurse manager arranged meeting times for both shifts that could be attended by as many providers (nurses, physicians, respiratory therapists, chaplain) as possible. After listening to the views of the participants, Ms. Sauerland discussed the difference between a moral dilemma and moral distress (Box 4.1). She observed that moral distress is a highly personal experience rooted in personal and profes-

(continued)

Box 4.6

**Moral Distress—Unit-Based
Discussion/Consultation** *(continued)*

sional values, and, for nurses, relieving pain and suffering is a primary professional value. The primary value for Mr. S, however, is perhaps not to disappoint or abandon his wife by "giving up"—as this may be more emotionally and physically painful for him than enduring continued interventions. Ms. Sauerland suggested to the providers that they step back and acknowledge both their pain and that of the patient and his wife. She reminded them that family dynamics are deeply entrenched and few of us know how we would respond if a similar situation involved someone we love. Ms. Sauerland stated, "When we've hit that 'it was just wrong' button, we need to talk about the situation. What felt right, what felt wrong, and what we would do differently the next time. We have to support each other." Sharing, understanding, and respecting each other's stories, those of the patient, his wife, and the providers, may not result in a solution or prevent moral distress but allows us to imagine the best possible way to act in the situation (Frank, 2014).

CONCLUSION

The night shift nurse caring for Mr. S encouraged Mrs. S to participate in care activities, as she (the nurse) believed it might enable her to see and experience his continual pain and suffering (Adams, Bailey, Anderson, & Docherty, 2011). This strategy resulted in a turning point, a reframing of hope, and a revision of their stories, as Mrs. S was able to let go and aggressive care was stopped.

Ms. Sauerland followed up with the unit nurse manager and made several recommendations that addressed aspects of the three levels of moral distress: the patient/family, the unit/team, and the organization (Epstein & Hamric, 2009; Hamric, 2014):

- Encourage early family meetings between days 3 and 5 of the patient stay to begin discussions about the goals of care and provide frequent, consistent communication with patients/family members.
- Provide education to the interprofessional team regarding how to recognize and speak up about moral distress.
- Empower all team members to initiate ethics consults and/or seek assistance to work through situations of moral distress.
- Encourage communication and collaboration with palliative care services.
- Strengthen the unit ethical climate.
- Identify root causes of moral distress and develop strategies to address them.

Building organizational competencies to address moral distress contributes to development of an ethical climate and a moral community. An individual nurse may feel that this organizational challenge is beyond his or her level of duty or influence. The NEC and unit-based ethics steward program discussed in this chapter and Chapter 2, however, demonstrates that this transformation can begin with one or more motivated individuals. In discussing organizational civility, Clark (2013) likens this process to that of a single seedling in an aspen grove; however, this metaphor can also be applied to developing a moral community:

> [T]he workplace is a constant flow of interaction and relationships between and among individuals. We continuously affect one another as well as being affected by the organizations in which we work. Organizations are living systems and, fostering change is an organic process that ultimately proliferates and thrives. Like an aspen grove, the process for fostering organizational civility might begin with one seedling of change that grows and spreads by sending runners that take deep root to fortify and reinforce the strength of the system. (pp. 180–181)

CONCLUSION

This chapter identified and discussed four responses to ethical situations, including that of moral distress. The origin of the concept of moral distress was presented followed by a description of personal, professional, and organizational causes. Current interventions and strategies to address moral distress at the personal, professional, and organizational levels were explored. Table 4.2 provides a summary of moral distress causes and interventions/strategies to address them.

Table 4.2

Causes of Moral Distress and Interventions/Strategies

CAUSES OF MORAL DISTRESS

Personal and Professional Factors

Protecting position or reputation
Lack of ethical knowledge/sensitivity
Perceived powerlessness
Past experiences
Emotional stability

(continued)

Table 4.2

Causes of Moral Distress and Interventions/Strategies (continued)

Organizational Factors

Deficient ethical climate
Fear of reprisal for actions
Lack of ethical leadership
Limited ethics resources
Inadequate/incompetent staff
Bullying, lateral violence, incivility, workplace violence

MORAL DISTRESS INTERVENTIONS/STRATEGIES

Personal and Professional Competencies

Ethics education—formal courses and continuing education
Effective communication and conflict engagement skills
Self-care competencies

Organizational Competencies

Supportive, ethical leadership
Organizational policies
Support services

Critical Thinking Questions and Activities

1. What did you learn from the chapter Case Scenario?

2. Think of an ethical conflict you have experienced. Use the CUS (I am Concerned, I am Uncomfortable, this is a patient Safety issue) and DESC (Describe, Express, Suggest, Consensus) to replay your communication in these situations. What did you learn?

3. What would you do differently in your work place based on the principles and content presented in this chapter?

4. Use Figure 4.1 to assess your current self-care and identify ways to improve your self-care.

5. Use Figure 4.2 to reflect on your personal level of workplace civility.

6. Give suggestions as to how your workplace could increase its organizational civility using the pathway in Figure 4.3.

7. Explore the additional resources provided in Box 4.5. Choose one from each section and discuss its relevance to your practice with a class peer or colleague.

REFERENCES

Adams, J., Bailey, D., Anderson, R., & Docherty, S. (2011). Nursing roles and strategies in end of life decision making in acute care: A systematic review of the literature. *Nursing Research and Practice*. doi:10.1155/2011/527834. Retrieved from http://www.hindawi.com/journals/nrp/2011/527834

Agency for Healthcare Research and Quality. (2015). Successful outcome using TeamSTEPPS techniques. Retrieved from https://m.youtube.com/watch?v=yWd56QVL1VQ; https://m.youtube.com/watch?v=VX1kHduTHng

Agency for Healthcare Research and Quality. (2016). TeamSTEPPS: Strategies and tools to enhance performance safety. Retrieved from http://www.ahrq.gov/professionals/education/curriculum-tools/teamstepps/index.html

Alspach, G. (2007). Critical care nurses as coworkers: Are our interactions nice or nasty? *Critical Care Nurse*, 27(3), 10–14.

American Association of Colleges of Nursing QSEN Education consortium. (2012). *Graduate level QSEN competencies*. Washington, DC: AACN. Retrieved from http://www.aacn.nche.edu/faculty/qsen/competencies.pdf

American Association of Critical Care Nurses. (2004). *The 4 A's to rise above moral distress: Ask, affirm, assess, act*. Retrieved from http://www.aacn.org/wd/practice/docs/moral_distress.pdf

American Association of Critical Care Nurses. (2008). AACN position statement: Moral distress. Retrieved from http://www.aacn.org.WD/Practice/Docs/Moral_Distress.pdf

American Holistic Nurses Association. (2015). Holistic stress management for nurses. Retrieved from http://www.ahna.org/Resources/Stress-Management/Managing-Stress

American Nurses Association. (2012). *Principles for nurse staffing*. Silver Spring, MD: Author.

American Nurses Association. (2014). Executive summary: American Nurses Association health risk appraisal preliminary findings. Silver Spring, MD: Author. Retrieved from http://www.nursingworld.org/MainMenuCategories/WorkplaceSafety/Healthy-Nurse/HRA-Executive-Summary/ANA-HRA-Executive-Summary.pdf

American Nurses Association. (2015a). *Code of ethics for nurses with interpretive statements*. Silver Spring, MD: Nursebooks.org. Retrieved from http://www.nursingworld.org/MainMenuCategories/EthicsStandards/Tools-You-Need/Code-of-Ethics-For-Nurses.html

American Nurses Association. (2015b). Position statement on incivility, bullying, and workplace violence. Silver Spring, MD: Author. Retrieved from http://www.nursingworld.org/MainMenuCategories/Policy-Advocacy/Positions-and-Resolutions/ANAPositionStatements/Position-Statements-Alphabetically/Incivility-Bullying-and-Workplace-Violence.html

American Nurses Association. (2016a). Moral courage/distress. Retrieved from http://www.nursingworld.org/MainMenuCategories/EthicsStandards/Courage-and-Distress

American Nurses Association. (2016b). HealthyNurse initiative. Retrieved from http://www.nursingworld.org/healthynurse

American Nurses Association. (2016c). Incivility, bullying, and workplace violence. Retrieved from http://www.nursingworld.org/MainMenuCategories/WorkplaceSafety/Healthy-Nurse/bullyingworkplaceviolence

Archibald, M., Caine, V., & Scott, S. (2014). The development of a classification schema for arts-based approaches to knowledge transition. *Worldviews on Evidence Based Nursing*, 11(5), 316–324.

Augsberger, D. (1973). *Caring enough to confront*. Glendale, CA: Regal Books.

Azoulay, E., Timsit, J., Sprung, C., Soares, M., Rusinova, K., Lafabrie, A., . . . Schlemmer, B. (2009). Prevalence and factors of intensive care unit conflicts: The conflicus study. *American Journal of Respiratory Critical Care Medicine*, 180(9), 853–860.

Bartlett, J. (2013). Developing ethical competence: The perspective of nurse educators from pre-licensure baccalaureate programs accredited by the Commission on Collegiate Nursing Education (Unpublished doctoral dissertation). University of Nevada, Las Vegas.

Blum, C. (2014). Practicing self-care for nurses: A nursing program initiative. *The Online Journal of Issues in Nursing, 19*(3), Manuscript 3. Retrieved from http://www.nursingworld.org/MainMe nuCategories/ANAMarketplace/ANAPeriodicals/OJIN/TableofContents/Vol-19-2014/ No3-Sept-2014/Practicing-Self-Care-for-Nurses.html

Briles, J. (2007). Snakes at the nurses' station. *American Nurse Today, 2*(8), 52–53.

Clark, C. (2013). *Creating and sustaining civility in nursing education.* Indianapolis, IN: Sigma Theta Tau International.

Clark, C. (2014). Seeking civility. *American Nurse Today, 9*(7), 18–21.

Clark, C., Barbosa-Leiker, C., Gill, L., & Nguyen, D. (2015). Revision and psychometric testing of the incivility in nursing education (INE) survey: Introducing the INE-R. *Journal of Nursing Education, 54*(6), 306–315.

Corley, M. C., Elswick, R. K., Gorman, M., Clor, T. (2001). Development and evaluation of a moral distress scale. *Journal of Advanced Nursing, 33*(2), 250–256.

Cronenwett, L., Sherwood, G., Barnsteiner, J., Disch, J., Johnson, J., Mitchell, P., . . . Warren, J. (2007). Quality and safety education for nurses. *Nursing Outlook, 55*(3), 122–131. Retrieved from http://qsen.org/competencies/pre-licensure-ksas/

Davis, A., & Aroskar, M. (1978). *Ethical dilemmas and nursing practice.* New York, NY: Appleton-Century-Crofts.

Dellasega, C., & Volpe, R. (2013). *Toxic nursing: Managing bullying, bad attitudes, and total turmoil.* Indianapolis, IN: Sigma Theta Tau International.

Dent, B. (2015). Nine principles to improve nurse staffing. *Nursing Economics, 33*(1), 41–44.

Der Bedrosian, J. (2015, Summer). Nursing is hard: Unaddressed ethical issues make it even harder. *Johns Hopkins Magazine.* Retrieved from http://hub.jhu.edu/magazine/2015/summer/nursing -ethics-and-burnout

De Veer, A., Francke, A., Struijs, A., & Willems, D. (2013). Determinants of moral distress in daily nursing practice: A cross sectional correlational questionnaire survey. *International Journal of Nursing Studies, 50*(1), 100–108.

Dolansky, M., & Moore, S. (2013). Quality and safety education for nurses (QSEN): The key is systems thinking. *The Online Journal of Issues in Nursing, 18*(3), Manuscript 1. Retrieved from http://www.nursingworld.org/Quality-and-Safety-Education-for-Nurses.html

Dyess, S., & Sherman, R. O. (2010). Developing a leadership mindset in new graduates. *Nurse Leader, 8*(1), 29–33.

Edmonson, C. (2015). Strengthening moral courage and the nurse leader. *The Online Journal of Issues in Nursing, 20*(2). Retrieved from http://www.nursingworld.org/MainMenuCategories/ EthicsStandards/Courage-and-Distress/Moral-Courage-for-Nurse-Leaders.html

Emergency Nurses Association. (2010). Workplace Violence Toolkit. Retrieved from https://www .ena.org/practice-research/Practice/ViolenceToolKit/Documents/toolkitpg1.htm

Epstein, E., & Delgado, S. (2010). Understanding and addressing moral distress. *The Online Journal of Issues in Nursing, 15*(3), Manuscript 1. Retrieved from http://www.nursingworld.org/Main MenuCategories/ANAMarketplace/ANAPeriodicals/OJIN/TableofContents/Vol152010/ No3-Sept-2010/Understanding-Moral-Distress.html

Epstein, E., & Hamric, A. (2009). Moral distress, moral residue, and the crescendo effect. *Journal of Clinical Ethics, 20*(4), 330–342.

Farouque, K., & Burgio, E. (2013). The impact of bullying in health care. *The Quarterly, The Royal Australasian College of Medical Administrators.* Retrieved from http://racma.edu.au/index.php ?option=com_content&view=article&id=634&Itemid=362

Fink-Samnick, E. (2015). The new age of bullying and violence in healthcare: The interprofessional impact. *Professional Case Management, 20*(4), 165–174.

Fowler, M. (2015). *Guide to the code of ethics for nurses with interpretive statements.* Silver Spring, MD: ANA.

Frank, A. (2014). Narrative ethics as dialogical story telling. *Hastings Center Report, 44*(1), S16–S20.

Galletta, M., Portoghese, I., Battistelli, A., & Leiter, M. (2013). The roles of unit leadership and nurse-physician collaboration on nursing turnover intention. *The Journal of Advanced Nursing, 69*(8), 1771–1784.

Garon, M. (2012). Speaking up, being heard: Registered nurses' perceptions of workplace communication. *Journal of Nursing Management, 20*, 361–371.

Glod, C. (1998). *Contemporary psychiatric-mental health nursing: The brain behavior connection.* Philadelphia, PA: F. A. Davis.

Grady, A. (2014). Experiencing moral distress as a nursing student. *Imprint, 61*(2), 40–42.

Griffin, M. (2004). Teaching cognitive rehearsal as a shield for lateral violence: An intervention for newly licensed nurses. *Journal of Continuing Education in Nursing, 35*(6), 257–263.

Griffin, M., & Clark, C. (2014). Revisiting cognitive rehearsal as an intervention against incivility and lateral violence in nursing: 10 years later. *Journal of Continuing Education in Nursing, 45*(12), 535–542.

Hamric, A. (2014). A case study of moral distress. *Journal of Hospice and Palliative Nursing, 16*(8), 457–463.

Hamric, A., Borchers, C., & Epstein, E. (2012). Development and testing of an instrument to measure moral distress in healthcare professionals. *American Journal of Bioethics Primary Research, 3*(2), 1–9.

Harvey, E., Wright, A., Taylor, D., Bath, J., & Collier, B. (2013). TeamSTEPPS simulation-based training: An evidence-based strategy to improve trauma team performance. *Journal of Continuing Education in Nursing, 44*(11), 484–485.

Houghtaling, D. (2012). Moral distress: An invisible challenge for trauma nurses. *Journal of Trauma Nursing, 19*(4), 232–237.

Institute for Healthcare Improvement. (2013a). Protecting 5 million lives from harm. Retrieved from www.ihi.org/offerings/Initiatives/PastStrategicInitiatives/5MillionLivesCampaign/Pages/default.aspx

Institute for Healthcare Improvement. (2013b). Transforming care at the bedside. Retrieved from www.ihi.org/offerings/Initiatives/PastStrategicInitiatives/TCAB/Pages/default.aspx

Institute for Healthcare Improvement. (2015). Web-based training: On demand: Improving skills to empower frontline nurses. Retrieved from http://www.ihi.org/education/WebTraining/OnDemand/NurseQI/Pages/default.aspx

Institute of Medicine. (1999). *To err is human: Building a safer health system.* Washington, DC: National Academies Press. Retrieved from http://iom.nationalacademies.org/~/media/Files/Report%20Files/1999/To-Err-is-Human/To%20Err%20is%20Human%201999%20%20report%20brief.pdf

Institute of Medicine. (2001). *Crossing the quality chasm.* Washington, DC: National Academy Press. Retrieved from http://iom.nationalacademies.org/~/media/Files/Report%20Files/2001/Crossing-the-Quality-Chasm/Quality%20Chasm%202001%20%20report%20brief.pdf

Jameton, A. (1984). *Nursing practice: The ethical issues.* Englewood Cliffs, NJ: Prentice-Hall.

Jameton, A. (2013). A reflection on moral distress in nursing together with a current application of the concept. *Journal of Bioethical Inquiry, 10*, 297–308.

Johns Hopkins University Health System. (2015). Safe at Hopkins. Retrieved from http://www.safeathopkins.org

Johnstone, M., & Hutchinson, A. (2015). "Moral distress": Time to abandon a flawed nursing construct? *Nursing Ethics, 22*(1), 5–15.

Jones, J. (2015). Walk forward with a strong ethical agenda. Retrieved from http://www.theamerican nurse.org/index.php/2015/08/31/walk-forward-with-a-strong-ethical-agenda-2/

Kramer, M. (1974). *Reality shock: Why nurses leave nursing.* St. Louis, MO: Mosby.

Kramer, M., Brewer, B., & Maguire, P. (2013). Impact of healthy work environments on new graduate nurses' environmental reality shock. *Western Journal of Nursing Research, 35*(3), 348–383.

Krautscheid, L., & Brown, M. (2014). Microethical decision making among baccalaureate nursing students: A qualitative investigation. *Journal of Nursing Education, 53*(3), S 19–S 25.

Kupperschmidt, B. (1994). Carefronting: Caring enough to confront. *The Oklahoma Nurse, 39*(4), 7–10.

Kupperschmidt, B. (2006). Addressing multigenerational conflict: Mutual respect and carefronting as strategy. *The Online Journal of Issues in Nursing, 11*(2), Manuscript 3. Retrieved from http://www .nursingworld.org/MainMenuCategories/ANAMarketplace/ANAPeriodicals/OJIN/Tableof Contents/Volume112006/No2May06/tpc30_316075.html

Kupperschmidt, B. (2008). Conflicts at work? Try carefronting. *Journal of Christian Nursing, 25*(1), 10, 17.

Laabs, C. (2015). Toward a consensus in ethics education for the Doctor of Nursing Practice. *Nursing Education Perspectives, 36*(4), 249–251.

Laschinger, H., & Smith, L. (2013). The influence of authentic leadership and empowerment on new graduate nurses' perceptions of interprofessional collaboration. *The Journal of Nursing Administration, 43*(1), 24–29.

Lipscomb, J., & London, M. (2015). *Not part of the job: How to take a stand against violence in the work setting.* Silver Spring, MD: Nursesbooks.org.

Makaroff, K., Storch, J., Pauly, B., & Newton, L. (2014). Searching for ethical leadership in nursing. *Nursing Ethics, 21*(6), 642–658.

Malloch, K. (2015). Measurement of nursing's complex health care work: Evolution of the science for determining the required staffing for safe and effective patient care. *Nursing Economics, 33*(1), 20–25.

Maxfield, D., Greeny, J., Lavandero, R., & Groah, L. (2011). The silent treatment: Why safety tools and checklists aren't enough to save lives. Retrieved from http://www.aacn.org/WD/hwe/docs/the-silent-treatment.pdf

Maxfield, D., Lyndon, A., Kennedy, H., O'Keefe, D., & Zlatnik, M. (2013). Confronting safety gaps across labor and delivery teams. *American Journal of Obstetrics and Gynecology, 209*(5), 402–408.

McCarthy, J., & Gastmans, C. (2015). Moral distress: A review of the argument-based nursing ethics literature. *Nursing Ethics, 22*(1), 131–152.

McPhaul, K., London, M., & Lipscomb, J. (2013). A framework for translating workplace violence intervention research into evidence-based programs. *The Online Journal of Issues in Nursing, 18*(1), Manuscript 4. Retrieved from http://www.nursingworld.org/MainMenuCategories/ANA Marketplace/ANAPeriodicals/OJIN/TableofContents/Vol-18-2013/No1-Jan-2013/A-Frame work-for-Evidence-Based-Programs.html

Milic, M., Puntillo, K., Turner, K., Joseph, D., Peters, N., Ryan, R., . . . Anderson, W. (2015). Communicating with patients' families and physicians about prognosis and goals of care. *American Journal of Critical Care, 24*(4), e56–e64.

Molloy, J., Evans, J., & Coughlin, K. (2015). Moral distress in the resuscitation of extremely premature infants. *Nursing Ethics, 22*(1), 53–63.

National Institute for Occupational Health and Safety. (2002). *Violence: Occupational hazards in hospitals.* Cincinnati, OH: NIOSH.

National Institute for Occupational Health and Safety. (2014). Workplace violence prevention for nurses. Retrieved from http://wwwn.cdc.gov/wpvhc/Course.aspx/Slide/Intro_1

National Institutes of Health. (2014). Nurse staffing and education linked to reduced patient mortality. Retrieved from https://www.nih.gov/news-events/news-releases/nurse-staffing-education-linked-reduced-patient-mortality

Needleman, J. (2015). Nurse Staffing: The knowns and unknowns. *Nursing Economics, 33*(1), 5–7.

Nikitas, D. (2014). Fostering civility: An interview with Cynthia Clark. *Nursing Economics, 32*(6), 306–311.

Nursing Solutions Incorporated. (2016). National healthcare and RN retention report. NSI Nursing Solutions. Lancaster, PA. Retrieved from http://www.nsinursingsolutions.com/Files/assets/library/retention-institute/NationalHealthcareRNRetentionReport2016.pdf

Okuyama, A., Wagner, C., & Bijnen, B. (2014). Speaking up for patient safety by hospital-based health care professionals: A literature review. *BMC Health Services Research, 14*(61), 1–8. Retrieved from www.ncbi.nim.nih.gov/pmc/articles/PMC4016383/pdf/1472-6963-14-61.pdf

Olson, L. (1998). Hospital nurses' perceptions of the ethical climate of their work setting. *Journal of Nursing Scholarship, 30*(4), 345–349.

Patterson, K., Grenny, J., Mc Millan, R., & Switzler, A. (2011). *Crucial conversations: Tools for talking when the stakes are high*. New York, NY: McGraw-Hill.

Pauly, B., Varcoe, C., & Storch, J. (2012). Framing the issues: Moral distress in health care. *HEC Forum, 24*, 1–11. Retrieved from http://link.springer.com/article/10.1007/s10730-012-9176-y/fulltext.html

Pavlish, C., Brown-Saltzman, K., Fine, A., & Jakel, P. (2015). A culture of avoidance: Voices from inside ethically difficult clinical situations. *Clinical Journal of Oncology Nursing, 19*(2), 1–7. Retrieved from https://cjon.ons.org/file/9831/download

Pavlish, C., Brown-Saltzman, K., So, I., & Wong, J. (2016). SUPPORT: An evidence-based model for leaders addressing moral distress. *The Journal of Nursing Management, 46*(6), 313–320.

Pavlish, C., Hellyer, J., Saltzman, M., Miers, A., & Squire, K. (2015). Screening situations for risk of ethical conflicts: A pilot study. *American Journal of Critical Care, 24*(3), 248–256.

Peter, E. (2015). Guest editorial: Three recommendations for the future of moral distress scholarship. *Nursing Ethics, 22*(1), 3–4.

Rainer, J. (2015). Speaking up: Factors and issues in nurses advocating for patients when patients are in jeopardy. *Journal of Nursing Care Quality, 30*(1), 53–62.

Rawson, J., Thompson, N., Sostre, G., & Deitte, L. (2013). The cost of disruptive and unprofessional behaviors in health care. *Academic Radiology, 20*(9), 1074–1076.

Registered Nurse Safe Staffing Act of 2015. Retrieved from https://www.congress.gov/114/bills/hr2083/BILLS-114hr2083ih.pdf

Rest, J. (1986). *Moral development: Advances in research and theory*. New York, NY: Prager.

Robert Wood Johnson Foundation. (2015). PACERS: Civility Toolkit: Resources to empower healthcare leaders to identify, intervene, and prevent workplace bullying. Retrieved from http://stopbullyingtoolkit.org

Robinson, E., Lee, S., Zollfrank, A., Jurchak, M., Frost, D., & Grace, P. (2014). Clinical ethics residency for nurses: An education mode to decrease moral distress and strengthen nurse retention in acute care. *Journal of Nursing Administration, 44*(12), 640–646.

Rosenstein, A. (2010). Measuring and managing the economic impact of disruptive behaviors in the hospital. *Journal of Healthcare Risk Management, 30*(2), 20–26.

Rushton, C., Batcheller, J., Schroeder, K., & Donohue, P. (2015). Burnout and resilience among nurses practicing in high intensity settings. *American Journal of Critical Care, 24*(5), 412–420. Retrieved from http://ajcc.aacnjournals.org/content/24/5/412.full.pdf+html?sid=b8128317-ce1b-4c3d-a94e-38c943956836

Rushton, C., Kasniak, A., & Halifax, J. (2013). Addressing moral distress: Application of a framework to palliative care practice. *Journal of Palliative Medicine, 16*(9), 1080–1088. Retrieved from https://www.upaya.org/wp-content/uploads/2013/12/JPM-application-of-framework-for-MD.pdf

Rushton, C., & Kurtz, M. (2015). *Moral distress and you.* Silver Spring, MD: American Nurses Association.

Sanchez-Reilly, S., Morrison, L., Carey, E., Bernacki, R., O'Neill, L., Kapo, J., Periyakoli, V., & Jde, T. (2013). Caring for oneself to care for others. *The Journal of Supportive Oncology, 11*(2), 75–81.

Sasso, L., Bagnasco, A., Bianchi, M., Bressan, V., & Carnevale, F. (2015, April 22). Moral distress in undergraduate nursing students: A systematic review. *Nursing Ethics.* pii: 0969733015574926. [Epub ahead of print].

Sauerlnd, J., Marotta, K., Peinemann, M., Berndt, A., & Robichaux, C. (2014). Assessing and addressing moral distress and ethical climate: Part 1. *Dimensions of Critical Care Nursing, 33*(4), 234–245. Retrieved from http://journals.lww.com/dccnjournal/Fulltext/2014/07000/Assessing_and_Addressing_Moral_Distress_and.9.aspx

Sauerland, J., Marotta, K., Peinemann, M., Berndt, A., & Robichaux, C. (2015). Assessing and addressing moral distress and ethical climate, part II: Neonatal and Pediatric Perspectives. *Dimensions in Critical Care Nursing, 34*(1), 33–46. Retrieved from http://journals.lww.com/dccn journal/Fulltext/2015/01000/Assessing_and_Addressing_Moral_Distress_and.8.aspx

Sayre, M., Mc Neese-Smith, D., & Leach, L. (2012). An educational intervention to increase the "speaking up" behaviors in nurses and improve patient safety. *Journal of Nursing Care Quality, 27*(2), 154–160.

Saxton, R. (2012). Communication skills training to address disruptive physician behavior. *AORN Journal, 95*(5), 602–611.

Schluter, J., Winch, S., Holzhauser, K., & Henderson, A. (2008). Nurses' moral sensitivity and hospital ethical climate: A literature review. *Nursing Ethics, 15*(3), 304–321.

Storch, J., Makaroff, K., Pauly, B., & Newton, L. (2013). Take me to my leader: The importance of ethical leadership among formal nurse leaders. *Nursing Ethics, 20*(2), 150–157.

Sullivan, P., Bissett, K., Cooper, M., Dearholt, S., Mammen, K., Parks, J., & Pulia, K. (2012, December). Grace under fire: Surviving and thriving in nursing by cultivating resilience. 7(12). Retrieved from http://www.americannursetoday.com/grace-under-fire-surviving-and-thriving-in-nursing -by-cultivating-resilience

The Joint Commission. (2015). Hospital national patient safety goals. Retrieved from http://www .jointcommission.org/hap_2015_npsgs

Theisen, J., & Sandau, K. (2011). Competency of new graduate nurses: A review of their weaknesses and strategies for success. *Journal of Continuing Education in Nursing, 44*(9), 406–414.

Thompson, M., & Davidson, S. (2014). National nursing specialty organizations with staffing standards. Oregon Nurses Association. Retrieved from http://c.ymcdn.com/sites/www.oregonrn.org/ resource/resmgr/Docs/ONA_NSOs_staffing.pdf

Trossman, S. (2015). It can make nurses sick: Aiming to prevent incivility, bullying, violence. *The American Nurse, 47*(3), 1, 6.

University of Kentucky College of Medicine. (2015). The Moral Distress Education Project. Retrieved from http://www.cecentral.com/moraldistress

Van Norman, G. (2015). Abusive and disruptive behavior in the surgical team. *AMA Journal of Ethics, 17*(3), 215–220.

Vanderbilt University Wellness Center. (2016). Retrieved from http://www.vanderbilt.edu/recrea tionandwellnesscenter/wellness

VitalSmarts. (2015). Case studies. Retrieved from https://www.vitalsmarts.com/case-studies

Webster, G., & Bayliss, F. (2000). Moral residue. In S. Rubin & L. Zoloth (Eds.), *Margin of error: The ethics of mistakes in the practice of medicine* (pp. 217–230). Hagerstown, MD: University Publishing Group.

West, E., Barron, D., Harrison, D., Rafferty, A., Rowan, K., & Sanderson, C. (2014). Nurse staffing, medical staffing, and mortality in intensive care: An observational study. *International Journal of Nursing Studies, 51*(5), 781–794.

Whitehead, P., Herbertson, R., Hamric, A., Epstein, E., & Fisher, J. (2015). Moral distress among healthcare professionals: Report of an institution-wide survey. *Journal of Nursing Scholarship*, *47*(2), 117–125.

Wilson, M., Goettemoeller, D., Bevan, N., & McCord, J. (2013). Moral distress: Levels, coping, and preferred interventions in critical care and transitional care nurses. *Journal of Clinical Nursing*, *22*(9–10), 1455–1466.

Witt, C. (2011). Continuing education: A personal responsibility. *Advances in Neonatal Care*, *11*(4), 227–228.

Wood, D. (2014, March 3). 10 Best practices for addressing ethical issues and moral distress. AMN Healthcare. Retrieved from http://www.amnhealthcare.com/latest-healthcare-news/10-Best-Practices-Addressing-Ethical-Issues-Moral-Distress

Yoes, T. (2012). Addressing moral distress: Challenges and strategies for nursing faculty. *The Oklahoma Nurse*, *57*(2), 14.

Zheng, D., Witt, L., Waite, E., David, E., van Driel, M., McDonald, D. P., . . . Crepeau, L. (2015). Effects of ethical leadership on emotional exhaustion in high moral intensity situations. *The Leadership Quarterly*. Retrieved from http://dx.doi.org/10.1016/j.leaqua.2015.01.006

Zook, E. (2014). Effective leadership promotes perioperative success. *AORN Journal*, *100*(1), 4–7.

Understanding the Process of Clinical Ethics: Committees and Consults

CRAIG M. KLUGMAN

Upon completion of this chapter, the reader will be able to:

- Explain the three functions of an ethics committee
- Describe the history of ethics committees
- Explain the process of a clinical ethics consultation
- Describe the history of clinical ethics consultation
- Understand the knowledge, skills, and experiences necessary to be a clinical ethics consultant
- Have awareness of the three forms of ethics consults
- Understand the process of ethics facilitation

In most hospitals, registered nurses and other clinicians faced with ethical dilemmas or issues can request an "ethics consult." As described in Chapter 1, these dilemmas and issues are problems where there is either a conflict of values or a question of what one ought to or ought not to do. The ethics consultant facilitates conversations and deliberations to determine what are the relevant ethical issues, what questions need to be asked, and to assist patients, families, and providers in resolving the issue. "Clinical ethics is a practical discipline that provides a structured approach for identifying, analyzing and resolving ethics issues in clinical medicine" (Jonsen, Siegler, & Winslade, 2006, p. 1).

As a registered nurse, you need to know when and how to call for an ethics consult where you are employed. You also need to understand the process of an ethics consultation and the role of ethics committee (EC) members. Finally, understanding ethical consult services and the skills necessary to conduct an ethics consult will assist you with your role in the process.

CASE SCENARIO

Mr. Ramirez is the youngest of nine children. Because of his developmental disability, at the chronological age of 32 he is at the developmental age of 8. He lives at home with his mother and his 34-year-old brother who are his primary caregivers. Mr. Ramirez has multiple health problems and now has a deep infection in the bones of his big toe that has not responded to antibiotics. His physicians have proposed amputating his toe to try to stop the infection from spreading. If the infection progresses further, it will enter his blood and long bones and kill him. Because of his inability to make choices, his mother is his legal guardian. However, she is in the hospital battling cancer and is unable to assist. His brother says that he wants nothing to do with providing care or making decisions. The majority of the siblings do not want the amputation saying that death would be preferable.

Not knowing who is the decision maker or what to do in this case, the attending physician requests an ethics consultation.

This opening Case Scenario demonstrates both a conflict of values and a question of what one ought to or ought not to do—a difference in values about amputation as well as an inability to move forward because of a lack of an identified decision maker.

Ethics consult services exist in 81% of U.S. hospitals and in 100% of hospitals with more than 400 beds (Fox, Myers, & Pearlman, 2007). However, only 8% of nurses have ever requested a consult (Gordon & Hamric, 2006). Those who conduct ethics consults have backgrounds in medicine (34%), nursing (31%), social work (11%), or chaplaincy (10%). Only 41% have formal training in ethics consultation (Fox et al., 2007).

Ethics consultation serves many purposes in a hospital. Such services increase patient satisfaction, improve employee morale, reduce costs, reduce risk of lawsuits, sustain corporate integrity, maintain the institution's brand identity, and improve the hospital's reputation (VA Ethics, n.d.). For nursing, ethics support services are part of professional practice, which is one aspect of the American Nurses Credentialing Center's Magnet® Model for excellence in nursing practice and for health care organizations seeking recognition through the Magnet program.

This chapter will examine the two main forms of clinical ethics in a hospital: ECs and ethics consultation services. After defining the history and function of each, the chapter examines the methods of ethics consultation.

Questions to Consider Before Reading On

1. Does your current place of work have an ethics consultation service?

2. Who can call for an ethics consult?

3. Only 8% of nurses have ever requested an ethics consult. What are some possible barriers to requesting an ethics consult?

4. As the nurse caring for Mr. Ramirez, which Quality and Safety Education for Nurses (QSEN) competencies (Box 5.1) are relevant to this opening Case Scenario?

Box 5.1

Process of Clinical ECs and Consults: Relevant QSEN Competencies

Acknowledge the tension that may exist between patient rights and organizational responsibility for professional, ethical care. (Attitudes)

Appreciate shared decision making with empowered patients and families even when conflicts occur. (Attitudes)

Communicate patient values, preferences, and expressed needs to other members of the health care team. (Skills)

Describe basic principles of consensus building and conflict resolution. (Knowledge)

Describe strategies to empower patients or families in all aspects of the health care process. (Knowledge)

Elicit patient values, preferences, and expressed needs as part of clinical interview, implementation of care plan, and evaluation of care. (Skills)

Engage patients or designated surrogates in active partnerships that promote health, safety and well-being, and self-care management. (Skills)

Explore ethical and legal implications of patient-centered care. (Knowledge)

Integrate understanding of multiple dimensions of patient-centered care: patient/family/community preferences/values; information, communication and education; involvement of families and friends. (Knowledge)

(continued)

Box 5.1

Process of Clinical ECs and Consults: Relevant QSEN Competencies *(continued)*

Participate in building consensus or resolving conflict in the context of patient care. (Skills)

Value continuous improvement of own communication and conflict resolution skills. (Attitudes)

Source: Cronenwett et al. (2007, pp. 123–129).

ETHICS COMMITTEES

ECs are groups composed of representatives of the disciplines and units at a hospital, which gather to address ethical problems in clinical practice. Ideally members of the committee are not involved with the cases they review. ECs often range in size from 10 to 40 people and may include physicians, nurses, social workers, lawyers, risk management specialists, and administrators. If the hospital has a trained clinical ethicist, then that person will also be a member. Some committees choose to have a community member who represents the morals and values of the community at large. In most cases, EC members are volunteers, not paid for their time or service. Historically, ECs developed as a result of case law and resource scarcity caused by technological development.

Questions to Consider Before Reading On

1. If you have an EC at your work place, who are the nurse members and other committee members?

2. How does one become a member of your ethics committee at your work place?

3. Do you have an interest in becoming a member of your EC? Why or why not?

History

Chapter 1 described the events and trends that led to the development of bioethics. Clinical ECs and consultation grew out of the same trends and interests: abuses in human subjects research, the Civil Rights movement, engagement with the public, and advances in life sciences and health care delivery technology. One such technology was kidney dialysis, a process that became available on a chronic basis with the invention of the Scribner shunt in 1960. However, with an expanded pool of eligible candidates, there was not an increase in the number of available artificial kidney machines. This begged the question as to who would get treatment—and thus live—and who would be turned away—and thus die. Swedish Hospital in Seattle convened the Admissions and Policies Committee of the Seattle Artificial Kidney Center (later known as the "God Committee"). Composed of community leaders, the committee was tasked with determining who would have access to dialysis. This group is considered the first modern EC. Similar committees formed at other hospitals as they were able to offer dialysis and soon thereafter, organ transplants.

In 1976, the New Jersey Supreme Court ruled on the case of Karen Ann Quinlan. Quinlan fell into a persistent vegetative state in 1975 after consuming alcohol and tranquilizers. A year later, her family sued the hospital, which had refused their request to remove her ventilator. In finding that there was indeed a right for the ventilator to be removed, the Court stated that the legal system was not the appropriate place for resolving ethical issues. Instead, the ruling recommended the use of ECs that had appeared in some hospitals:

> I suggest that it would be more appropriate to provide a regular forum for more input and dialogue in individual situations and to allow the responsibility of these judgments to be shared. Many hospitals have established an Ethics Committee composed of physicians, social workers, attorneys, and theologians . . . which serves to review the individual circumstances of ethical dilemma and which has provided much in the way of assistance and safeguards for patients and their medical caretakers. (The Supreme Court of New Jersey, 1976)

Functions

As shown in Box 5.2, ECs can have three functions: policy, education, and consultation (Hester & Schonfeld, 2012). In many hospitals, the EC develops, reviews, and implements institutional policies that deal with ethical concerns. For example, policies that deal with surrogate decision makers or advance directives may come under the EC. More recently, policies related to treating Ebola patients and whether staff members are required to assist or volunteer have required review. ECs meet at least monthly and should be supported by upper administration in order to be integrated into hospital operations and not exist just for show. Through this work, the committee supports the institution's mission, relations with patients, and treatment of employees.

The education role of the committee has two components: of the committee and by the committee. In the first sense, committee members need

Box 5.2

Three Functions of the Ethics Committee

1. Policy review and development

2. Education

3. Consultation

Source: Hester and Schonfeld (2012).

to be educated on ethics theories, issues, and methods. As stated at the outset, only 41% of committee members have formal training. It is the task of the EC chair and a clinical ethicist—if one exists—to provide continuing education opportunities. In the second sense, the members of the committee are local ethics experts for their discipline and their units. They are expected to take what they learn in the committee and spread that knowledge to their coworkers. Thus, they become a resource about hospital policies that deal with ethics and identify ethical challenges. Committee members can also help advise when a case should be referred for an ethics consult.

The third role of the EC is ethics consultation. In most hospitals, consults are done by a small subgroup of the committee or by a few individuals. The full committee, however, should regularly review such cases for quality improvement, education, and identifying when new policies may be needed or old ones may require revision. Thus, a case log and case discussion are a part of every scheduled EC meeting. The actual process and history of ethics consultation are addressed in the next section.

Questions to Consider Before Reading On

1. Do members of your EC provide ethics education opportunities?

2. What types of ethics education do you believe are needed in your facility/unit?

ETHICS CONSULTANTS

An ethics consultant (also known as *clinical ethics consultant* or *clinical ethicist*) is an individual with specific training who works with care providers and hospital staff to identify, analyze, and recommend resolutions to ethical dilemmas and issues in the course of clinical care. An ethics consultation service is a hospital-based program that assists in addressing ethical issues.

Often, ethics consults are requested for reasons that do not relate to clinical ethics. For example, some consult calls are reporting a colleague doing wrong, aiding someone who is having problems with a supervisor or peer, or helping a patient who "just does not understand how sick she is." None of these are ethical issues. This delineation is confusing, especially when posted signs tell people to call an "Ethics Hotline" if they see people stealing staplers, misusing resources, or treating patients badly. In some institutions, ethics services are located under the mission department and thus become connected with the idea of pastoral care. Ethics consultation is not medical or nursing review, risk management, compliance, palliative care, or pastoral care. The reason people call for an ethics consult with these concerns or questions is because there is often no clear information on how to deal with these issues or a designated department that has responsibility.

Ethics consultants are also not an "ethics police" out to catch people in wrongdoing. Ethics is about value disagreement. Consults are most often called because an uncertain situation is encountered. For example, for assistance in making a decision regarding patient care, for help interacting with a difficult patient or family, for advice on legal or administrative questions, for an "emotional trigger" in the case, or for help "thinking through an ethical issue" (DuVal, Sartorius, Clarridge, Gensler, & Danis, 2001). Consults are most often about end-of-life care (advance directives, do-not-resuscitate orders, futility, withholding or withdrawing treatment), identifying a surrogate decision maker, patient autonomy, informed consent, and conflicts between parties. Less common reasons for consults are questions of genetics, abortion, substance abuse, religious and cultural issues, professional misconduct, confidentiality, and truth-telling (DuVal et al., 2001; Fox et al., 2007; McClung, Kamer, DeLuca, & Barber, 1996).

Question to Consider Before Reading On

1. Ethics consults are most often called because an uncertain situation is encountered. Have you or a class peer or colleague experienced a situation in which a consult might have been helpful but was not initiated?

The next section examines the history of ethics consultation, the areas of core knowledge, and essential skills that a clinical ethics consultant brings to resolving a case.

History

As scholars from medicine, law, philosophy, and theology began studying the ethical issues raised by new medical technologies, they worked to incorporate this material into medical and nursing curricula. In 1972, only 17 medical schools offered ethics courses but by 1976 that number had risen to 56, although only 6 had a required course (Veatch & Sollitto, 1976). A 1977 survey found that two thirds of nursing schools integrated ethics into their teaching, but did not offer separate required or elective courses (Aroskar & Veatch, 1977). One of the reasons for the lack of stand-alone courses was the lack of nursing specific materials.

Once they were teaching in health professional education environments, these scholars found themselves interested in issues in real-world practice. Across the United States, bioethics scholars began entering the hospital and helping health care professionals to think about difficult ethical challenges. Among the early practitioners were two philosophers: Albert Jonsen at the University of California at San Francisco and Ruth Purtilo at the University of Nebraska (Aroskar & Veatch, 1977).

These new consultation services ran into early philosophical challenges. Physicians who also practiced ethics believed that only physicians could resolve these dilemmas. Nonphysicians, who included philosophers and theologians, believed that only outsiders could bring in ethical theory and neutral perspective. In 1982, a philosopher, attorney, and physician—all involved with clinical consultations—coauthored the first edition of *Clinical Ethics*, a book that described ethics consultation and suggested a method for thinking about these challenging cases (Tapper, 2013).

As of 1983, 4.3% of hospitals had ECs and all of those had over 200 beds (Jonsen et al., 2006). A 1983 report by the *President's Commission for the Study of Ethical Problems in Medicine and Biomedical and Behavioral Research* stated that hospital ECs should be an important body in making decisions for incapacitated patients (Youngner, Jackson, Colton, Juknialis, & Smith, 1983). In 1985, the Department of Health & Human Services called for the creation of "infant care committees" to facilitate decision making in care of impaired newborns. This action was a response to a series of cases involving the deaths of newborns with severe health problems where parents refused treatment. Ultimately, this led to the Baby Doe rules and established an abuse hotline to report when newborns were not given care.

Also in 1985, a group of individuals who identified themselves as ethics consultants gathered at the National Institutes of Health. This meeting led to the formation of the first professional organization, the Society for Bioethics Consultation (now part of the American Society for Bioethics & Humanities), and defined the function of the clinical ethics consultant.

In 1992, the Joint Commissions for the Accreditation of Hospital Organizations (now The Joint Commission) released a statement that all hospitals should have a mechanism for resolving ethical issues. Today, Joint Commission accreditation has 24 standards related to ethics, patient rights, and organizational responsibilities. The American Medical Association adopted a statement in support of ethics consultation in 1997. And in 1999, Medicare regulations (64 Fed Reg 36060) required that institutions that receive federal funding had to inform patients of the availability of ethics consultation.

As a result of these events, 81% of all U.S. hospitals now offer these services.

Questions to Consider Before Reading On

1. Have you or a class peer or colleague participated in an ethics consultation?

2. Describe the skills and knowledge used by the consultant(s) in the case:

   ▪ For example, did he or she assist in clarifying the major issues?

   ▪ Discuss relevant prior cases.

   ▪ Use mediation skills to resolve a conflict.

CONSULTANT CREDENTIALING

In hospitals that have a dedicated clinical ethics consultant, that individual is likely to have many responsibilities. Beyond chairing or being a leader in the EC, the consultant will attend rounds on patients, organize educational sessions, serve on other hospital committees as an ethics liaison and expert, and be involved with clinical ethics consultation.

Although there are currently no accreditation standards for people who do ethics consultations, some standards are being established. The American Society for Bioethics and Humanities is developing a method of credentialing that requires a person to have (a) an advanced degree in bioethics or related field, (b) completed a fellowship in clinical ethics consultation, (c) completed mediation training, (d) familiarity with the proposed code of ethics and professional responsibilities for health care ethics consultants (see Box 5.3), (e) demonstrated experience in a clinical setting, and (f) undergone quality attestation review.

Box 5.3

Code of Ethics and Professional Responsibilities for Health Care Ethics Consultants

1. Be competent

2. Preserve Integrity

3. Manage conflicts of interest and obligation

4. Respect privacy and maintain confidentiality

5. Contribute to the field

6. Communicate responsibly

7. Promote just health care

Source: ASBH (2014).

The last is a process in development. The quality attestation review will most likely consist of a written examination on core knowledge as well as a demonstration of skills through presentation of a case portfolio and an oral examination.

A clinical health care ethicist needs to have a broad range of knowledge to bring to the consult. This includes knowing about ethical theories, communication skills, law, mediation, process of a consult, religion, as well as history of bioethics and clinical ethics consultation. In addition, a consultant should know major cases that have influenced thinking in clinical ethics and the debates surrounding major issues:

- Decision-making capacity

- Informed consent

- Surrogate decision making

- Advance care planning and advance directives

- End-of-life decision making

- Privacy and confidentiality

- Pregnancy and perinatal issues

- Difficult patients

- Culture (anthropology, sociology, and ethnography)

- Minors (best interest, assent, parental limits)

- Newborns, infants and children (delivery room, neonatal intensive care unit (NICU)/pediatric intensive care unit (PICU), Baby Doe regulations, sterilization)

- Adolescents (mature minor, emancipated minor) (ASBH Clinical Ethics Task Force, 2009)

A consultant must also possess the skills necessary to conduct a clinical ethics consultation. This expertise includes communication, mediation, research, ethical analysis, issue identification and clarification, implementation science, and evaluation.

FORMS OF CONSULTS

Consult services may differ in how they structure the consultation response based on institutional history and available resources. Consultations may be done by individuals, teams (or EC subcommittee), or the full committee. Small hospitals may not have enough resources to have a consultant or an EC. In those situations, the hospital may consult with an academic medical center's ethics program or be part of a regional or state-wide clinical ethics network that serves as an ethics education and consultation service.

A large hospital may have a clinical ethicist on staff. In this situation, the ethicist may do consultations alone or as the leader of a small team. A solo consultant is a highly trained professional who can respond quickly. However, given that ethics consultation is not reimbursable by insurance, this model is a cost center for the hospital and thus not as common.

If a clinical ethicist is not on staff, then consults may be done by a subset of the EC who are trained in conducting consults. In the team approach, two to three individuals may be involved in the case. The team approach allows for a division of duties, as well as offering several different perspectives and areas of expertise. This larger group, though, makes scheduling and responsiveness more challenging.

A full EC consult is the norm in a few places, but in most circumstances, this approach is reserved for cases that present novel situations, is required by law, or where the decision to be made is controversial. The full committee model requires coordinating schedules of a large number of people and makes reaching decisions more difficult. Thus, this approach should be used only in the circumstances outlined previously.

PROCESS OF A CONSULT

Many different methods have been developed for performing a consult including CASES (clarify, assemble information, synthesize information, explain, support the process) by the Veteran's Administration National Center for Ethics in Health Care, clinical ethics mediation, clinical ethics, facilitation, and more (see Chapter 1). Each of these approaches has its advantages and disadvantages.

The process for ethics consultation that has been endorsed by the American Society for Bioethics and Humanities is known as "bioethics facilitation." This is a process where the consultant helps create a safe space for discussion that ensures that all voices are heard. The consultant works with interested parties (health care team, patient, family) to guide them in reaching an acceptable solution.

Bioethics facilitation is a five-step process for completing the consult:

1. Gather information

2. Analyze

3. Negotiate options

4. Document

5. Evaluate (Spike, 2012)

These steps are not necessarily sequential and any one step may be revisited multiple times. Similarly, several could happen at once. For example, at a family meeting, one might be gathering new information, analyzing, and negotiating options simultaneously.

Request

The first step of an ethics consult is that someone has to request it. As a consulting service in the hospital, an ethics consultant does not have any patients, but rather assists other health care providers in caring for their patients. Hospital policy determines who is permitted to request a consult. In many hospitals, anyone can request. In others, all requests must go through the attending physician. The hospital may have a consult pager or phone number that one calls to request ethics assistance while others enable one to make the request through the electronic medical record.

Unfortunately, few people in a hospital are aware of the availability of this service or how to contact it. Studies show that most house staff have never requested a consult and that only in half of hospitals do nurses have access to them or to request them (Danis et al., 2008; Gacki-Smith & Gordon, 2005). Consider that only 8% of nurses have requested consults while 15% expressed a desire to ask for one but did not. This difference between knowledge and action is explained by the reasons nurses give for not requesting consults:

1. Lack of awareness or not knowing how to request

2. Fear of adverse repercussions

3. Case resolved on its own

4. Emergency situations created time constraints

5. Lack of availability on the night shift (Gordon & Hamric, 2006)

Fear of repercussions includes concerns about angering physicians, injuring peer relationships, and worries that such a request could lead to dismissal. Nearly half of nurses have experienced or observed retaliation for an ethics consult request (Danis et al., 2008). Ideally, all individuals including patients and families should have access to an ethics consultation request.

Questions to Consider Before Reading On

1. Discuss the process used to request an ethics consultation in your facility and/or that of a class peer or colleague. What are the similarities and differences in the process?

2. How do the provisions and relative statements from the Code of Ethics in Box 5.4 support the nurse's role in ethics consultation?

Once contact has been made, the requestor will be asked several questions: What is the ethical issue? What has happened so far to resolve the situation? Who should be part of the discussion? Does the attending physician know of this request? Who is the patient? And what is the urgency? Some requests

Box 5.4

Process of Clinical Ethics: Committees and Consults—Provisions and Relative Statements From the Code of Ethics

PROVISION 1

The nurse practices with compassion and respect for the inherent dignity, worth, and unique attributes of every person.

PROVISION 6

The nurse, through individual and collective effort, establishes, maintains, and improves the ethical environment of the work setting and conditions of employment that are conducive to safe, quality health care.

FROM INTERPRETIVE STATEMENT, 1.4

Respect for human dignity requires the recognition of specific patient rights, in particular, the right to self-determination. Patients have the moral and legal rights to determine what will be done with and to their own person; to be given accurate, complete, and understandable information in a manner that facilitates an informed decision; and to be assisted with weighing the benefits, burdens, and available options in their treatment, including the choice of no treatment. They also have the right to accept, refuse, or terminate treatment without deceit, undue influence, duress, coercion, or prejudice and to be given necessary support throughout the decision-making and treatment process.

FROM INTERPRETIVE STATEMENT, 6.1

- Virtues are universal, learned, and habituated attributes of moral character that predispose persons to meet their moral obligations, that is, *to do* what is right.
- Virtues are what we are *to be* and make for a morally "good person."

FROM INTERPRETIVE STATEMENT, 6.2

- Obligations focus on what is *right and wrong* or what we are *to do* as moral agents.
- Obligations are often specified in terms of principles such as beneficence or doing good; nonmaleficence or doing no harm; justice or treating people fairly; reparations, or making amends for harm; fidelity, and respect for persons.

FROM INTERPRETIVE STATEMENT, 6.3

Nurses are responsible for contributing to a moral environment that demands respectful interactions among colleagues, mutual peer support, and open identification of difficult issues, which includes ongoing professional development of staff in ethical problem solving.

Source: American Nurses Association (2015).

are time sensitive and need immediate response. Others have longer time scales of days or weeks. This information is important for the consultant to know how much time he or she has to respond.

Question to Consider Before Reading On

Recall a recent situation in which you or a class peer/colleague believed an ethics consultation should have been requested.

1. As the requestor, how would you respond to the questions in the previous section?

Gather Information

After receiving the request, an individual consultant or consultation team will be assigned to the case (for this discussion we will assume an individual consultant). Information gathering requires looking at records, making phone calls, visits to the ward, and possibly a family meeting. The consultant will contact the individual who initiated the request for further information. The consultant will review the patient chart and interview the care team (nurses, physicians, social workers, and other allied health specialists, if relevant). Conversations will also be held with the patient, surrogate decision maker, and family.

Analyze

The analysis step is where the consultant applies ethical theories, health law, hospital policies, and community standards to identify the ethical issue—which may or may not be what was reported—and to examine the issues in the case. This step requires research, referring to similar previous cases, discussion, and reflection.

NEGOTIATE OPTIONS

An ethics consultant in discussion with all relevant parties will identify the options available for dealing with the issue at hand. Each option will be examined for its potential positive and negative outcomes in order to assess the viability of the choices. The consultant can then work with the health care team, patient, and family to reach a consensus choice and/or can make a recommendation. Note that ethics consultants can only offer recommendations. Since the health care team has the fiduciary relationship with the patient and thus is responsible for providing care, the consultant's suggestion can be followed or not.

DOCUMENT

Like all consult services, the consultation process and recommendation will be entered into the patient's chart. Some hospitals even have separate ethics notes. These notes outline the facts of the case, the steps taken, the analysis done, and the recommendation made.

EVALUATE

After the consult, the ethics service will request that the health care team, patient, and family provide feedback on the consult and how helpful it was. Through this step, the ethics consult program performs continual quality improvement and makes sure that the services meet the needs of its users. Most studies of physicians and nurses show strong satisfaction with ethics consult services in helping to resolve an ethical issue or dilemma (Schneiderman et al., 2003). Clinical ethics consults are correlated with shorter hospital stays and shorter ICU stays (Chen et al., 2014).

Ethics Consult for Mr. Ramirez

CASE SCENARIO *(CONTINUED)*

*Using the facilitation method discussed here, we will examine the opening case of Mr. Ramirez to demonstrate how these steps transpire in a case. The consultation request for Mr. Ramirez's case came from the patient's primary nurse. A consultation team of two people (one ethicist and one attorney) then began **gathering** information by reading through his chart, talking to the nurse who requested the consult, talking to the physicians (in this case a general medicine physician, podiatrist, and psychiatrist), and talking to other team members (nursing, social work). The consult team visited the patient in his room and was able to talk to his two sisters who were the only siblings able to visit. The other siblings were working, taking care of their children, or dealing with their mother who was a patient at another hospital. The ethics team realized that a family meeting was necessary. The medical team in charge of the patient's care organized this meeting.*

One of the most shocking events at this meeting was when the various doctors and health care providers introduced themselves. Despite the complicated nature of this case requiring several specialties, none of the care providers had spoken to each other before. Their only contact had been from reading notes in the chart, if that even happened. For 45 minutes, the ethics team acted as facilitator, making sure that each member of the health care team had an

(continued)

opportunity to speak. For many of them, it was the first time they had heard about some of the issues involved. With all of the information on the table, it was time to hear from the family and then **negotiate** *the options. However, when the social worker turned to the family and asked, "Do you understand what has been said," the two sisters turned to each other and spoke in Spanish. Then one sister said haltingly, "No, we do not speak English." No one had thought to ask if the family spoke English. Thus began a period of time where the family was told what had happened in their own language. While the ethics group spoke Spanish and participated, none of the care providers did. Their body language made it apparent that they were not interested in the language issue.*

At this point, the ethics group offered a summary **analysis** *of the conflicting values. For the physicians, patient autonomy was important and lacking that, they wanted a decision maker to make the choices for the patient. The family was going through a great deal at the time and none of the siblings felt they could take responsibility for making a choice, nor could they agree. They believed that the amputation was unnecessary because a family member with diabetes had a similar infection on her hand and was told that she would have to lose a finger. After much prayer and family folk healing, she was healed and the amputation was not necessary. Thus, their lived experience was that the doctors were wrong. Underlying this conversation was a desire to honor beneficence, that is, to do what was best for Mr. Ramirez. The medical truth was that his spreading infection was life threatening.*

Part of **analysis** *is understanding the law and hospital policies. Under the law of this state, lacking a medical power of attorney and a spouse meant that decision-making power fell to the parents. His father was deceased and his mother was unavailable.*

According to statute, next in line were the siblings: Not one sibling, or the loudest sibling, or the eldest sibling, but all siblings. They had to agree and in this family, there was no agreement. It was medically clear that the toe needed to be amputated—that was in the patient's best interest. What was not clear was who could decide for the patient. The **negotiation** *became about this issue. In the end, the ethics group told the family that one sibling had to be the spokesperson for the family and tell the group the decision. In return for that person taking on the responsibility, the rest of the siblings should support him or her even if they disagree. The family needed to come together.*

The next day one of the sisters called to say that the family had talked. She was to be the decision maker and she said to do the surgery. This information was **documented***. Ethics detailed the process in the patient's chart and contacted all of the physicians working on the case. In follow-up* **evaluation** *conversations with the health care team, the ethics group learned that the ethics consultation process was helpful in elucidating the issues, making sure everyone was heard, and in recommending a solution.*

Questions to Consider Before Reading On

1. None of the care providers had communicated with each other prior to the meeting. As the nurse caring for Mr. Ramirez, how could you have facilitated this communication process earlier in his care? Which QSEN competencies and Code provisions/statements would support your role as facilitator?

2. What would you share in the follow-up evaluation conversation with the ethics consultation team?

CONCLUSION

Clinical ethics is a method for "identifying, analyzing and resolving ethics issues in clinical medicine" (Jonsen et al., 2006). A method for resolving ethical issues is required by The Joint Commission, Medicare, case law, and professional organizations. The most common methods found in hospitals are ECs and clinical ethics consultation services.

ECs are interdisciplinary groups composed of experts from various health disciplines and hospital units. The committee can have three functions: policy, education, and consultation.

Ethics consultants are trained in ethical theories, mediation, facilitation, and communication. They also have an advanced degree, clinical experience, and knowledge of relevant laws and policies. Accreditation of consultants will likely include written and oral exams and maintenance of a case portfolio.

Ethics consultation can be done by individuals, teams, or the full EC. The American Society for Bioethics & Humanities recommends a process of bioethics facilitation that includes (a) gathering information, (b) analyzing, (c) negotiating options, (d) documenting the process and recommendations, and (e) evaluating the process.

Ethics consultation helps support the care of patients as well as the well-being of health care practitioners by providing assistance in difficult cases. A strong consult service can improve patient satisfaction, reduce costs, reduce the risk of lawsuits, and improve the hospital's reputation.

Box 5.5

Exemplar—Case Study

Mark is a 70-year-old man with multiple myeloma in the hospital. Mark has no family. Two years ago, he completed a medical power of attorney document naming Daniel, his 17-year-old neighbor, as his proxy decision maker and Daniel's mother as the second agent. At the

(continued)

Box 5.5

Exemplar—Case Study *(continued)*

time, Mark chose that he wanted all efforts made to prolong his life as long as possible. This decision has meant considerable time in the hospital and undergoing uncomfortable treatments. Now Mark is significantly more debilitated. In a conversation with his nurse he has stated that he was done and that if his heart stopped, he did not want any further treatment. He then completed an advance directive and requested a do not resuscitate (DNR) order. Daniel has not visited Mark nor is Daniel aware of the new advance directive. When Mark declines further and slips into unconsciousness, a decision needs to be made to intubate him. Daniel (who is now 19 years old) is called and says, "He wanted everything done. Yes, you must intubate Mark."

1. What are the ethical issues in this case?

2. How can an ethics committee assist in this situation?

3. How can the patient's voice be represented?

4. What information needs to be gathered? Who needs to be involved in conversation?

5. What are the action options in this case?

6. Should Daniel still be the decision maker?

7. How does a nurse best care for Mark?

8. What recommendation should the ethics committee make?

Box 5.6

Evidence-Based Practice Resources

Chen, Y. Y., Chu, T. S., Kao, Y. H., Tsai, P. R., Huang, T. S., & Ko, W. J. (2014). To evaluate the effectiveness of health care ethics consultation based on the goals of health care ethics consultation: A prospective cohort study with randomization. *BMC Medical Ethics, 15*, 1. doi: 10.1186/1472-6939-15-1

Danis, M., Farrar, A., Grady, C., Taylor, C., O'Donnell, P., Soeken, K., & Ulrich, C. (2008). Does fear of retaliation deter requests for ethics consultation? *Medicine, Health Care, and Philosophy, 11*(1), 27–34. doi: 10.1007/s11019-007-9105-z

(continued)

Box 5.6

Evidence-Based Practice *(continued)*

DuVal, G., Sartorius, L., Clarridge, B., Gensler, G., & Danis, M. (2001). What triggers requests for ethics consultations? *Journal of Medical Ethics*, 27(Suppl. 1), i24–i29.

Fox, E., Myers, S., & Pearlman, R. A. (2007). Ethics consultation in United States hospitals: A national survey. *The American Journal of Bioethics*, 7(2), 13–25. doi:10.1080/15265160601109085

Gordon, E. J., & Hamric, A. B. (2006). The courage to stand up: The cultural politics of nurses' access to ethics consultation. *Journal of Clinical Ethics*, 17(3), 231–254.

McClung, J. A., Kamer, R. S., DeLuca, M., & Barber, H. J. (1996). Evaluation of a medical ethics consultation service: Opinions of patients and health care providers. *American Journal of Medicine*, 100(4), 456–460. doi:10.1016/S0002-9343(97)89523-X

Schneiderman, L. J., Gilmer, T., Teetzel, H. D., Dugan, D. O., Blustein, J., Cranford, R., . . . Young, E. W. (2003). Effect of ethics consultation on nonbeneficial life-sustaining treatments in intensive care setting: A randomized controlled trial. *Journal of the American Medical Association*, 290(9), 1166–1172.

Veatch, R. M., & Sollitto, S. (1976). Medical ethics teaching. Report of a National Medical School Survey. *Journal of the American Medical Association*, 235(10), 1030–1033.

Youngner, S. J., Jackson, D. L., Colton, C., Juknialis, B. W., & Smith, E. (1983). *A National Survey of Hospital Ethics Committees*. (83–600503). Washington, DC: U.S. Government Printing Office.

Critical Thinking Questions and Activities

1. As in the Case Scenario, providers may not be communicating with each other or with the patient/family about the patient's status. Nurses are in a unique position to facilitate this communication process. Discuss the strategies proposed to improve this process in the article by Milic et al. (2014), with a class peer or colleague.

http://ajcc.aacnjournals.org/content/24/4/e56.full.pdf+html

2. Review the roles for bedside nurses in discussions of prognosis and goals of care with patients' families and physicians in Figure 1 of the Milic article. Do nurses perform these roles in your current practice? If not, how could they be implemented?

(continued)

Critical Thinking Questions and Activities *(continued)*

3. Identify how the communication skills and example statements presented in Table 1 of the Milic article could have been utilized in a recent (or future) patient situation.

4. Choose one of the evidence-based articles in Box 5.6 and discuss with a class peer or colleague.

REFERENCES

American Nurses Association. (2015). *Code of ethics for nurses with interpretive statements*. Silver Spring, MD: Nursebooks.org.

American Society for Bioethics & Humanities. (2014). Code of ethics and professional responsibilities for healthcare ethics consultants. Retrieved from http://asbh.org/uploads/publications/ASBH%20Code%20of%20Ethics.pdf

Aroskar, M., & Veatch, R. M. (1977). Ethics teaching in nursing schools. *Hastings Center Report*, 7(4), 23–26.

ASBH Clinical Ethics Task Force. (2009). *Improving competencies in clinical ethics consultation: An education guide*. Chicago, IL: American Society for Bioethics and Humanities.

Chen, Y. Y., Chu, T. S., Kao, Y. H., Tsai, P. R., Huang, T. S., & Ko, W. J. (2014). To evaluate the effectiveness of health care ethics consultation based on the goals of health care ethics consultation: A prospective cohort study with randomization. *BioMed Central Medical Ethics*, 15, 1. doi: 10.1186/1472-6939-15-1

Cronenwett, L., Sherwood, G., Barnsteiner, J., Disch, J., Johnson, J., Mitchell, P., . . . Warren, J. (2007). Quality and safety education for nurses. *Nursing Outlook*, 55(3), 122–131.

Danis, M., Farrar, A., Grady, C., Taylor, C., O'Donnell, P., Soeken, K., & Ulrich, C. (2008). Does fear of retaliation deter requests for ethics consultation? *Medicine, Health Care, and Philosophy*, 11(1), 27–34. doi:10.1007/s11019-007-9105-z

DuVal, G., Sartorius, L., Clarridge, B., Gensler, G., & Danis, M. (2001). What triggers requests for ethics consultations? *Journal of Medical Ethics*, 27(Suppl. 1), i24–i29.

Fox, E., Myers, S., & Pearlman, R. A. (2007). Ethics consultation in United States hospitals: A national survey. *The American Journal of Bioethics*, 7(2), 13–25. doi:10.1080/15265160601109085

Gacki-Smith, J., & Gordon, E. J. (2005). Residents' access to ethics consultations: Knowledge, use, and perceptions. *Academic Medicine*, 80(2), 168–175.

Gordon, E. J., & Hamric, A. B. (2006). The courage to stand up: The cultural politics of nurses' access to ethics consultation. *Journal of Clinical Ethics*, 17(3), 231–254.

Hester, D. M., & Schonfeld, T. (Eds.). (2012). *Guidance for healthcare ethics committees*. New York, NY: Cambridge University Press.

Jonsen, A. R., Siegler, M., & Winslade, W. J. (2006). *Clinical ethics* (6th ed.). New York, NY: McGraw-Hill.

McClung, J. A., Kamer, R. S., DeLuca, M., & Barber, H. J. (1996). Evaluation of a medical ethics consultation service: Opinions of patients and health care providers. *The American Journal of Medicine*, 100(4), 456–460. doi:10.1016/S0002-9343(97)89523-X

Milic, M. M., Puntillo, K., Turner, K., Joseph, D., Peters, N., Ryan, R., . . . Anderson, W. (2015). Communicating with patients' families and physicians about prognosis and goals of care.

American Journal of Critical Care, 24(4):e56–e64. Retrieved from http://ajcc.aacnjournals.org/content/24/4/e56.full.pdf+html

Schneiderman, L. J., Gilmer, T., Teetzel, H. D., Dugan, D. O., Blustein, J., Cranford, R., . . . Young, E. W. (2003). Effect of ethics consultation on nonbeneficial life-sustaining treatments in intensive care setting: A randomized controlled trial. *Journal of the American Medical Association, 290*(9), 1166–1172.

Spike, J. (2012). Ethics consultation process. In D. M. Hester & T. Schonfeld (Eds.), *Guidance for healthcare ethics committees* (pp. 41–47). New York, NY: Cambridge University Press.

The Supreme Court of New Jersey. (1976). In Re Quinlan. 70 NJ 10 (355 A.2d 647).

Tapper, E. B. (2013). Consults for conflict: The history of ethics consultation. *Proceedings (Baylor University Medical Center), 26*(4), 417–422.

VA Ethics. (n.d.). A brief business case for ethics. Retrieved from http://www.ethics.va.gov/businesscase.pdf

Veatch, R. M., & Sollitto, S. (1976). Medical ethics teaching. Report of a National Medical School Survey. *Journal of the American Medical Association, 235*(10), 1030–1033.

Youngner, S. J., Jackson, D. L., Colton, C., Juknialis, B. W., & Smith, E. (1983). *A National Survey of Hospital Ethics Committees.* (83-600503). Washington, DC: U.S. Government Printing Office.

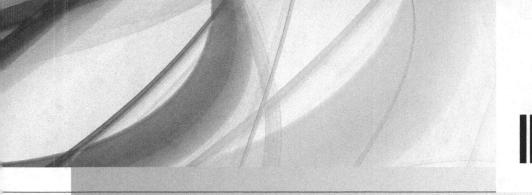

Emerging Ethical Issues in Nursing Practice

6

Exploring Ethical Issues Related to Person- and Family-Centered Care

MARY K. WALTON

LEARNING OBJECTIVES AND OUTCOMES

Upon completion of this chapter, the reader will be able to:

- Identify three ethical issues arising for clinical nurses in the provision of person- and family-centered care (PFCC)
- Describe three nursing competencies that support PFCC in the acute care setting
- Describe one approach to eliciting the preferences, values, and needs of patients

As a registered nurse, you have seen the degree of patient and family involvement in decision making regarding nursing care varies depending on the patient's individual needs, preferences, and values. Nursing practice has always centered on the care of the patient, although the relationship has varied, ranging from the nurse providing total care and making all the decisions to one that can be accurately characterized as a full partnership where the expertise of the patient and family, if the patient wishes, is valued equally with that of the nurse. In such a partnership the patient and nurse jointly identify the problem, establish goals, create a plan of care, and evaluate the success of the plan. The term *patient centeredness*, introduced in medical literature (Balint, 1969) to characterize the concept of understanding each patient as a unique human being, is now recognized as an essential concept to achieve quality in health care (IOM, 2001). As you read this chapter, think about relationships and concerns you have experienced in caring for patients and families regarding decision making in their nursing care.

CASE SCENARIO

Mr. Charles Jones is 35 years old and hospitalized for a severe genetic cardiopulmonary condition. He has survived long past the average life expectancy for an individual with his diagnosis. Hospitalizations are increasingly necessary as his disease has progressed and nighttime ventilator support became part of his home routine 5 years ago. His father is his primary caregiver. They share a home and both describe the importance of their faith throughout the long journey with his progressive and life-limiting condition. Admitted for worsening heart failure symptoms, nurses express frustration with his care, primarily related to maintaining his oral fluid limits and his nighttime ventilation routine. Physicians express annoyance when the very limited oral fluid allowance is not maintained. Some nurses "give in" to his requests to quench his ever present thirst, leaving fluids at his bedside where he can access them as needed; other nurses describe an obligation to follow physician orders, posting signs alerting staff to not respond to the patient's request for beverages. Respiratory therapists resist his requests to veer from their standard hospital routine; he wants to follow his home schedule for nighttime ventilation. Since Mr. Jones's home routine for sleep is much later than the 9 p.m. hospital standards, he objects to going on the ventilator when the therapists make their evening rounds, he enjoys late night TV with a snack before going on the ventilator and wants to start his morning routine much later than the hospital's 6 a.m. routine. The nurse manager, recognizing the ethical aspects to this situation, consults the nurse ethicist for assistance in addressing the care issues for the patient and the emerging conflict among the nurses and between physicians and nurses.

BACKGROUND

Societal changes marked by the quality and patient safety movement, consumer demand, and regulatory and accrediting bodies are forcing health care settings to shift the culture to one truly centered on the needs of patients and families rather than on the preferences of providers. Furthermore, provisions in the American Nurses Association (ANA) Code of Ethics for Nurses, the ethical standard for professional practice, mandate attention to the primacy of the patient's interests, the right to self-determination, and the recognition of the unique needs of the individual (ANA, 2015a).

Clinical nurses practicing in acute care settings are likely to be challenged to provide PFCC as patient values and preferences may be invisible or alternately not honored as they conflict with clinician or organizational values. However, their proximity to the patient in a therapeutic relationship places them in a pivotal position to promote this cultural transformation albeit requiring significant changes in nursing practice. Ethical concerns will likely arise for clinical nurses with the recognition of professional obligations as well as honoring personal values, the values of their organization, and those of the patient and family. In this chapter, several ethical issues will be identified along with the requisite knowledge, skills, and attitude (KSA) that support the provision of PFCC.

Question to Consider Before Reading On

1. How would you define PFCC in your current practice setting?

WHAT IS PFCC?

The Institute of Medicine, in its landmark report *Crossing the Quality Chasm,* identified one of six imperatives for quality as patient-centered care, defined as "providing care that is respectful of and responsive to individual patient preferences, needs and values and ensuring that patient values guide all clinical decisions" (IOM, 2001, p. 40). An extension of the IOM definition of patient-centered care developed for the Quality and Safety Education for Nurses (QSEN) work highlights both nursing's obligations to patients and the importance of partnership, "recognizing the patient or designee as the source of control and full partner in providing compassionate and coordinated care based on respect for patient's preferences, values and needs" (Cronenwett et al., 2007, p. 123).

Partnership and engagement are central to achieving an exceptional experience in the inpatient setting:

- Every care interaction is anchored in a respectful partnership, anticipating and responding to patient and family needs (e.g., physical comfort, emotional, informational, cultural, spiritual, and learning).

- Patients are part of the care team and participate at the level the patient chooses.

- Care for each patient is based on a customized interdisciplinary shared care plan with patients educated, enabled, and confident to carry out their care plans. (Balik, Conway, Zipperer, & Watson, 2011, p.14)

Question to Consider Before Reading On

1. How are the these aspects of partnership and engagement integrated in your current practice?

An analysis of the concept of patient centeredness through the formal theories of ethics justifies the concept as the ethical approach to care (Duggan et al., 2005)

Although the QSEN competency reads *patient-centered care*, the term *person- and family-centered care* is more representative of the concept. Many experts have brought forth the idea that in order to treat the patient, one must see the person (Barnsteiner, Disch, & Walton, 2014; Koloroutis & Trout, 2012; Schenck & Churchill, 2012). Moreover, individuals are engaging in health care beyond the hospital walls and family plays a significant role in health care experiences.

ETHICAL ISSUES ARISING IN PFCC

The Code of Ethics for Nurses embraces the ethical demands of respecting the wholeness of the person dwelling in a family and community (ANA, 2015a). However, models of ethical decision making in clinical practice traditionally focus on quandary ethics using formal biomedical principles and theories to examine dilemmas and conflicts often to the exclusion of the importance of everyday skillful ethical comportment (Dreyfus, Dreyfus, & Benner, 2009).

Ethical dilemmas often present with the dramatic events in health care where decisions may have an immediate and irreversible impact on patients and their loved ones—listing for transplant, whether to use invasive life-sustaining technology, or whether to limit or withdraw aggressive care. However, the attention given to these momentous decisions characterized as "quandary ethics" draws attention away from the everyday ethical issues embedded in nursing practice:

> Doctors and nurses make "constant small ethical decisions [in their] everyday clinical work" like whether to make eye contact with a patient or take seriously a patient's complaints about treatment side effects. Their choices have a major impact on patients and caregivers. Concepts like beneficence and respect for persons are as relevant to these interactions as they are to conventional ethics concerns like decision-making about life-sustaining interventions." (Dresser, 2011, p.15)

Although the challenges that face patients, families, and clinicians at the margins of life require skilled analysis, as the field of bioethics has matured, there is increasing recognition of the ethical aspects of everyday clinical practice—microethics rather than quandary ethics (Churchill, Fanning, & Schenck, 2013; Truog et al., 2015). The constant small decisions made in routine, everyday interactions are inherently ethical in nature; they have significant impact on vulnerable patients and families. Every clinical encounter between a nurse and a patient or his or her family member is an opportunity to care; the act of caring is a moral ideal and foundational to the practice of nursing (ANA, 2015b).

Looking at nursing practice through the lens of PFCC reveals opportunities that arise for ethical issues and conflicts for clinical nurses in the acute care setting. Three ethical issues related to the introductory Case Scenarios for analysis are:

1. Ensuring that the patient's voice has primacy over that of the nurse

2. Honoring the choices of the patient even when they conflict with those of the nurse

3. Engaging with family as the patient directs

Questions to Consider Before Reading On

1. What are some microethics issues you have encountered in your daily practice?

2. How did you identify these as ethical in nature?

Primacy of the Patient's Voice

The need for patient-centered care is recognized in the Institute of Medicine report *The Future of Nursing: Leading Change, Advancing Care*, "yet practice still is usually organized around what is most convenient for the provider, the payer, or the health care organization and not the patient. Patients are repeatedly asked, for example, to change their expectations and schedules to fit the needs of the system" (IOM, 2010, p. 51). PFCC calls for clinicians to re-envision how work is accomplished by shifting the power base from the clinician to the patient toward establishing a partnership for safe, high-quality care. In fact, no longer is the clinician's evaluation of the quality of care considered the ultimate measure of quality. How the individual person experiences care is now a recognized quality metric; patient experience is broadly defined as "the sum of all interactions, shaped by an organization's culture, that influence patient perceptions across the continuum of care" (Wolf et al., 2014). However, in the acute-care setting, where professionals from many disciplines are responsible for accomplishing myriad tasks in set chronological 24-hour time blocks, staff schedules and unit routines hold higher priority than patient preferences and dictate practices to achieve standardization, efficiency, and safety. For clinical nurses, individualizing care presents challenges; furthermore, seeing the patient as the source of control and a full partner may seem virtually impossible. Nurses often describe their own inability to have control over schedules, let alone more complex care issues. While standardization can promote safety and efficiency, it is blind to individual needs and preferences. Nurses are uniquely positioned to engage patients in articulating their values and preferences and creating partnerships to ensure clinical decisions reflect the same.

CASE SCENARIO (*CONTINUED*)

In our opening Case Scenario, although Mr. Jones has successfully managed a complex care regimen in his home with the help of his father, the schedule for nighttime ventilation is based on hospital routine. The patient's preferences are not honored; his request to enjoy a snack and TV before going back on the ventilator for the night is not considered of importance. The needs of the respiratory therapy department trump those of the patient. Among the many voices in the care discussions, those of the nurses, physicians, and therapists are given priority over that of the individual patient. Care provided is neither coordinated nor compassionate as described in the Case Scenario.

Valuing Patient and Family Choices Over Those of Nurse and/or Organization

For inpatient experiences to be both satisfactory to the patient and achieve quality health outcomes, patients need to be actively engaged in their care. The Nursing Alliance for Quality Care (NAQC), which includes both nursing and patient/consumer representatives, endorses the vision of partnership, competent decision making, and ethical behavior to achieve high-quality and safe care. Nurses must support patients not only in making competent, well-informed decisions, but also in supporting their actions in carrying out those decisions (Sofaer & Schumann, 2013). The nurse is in the ideal position among health care providers to experience the patient as a unique human being with individual strengths and complexities in order to advocate from a patient rather than a provider-centric stance. Gadow's concept of existential advocacy expresses the ideal that advocacy is "the effort to help persons *become clear about what they want* to do, by helping them discern and clarify their values in the situation, and on the basis of that self-examination, to reach decisions which express their reaffirmed, perhaps recreated, complex of values" (Gadow, 1980, p. 44). This approach to nursing's advocacy role can ensure that a patient's decision is actually self-determined rather than a decision that a clinician would choose for him or her.

The Case Scenario illustrates a lack of coordination and continuity of care among the bedside nurses as well as open conflict about one of the strategies to treat the patient's cardiac symptoms. The nursing staff is not in agreement about honoring the medical orders and there is no evidence of any collaboration with the patient and/or the interprofessional team about this aspect of care. Given the patient's years of experience—in fact, his established expertise—the Case Scenario does not indicate that the patient's perspective on this issue is sought. Clinical nurses will appreciate the frustration of working with physicians who expect medical orders followed; however, can they imagine how a person with an intense thirst feels when begging for fluids? In the Case Scenario, Mr. Jones is clearly not the source of control nor does it seem decisions are based on his preferences and values. Exploring the patient's experience with managing his cardiac condition and his goals not only for the hospitalization but also for his future is indicated. Did he participate in and agree to the plan for fluid restriction? Is his refusal to adhere to medical recommendations a signal that he wants to renegotiate goals? Is he evaluating the risk/benefit equation and deciding the burden of tight fluid control is not worth the benefit of reduced symptoms? Perhaps he does not believe fluid restriction is effective. Could a care-planning discussion with the patient and the clinical team reveal new goals and/or strategies that the patient can support? Can nurses and physicians accept and honor decisions that Mr. Jones makes based on his values and goals, even if they do not represent standard medical practices?

Questions to Consider Before Reading On

1. Recognizing the variation in the clinical nurses' response to Mr. Jones's requests for fluids, how might you engage your colleagues in coordinating the plan for fluid restriction *with* the patient? Who could be an ally?

2. Do you think "giving in" accurately characterizes professional practice? Alternately do you believe following medical orders against the patient's wishes reflects ethical practice?

Engaging Family in Care

Recognizing the inherent vulnerability of any individual who is hospitalized, regulations and standards issued in 2010 by Centers for Medicare & Medicaid Services (CMS) and The Joint Commission specify the patient's right to have a support person present in the inpatient setting, including critical care settings, at all times. As family presence and participation is increasingly recognized as essential for patient safety and quality, clinical staff is challenged to shift from doing for or *to* patients to doing *with* patients and their families. Nurses must work with patients and their family if the patient so directs; these loved ones offer invaluable knowledge of the patient as a person as well as home and community resources. They can offer history and assistance with plans for transitions to home or other care settings. Recognition of the important role of the patient's support person is essential for PFCC.

Family is defined by the patient, not solely by blood or legal relationships, and can be characterized as "those for whom it matters." Ethical concerns about protection of the rights of privacy and confidentiality must be carefully addressed; confusion about legal considerations related to Health Insurance Portability and Accountability Act (HIPAA) regulations should not prevent sharing information and working with family members as directed by the patient.

KSA to Achieve PFCC

There are 39 QSEN graduate-level KSAs associated with the QSEN patient-centered care competency. Eleven are selected here to illustrate how the KSAs relate to the scenario.

Knowledge

- Analyze multiple dimensions of patient-centered care including patient/family/community preferences and values, as well as social, cultural, psychological, and spiritual contexts

- Analyze patient-centered care in the context of care coordination, patient education, physical comfort, emotional support, and care transitions.

- Analyze ethical and legal implications of patient-centered care.

Skills

- Based on active listening to patients, elicit values, preferences, and expressed needs as part of clinical interview, diagnosis, implementation of care plan as well as coordination and evaluation of care.

- Work to address ethical and legal issues related to patients' rights to determine their care.

- Work with patients to create plans of care that are defined by the patient.

- Assess patients' understanding of their health issues and create plans with the patients to manage their health.

Attitudes

- Commit to the patient being the source of control and full partner in his or her care.

- Commit to respecting the rights of patients to determine their care plan to the extent that they want.

- Respect the complexity of decision making by patients.

- Value the involvement of patients and family in care decisions (QSEN, 2012).

Question to Consider Before Reading On

1. How could one of the nursing actions related to knowledge, skill, or attitude be used by the nurse in the chapter Case Scenario?

Skills and Practices Using Selected Key PFCC Practices

Among the many recognized practices that support a culture of PFCC (Herrin et al., 2016), there are two that clinical nurses have significant authority to influence/implement: (a) recognizing the patients' right to specify which family members will be actively involved in their care, and (b) encouraging patients and family to participate in nurse-shift change report. Two routine nursing practices, the admission assessment and nurse-shift change report, serve to illustrate how the QSEN competencies are demonstrated.

The Admission Assessment

Nurses interview all patients on admission to the hospital. Assessing the patient's physical and emotional condition, learning needs and orienting the patient to the care environment are well-established nursing responsibilities. Integral to this activity is recognizing the impact of first impressions, identifying communication needs and a support person, and beginning role negotiation (Walton, 2011). Engaging patients or their support persons in expressing their goals as well as discussing the role they want to play in this health care experience lays the foundation for a positive experience. Nurses should first learn about goals for the hospitalization from the patient's perspective. Prompting the patient to describe personal expectations is informative; goals of care are concepts patients recognize and may be more helpful than focusing solely on interventions (Kaldjian, Curtis, Shinkunas, & Cannon, 2009). For example, whether a patient is being admitted for an elective procedure or an exacerbation of a medical condition, nurses can elicit not only the intervention(s) planned or underway but also the patient's understanding of what these measures will achieve. Understanding patient expectations may highlight important distinctions from the clinician's perspective and should inform the consent process. Orienting patients to the team and hospital routine should also include a discussion of the role the patient and support person hope or want to play in shaping the care plan and achieving the goals as the patient sees them. The phrase "nothing about me without me" serves to remind clinicians that the voice of the patient is essential in all aspects of inpatient care (Delbanco et al., 2001).

CASE SCENARIO *(CONTINUED)*

Examples of prompts that could be used to elicit the patient's goals, care preferences, and preference of family involvement in the Case Scenario of this chapter are:

(continued)

CASE SCENARIO (*CONTINUED*)

- *Mr. Jones, since you have been hospitalized in the past, I consider you an expert in your own care. It is important that we have your guidance and direction.*
- *Can you share with me your goals for this admission? Tell me a little about how the decision for admission was made and what you hope will be achieved.*
- *Mr. Jones, can you tell me about your home routine for your nighttime ventilation program? Please highlight what you know works best and why.*
- *We recognize the value of having a family member or friend as a support person while in the hospital. We welcome them as you wish. Are there people (there may be more than one) you want us to include in your care?*
- *What approaches have been used in previous hospital stays that worked? How have nurses helped you be successful in managing treatment interventions that are challenging for you? What is most important for us to know about your care or hopes for this inpatient stay?*

Prompts such as these signify a desire to work with the patient and, if he desires, family members/support persons. It also creates a clear opportunity for the patient to set his standards for care. This approach validates his success in managing a complex care routine and conveys respect and dignity for his role in self-care. Clinical nurses practicing in the acute care setting will likely learn successful home care strategies when patients have the opportunity to share their knowledge and skills and teach the nurse. Here, the nurse would learn more about Mr. Jones as an individual, managing his health care at home in contrast to learning about his care when he objects to plans based on clinician and organizational needs. Additionally, engaging a family member in developing a plan will likely introduce both knowledge and skill based on experience for this patient as well as emotional support.

Nurse Bedside Shift Report

The goal of bedside shift report is to ensure the safe handover of care between nurses by exchanging accurate information, providing for continuity, and involving the patient and family in the process. Here the patient and family have the opportunity to hear what has happened throughout the shift and the next steps in their care. It also offers the opportunity for them to ask questions and provide input into the care process; it is a visible symbol of patient-centered care as nurses are engaging *with* the individual in evaluating care and establishing goals. Engaging patients in rounds refocuses the exchange of information to include the patient and family (Radtke, 2013). Exchanging information in the presence of the patient without their participation in the process is not patient/family centered. This is an important distinction. Learning how to accomplish effective and efficient bedside shift report requires planning and practice. An implementation handbook published by Agency for Healthcare Research and Quality (AHRQ) as part of a Guide to Patient and Family Engagement offers strategies and resources as well as case examples (AHRQ, 2014). While nurse-to-nurse handover is a well-established ritual, the various methods for accomplishing the goals of it are not evidence based and practices vary widely. However, the need to ensure patients have the information is evident (Staggers & Blaz, 2012). Given variation in practices, orienting patients and family members to the unit's shift report routines is important.

CASE SCENARIO (CONTINUED)

Suggested prompts for the Case Scenario of this chapter to orient the patient and family to bedside shift report:

- *Mr. Jones, can you tell us how you participated in your care on previous hospitalizations? I am interested in knowing how you have worked with the nurses on planning your care.*
- *It is important for us to work together during your hospitalization. When the nursing shift change happens between 7 and 7:30 a.m. and 7 and 7:30 p.m., we will invite your participation. We hope if you feel able you will share how you feel your care is progressing and your goals for the next shift/time period. We want to be sure we understand your needs and goals and how best to meet them. You will also meet the nurse who will be assuming your care on the oncoming shift.*

STRATEGIES TO ELICIT PATIENT'S PREFERENCES, VALUES, AND NEEDS

The desire to create partnerships with patients is essential; however, developing partnership requires significant communication skills in order to create a safe space for patient preferences, values, and needs to be expressed and discussed. Values may best be thought of in the broadest sense as the preferred events that people seek, arising from needs and wants; values are evident in the everyday life experiences of individuals (Glen, 1999). Nurses must recognize that health care is not a value-neutral science and expert clinicians are. . .

> more than repositories of facts and technical skills—they become experts at a set of activities that can only be described as governed and constituted by particular values and ends: the badness of pain, a picture of human flourishing and wellness, the nature of dignity and more. . . . There is no extractable core of value neutral knowledge that forms the essence of the clinician's skilled expertise. (Kukla, 2007, p. 32)

If care is to be truly centered on the values of the person who is the patient rather than those of the clinician, there needs to be both a recognition of the values of both and clarity about the primacy of the patient's values over those of the clinician. Developing communication skills to elicit and discuss values is as essential to safety and quality as are the myriad technical skills that nurses are required to demonstrate competency. How patients conceptualize their health and illness and their explanatory framework is likely to vary from that of the clinician, given the diversity of human experience. Eliciting the patient's explanatory framework, active listening, and responding to emotion are all communication skills that take time and experience to develop.

Active listening is an essential skill to elicit values, preferences, and expressed needs as part of clinical interviews to determine how to deliver, coordinate, and evaluate care (Cronenwett et al., 2009). Although typically portrayed as a simple skill, listening actually takes energy and concentration. It is a way of focusing and giving attention and communicates, "You are worth my time. I think this interaction with you is important. I am willing and able to be with you rather than somewhere else" (Churchill et al., 2013, p. 60). Nurses routinely ask patients for a great deal of information, such as medication history, symptoms, and functional level. This information is most often elicited through closed-ended questions in order to populate standardized forms and may inhibit revealing unique aspects of the patient's story. This process can become rote rather than an opportunity for the nurse to learn from the patient and begin building the trust necessary for the therapeutic relationship. Curiosity and a genuine interest in learning about the patient as a person with a life story that is not solely grounded in his or her health and illness journey will convey respect for the dignity of the person and enrich the work life of the nurse. Numerous tools are recognized in the literature as valuable in helping clinicians elicit health beliefs that patients hold and will likely influence how they make decisions about their care and shape their expectations of care providers. Two that support PFCC are Kleinman's Questions (Box 6.1; Kleinman, Eisenberg, & Good, 1978) and LEARN (Berlin & Fowkes, 1983). Selecting a few of the eight Kleinman's Questions to explore aspects of care with Mr. Jones could reveal valuable insight into what matters to the patient. They are included in The Joint Commission Roadmap (TJC, 2010).

Question to Consider Before Reading On

1. How would you use the LEARN framework (Box 6.2) in a past experience you have had with a patient to improve communication of both your and the patient's perspectives and perceptions of the situation?

Using the LEARN framework in a discussion about the patient's preferences and the medical recommendations for heart failure highlights the need for the clinician and patient to explore each other's perspective in order to develop a mutually agreed upon plan for the inpatient stay.

Responding to Emotion

Sometimes in eliciting patient values and preferences, nurses will have an internal emotional response as the patient's values and preferences may differ

Kleinman's Questions

1. What do you think has caused your problem?

2. Why do you think it started when it did?

3. What do you think your sickness does to you? How does it work?

4. How severe is your sickness? Will it have a short or long course?

5. What kind of treatment do you think you should receive?

6. What are the most important results you hope to receive from this treatment?

7. What are the chief problems your sickness has caused for you?

8. What do you fear most about your sickness?

Adapted from Kleinman et al. (1978).

Box 6.2

LEARN

L *Listen* with sympathy and understanding to the patient's perception of the problem

E *Explain* your perceptions of the problem

A *Acknowledge* and discuss the differences and similarities

R *Recommend* treatment

N *Negotiate* Agreement

Adapted from Berlin and Fowkes (1983, p. 934).

from theirs. Given the inherent vulnerability of patients and their loved ones in the acute care environment and the goal of providing compassionate care, nurses must develop skill in responding to emotions. A tendency to withdraw from intense and challenging emotions will inhibit a sense of partnership and prevent the healing benefits of therapeutic presence. Nurses who develop an accepting response to expressions of emotion will learn about the patient's thoughts and feelings. Rather than providing immediate reassurance, rebuttal, or agreement, the accepting response accepts what the patient says without judgment, acknowledges that patients ought to hold their own views and feelings, and validates the importance of the patient's contributions in a therapeutic relationship. This is distinct from agreeing with the patient's hopes or beliefs. NURSE is a useful mnemonic corresponding to and accepting patient emotions.

Questions to Consider Before Reading On

1. Think about your previous experiences with patients' family members (Box 6.3). Were you able to accept their emotional expressions and validate their right to those feelings even if they were critical of your work or your organization?

2. Reflect on family members' response to your interventions—were you an active listener or alternately did you correct, dismiss, or ignore their emotional expressions?

3. How did your interactions engage them or alternately distance them from supporting the patient's care?

Box 6.3

Responding and Accepting Patient Emotions

NURSE:

N = Name the emotion
   Naming, restating, and summarizing are ways to begin.
   I wonder if you're feeling angry. Some people in this situation would be angry; not *I can see you are angry.*
   What is the difference between the two examples from patient perspective?

U = Understanding
   My understanding of what you are saying is . . . .
   This gives the patient an opportunity to clarify or correct if the restatement does not capture the emotion that is felt and offers confirmation of being accurately heard.

R = Respecting
   Can be nonverbal response—facial expression, touch, change in posture.

S = Supporting
   I will be with you; express willingness to help. Think presence.

E = Exploring
   Tell me more; clues offered with emotions. Asking to elaborate.

Adapted from Back et al. (2005).

CONCLUSION

Appreciating the vulnerability of individuals when hospitalized and in need of nursing care is foundational to developing the therapeutic nurse–patient relationship and ethical practice. Engaging patients and their families as full partners in care requires specific KSAs as described in the QSEN KSAs for patient-centered care. Embracing these beliefs and developing these skills will reshape the care experience to one truly centered on the values and preferences of the individuals and families receiving nursing care. In the introductory Case Scenario, partnership has not been established and the patient is not the source of control. If clinical nurses worked to create a partnership with Mr. Jones, starting with the admission assessment and continuing with the bedside shift report, the impasses described would likely be prevented. On admission, the patient's goals and expectations could have been explored and a plan negotiated; physicians and therapists could have been consulted before the plan the patient objected to was enacted. Realistic and feasible approaches needed to be agreed upon in collaboration with physicians and therapists. Clinicians needed to value the patient's reasons for maintaining the home time schedule for ventilation such as the pleasure he experiences with late night TV and knowing he will not have to readjust his schedule when he returns home. Or alternately, does the clinical condition that necessitated hospitalization support a rationale for a different, perhaps longer time on the ventilator? These are components of the benefit/burden analysis that should be discussed rather than requiring conformity with departmental standard routine. Given Mr. Jones's expertise in living with his condition with multiple hospitalizations, it is likely he has ideas and approaches that are workable. Working *with* Mr. Jones about the recommended strategies will reveal his beliefs about what caused his current exacerbation and what will improve it. If he believes fluid restriction is a successful strategy, he can direct nurses in how to help him follow it. If he does not believe fluid restriction is important, together with nurses and physicians, a compromise or alternative strategy must be developed including perhaps even considering discharge if there is not a care plan that warrants an impatient stay.

Using strategies to elicit the patient's values, beliefs, and care preferences, negotiating plans and providing emotional support are all within the purview of the clinical nurse. Informed consent is an ethically relevant principle for the everyday aspects of care, not only those that require documentation of the informed consent process. Engaging *with* patients from the time of admission and consistently in nurse bedside shift report will support PFCC in the acute care setting. Inpatient nurses are central to the quality of the inpatient experience of care and are well positioned to establish partnerships with patients and their family members. Nurses are also influential in promoting other disciplines to work more collaboratively with patients and family members given their central role in the acute care setting. A culture of PFCC is based on mutual respect of knowledge and skills among all stakeholders in the care relationship and values multiple points of view.

Critical Thinking Questions and Activities

1. Since many individuals successfully manage complex chronic illnesses in their homes, and may in fact have greater expertise than nurses and physicians with some aspects of their care, identify strategies to engage patients in teaching clinicians.

2. Explain how you could have acknowledged the need to learn from a patient to your colleagues. Was this or would this type of acknowledgment be viewed in your current workplace within your practice group as a strength or a weakness? Explain.

3. Explain how your acknowledgment could or did influence the development of a therapeutic relationship with your patient.

4. Explore the resources and assessment tools available on the Institute for Patient- and Family-Centered Care website: www.ipfcc.org/tools/downloads-tools.html. Describe a situation in which you could use some of these resource tools in your nursing practice.

REFERENCES

Agency for Healthcare Research and Quality. (2014). Guide to patient and family engagement. Exhibit 9. Strategies to engage patients and families as part of the health care team. Environmental Scan Report. Agency for Healthcare Research and Quality, Rockville, MD. Retrieved from http://www.ahrq.gov/research/findings/final-reports/ptfamilyscan/ptfamilyex9.html

American Nurses Association (ANA). (2015a). *Code of ethics for nurses with interpretative statements*. Silver Spring, MD: Nursebooks.org

American Nurses Association. (2015b). *Nursing scope and standards of practice* (3rd ed.). Silver Spring, MD: Nursebooks.org.

Back, A. L., Arnold, R. M., Baile, W. F., Tulsky, J. A., & Fryer-Edwards, K. (2005). Approaching difficult communication tasks in oncology. *CA: A Cancer Journal for Clinicians, 55*(3),164–177.

Balik, B., Conway, J., Zipperer, L., & Watson, J. (2011). *Achieving an exceptional patient and family experience of inpatient hospital care*. IHI Innovation Series white paper. Cambridge, MA: Institute for Healthcare Improvement. Retrieved from http://www.ihi.org/resources/Pages/IHIWhitePapers/AchievingExceptionalPatientFamilyExperienceInpatientHospitalCareWhitePaper.aspx

Balint, E. (1969). The possibilities of patient-centered medicine. *Journal of the Royal College of General Practitioners, 17*, 269–276.

Barnsteiner, J., Disch, J., & Walton, M. K. (Eds.). (2014). *Person and family centered care*. Indianapolis, IN: Sigma Theta Tau International.

Berlin, E. A., & Fowkes, W. C. (1983). A teaching framework for cross-cultural health care. *The Western Journal of Medicine,139*(6), 934–938.

Centers for Medicare & Medicaid Services. (2010). Medicare and Medicaid programs: Changes to the hospital and critical access hospital conditions of participation to ensure visitation rights for all patients. *Federal Register, 75*, 70831–70844.

Churchill, L. R., Fanning, J. B., & Schenck, D. (2013). *What patients teach: The everyday ethics of health care.* New York, NY: Oxford University Press

Cronenwett, L., Sherwood, G., Barnsteiner, J., Disch, J., Johnson, J., Mitchell, P., . . . Warren, J. (2007). Quality and safety education for nurses. *Nursing Outlook, 55*(3), 122–131.

Cronenwett, L., Sherwood, G., Pohl, J., Barnsteiner, J., Moore, S., Sullivan, D., . . . Warren, J. (2009). Quality and safety education for advanced nursing practice. *Nursing Outlook, 57*(6), 338–348.

Delbanco, T., Berwick, D. M., Boufford, J. I., Edgman-Levitan, S., Ollenschlager, G., Plamping, D., & Rockefeller, R. G. (2001). Healthcare in a land called PeoplePower: Nothing about me without me. *Health Expectations, 4*(3), 144–150.

Dresser, R. (2011). Bioethics and cancer: When the professional becomes personal. *Hastings Center Report, 41*(6), 14–18.

Dreyfus, H. L., Dreyfus, S. E., & Benner, P. (2009). Implications of the phenomenology of expertise for teaching and learning everyday skillful ethical comportment. In P. Benner, C. Tanner, & C. Chesla (Eds.). *Expertise in nursing practice: Caring, clinical judgment and ethics* (2nd ed.). New York, NY: Springer.

Duggan, P. S., Geller, G., Cooper, L. A., & Beach, M. C. (2005). The moral nature of patient-centeredness: Is it "just the right thing to do"? *Patient Education and Counseling, 62*, 271–276.

Gadow, S. (1980). Existential advocacy: Philosophical foundations of nursing. In S. F. Spicker & S. Gadow (Eds.). *Nursing images and ideals: Opening dialogue with the humanities.* New York, NY: Springer.

Glen, S. (1999). Educating for interprofessional collaboration: Teaching about values. *Nursing Ethics, 6*(202), 202–213. doi:10.1177/096973309900600303

Herrin, J., Harris, K. G., Kenward, K., Hines, S., Joshi, M. S., & Frosch, D. L. (2016). Patient and family engagement: A survey of US hospital practices. *BMJ Quality & Safety, 25*(3), 182–189. doi:10.1136/bmjqs-2015-004006

Institute for Patient- and Family-Centered Care. Tools to foster the practice of patient- and family-centered care. Retrieved from www.ipfcc.org/tools/downloads-tools.html

Institute of Medicine (IOM). (2001). *Crossing the quality chasm: A new health system for the 21st century.* Washington, DC: National Academies Press.

Institute of Medicine. (2010). *The future of nursing: Leading change, advancing health.* Washington, DC: National Academies Press.

Kaldjian, L. C., Curtis, A. E., Shinkunas, L. A., & Cannon, K. T. (2009). *American Journal of Hospice and Palliative Medicine, 25*(6), 501–511.

Kleinman, A., Eisenberg, L., & Good, B. (1978). Culture, illness and care. *Annals of Internal Medicine, 88*, 251–258.

Koloroutis, M., & Trout, M. (2012). *See me as a person: Creating therapeutic relationships with patients and their families.* Minneapolis, MN: Creative Health Care Management.

Kukla, R. (2007). How do patients know? *Hastings Center Report, 37*(5), 27–35.

Radtke, K. (2013). Improving patient satisfaction with nursing communication using bedside shift report. *Clinical Nurse Specialist, 27*(1), 19–25.

Schenck, D., & Churchill, L. (2012). *Healers: Extraordinary clinicians at work.* New York, NY: Oxford University Press.

Sofaer, S., & Schumann, M. J. (2013). *Fostering successful patient and family engagement: Nursing Critical Role.* Washington, DC: Nursing Alliance for Quality Care.

Staggers, N., & Blax, J. W. (2012). Research on nursing handoffs for medical and surgical settings: An integrative review. *Journal of Advanced Nursing, 69*(2), 247–262.

The Joint Commission. (2010). *Advancing effective communication, cultural competence, and patient- and family-centered care: A roadmap for hospitals.* Oakbrook Terrace, IL. Retrieved from http://www .jointcommission.org/assets/1/6/ARoadmapforHospitalsfinalversion727.pdf

Truog, R. D., Brown, S. D., Browning, D., Hundert, E. M., Rider, E. A., Bell, S. K. & Meyer, E. C. (2015, January–February 11–16). Microethics: The ethics of everyday clinical practice. *Hastings Center Report, 45*(1), 11–17.

Walton, M. K. (2011). Supporting family caregivers: Communicating with family caregivers. *American Journal of Nursing, 111*(12), 47–53.

Wolf, J. A., Niederhauser, V., Marshburn, D., & LaVela, S. L. (2014). Defining patient experience. *Patient Experience Journal, 1*(1), Article 3. Retrieved from http://pxjournal.org/journal/vol1/ iss1/3

7

Applying Ethics in Research and Evidence-Informed Practices

CATHERINE ROBICHAUX

LEARNING OBJECTIVES AND OUTCOMES

Upon completion of this chapter, the reader will be able to:

- Describe the nurse's role in promoting ethical research and evidence-informed practice
- Discuss the historical events that resulted in development of ethical research guidelines
- Use criteria to determine the ethical nature of research studies
- Explain how to promote ethical nursing practices based on research evidence

Nurses are advocates for patients involved in research studies and their role in ensuring adequate informed consent for participation is well documented (Judkins-Cohn, Kielwasser-Withrow, Owen, & Ward, 2014). This role has expanded dramatically, however, with recommendations from the Institute of Medicine (IOM; 2011) and the American Nurses Credentialing Center (ANCC, 2014) Magnet® program requirements, among other regulatory and accrediting bodies. As seen in Box 7.1, Provision 7 of the Code of Ethics also states, "The nurse, in *all* roles and settings advances the profession through research and scholarly inquiry . . ." (2015).

As nurses' participation in research has increased, so has the number of alternatives sites in which research is conducted such as special clinics and private offices. Nurses may be involved in offering research information, recruiting and monitoring participants, obtaining/maintaining data, and writing and/or presenting results. They may be primary or coinvestigators or be

Box 7.1

Ethics in Research and Evidence-Informed Practice—Provision 7 and Relevant Statements From the Code of Ethics (2015)

PROVISION 7

The nurse, in all roles and settings, advances the profession through research and scholarly inquiry, professional standards development, and the generation of both nursing and health policy.

FROM INTERPRETIVE STATEMENT 7.1

Whether the nurse is data collector, investigator, member of an institutional review board, or care provider, patients' rights and autonomy must be honored and respected.

Patients'/participants' welfare must never be sacrificed for research ends.

Care is taken that research is soundly constructed, significant, and worthwhile.

Dissemination of research findings, regardless of results, is an essential part of respect for the participants.

Research utilization and evidence-informed practice is expected of all nurses.

Source: American Nurses Association (2015).

involved in critiquing research, quality improvement studies, and clinical practice guidelines. Nurses are also required to provide safe, effective nursing interventions using current research findings and evidence-based outcomes. In all these roles and settings, nurses are responsible for understanding the principles and issues underlying the ethical conduct of research and evaluate the ethical components of research studies and evidence-based practice recommendations/guidelines (Barrett, 2010; Grady & Edgerly, 2009). The purpose of this chapter is to provide you as a practicing nurse with a clear understanding of your role responsibilities in research and related issues.

You will see the terms "evidence-based" and "evidence-informed" practice used in this chapter and in others. The former is the more frequently used term, originally defined as the "conscientious, explicit use of current best evidence in making decisions about the care of individual patients" (Sackett et al., 1996, p. 71). Although this definition has been expanded, evidence-informed practice, as described in the Code of Ethics (2015, p. 43) and by Fowler (2015), reflects a more comprehensive understanding:

> Evidence-informed practice, then, utilizes a diversity of forms of knowledge including clinical expertise; ethical understanding;

patient and family values, beliefs, and preferences; theories, health-care resources and practice environments; and even nurse practice or DHHS regulations. While it includes evidence-based practice, *evidence-informed practice* is a more encompassing term. (Fowler, 2015, p. 124)

Fowler (2015) also notes that this interpretation and application influences not only direct patient care but ultimately affects health systems worldwide. In so doing, evidence-informed practice works to reduce inequalities in care and is a matter of justice. The difference in understanding between these two terms is discussed further in the section Ethics and Evidence-Informed Practice. Additional interpretive statements relevant to ethics in research and evidence-informed practice are included in Box 7.1.

Question to Consider Before Reading On

1. Have you participated in a research study? What was your role? Discuss your experience with a class peer or colleague.

CASE SCENARIO

Jeanie, who has worked in a large medical surgical unit in an academic medical center for 5 years, recently transferred to the oncology unit after receiving her BSN. Several patients on this unit are participants in various clinical trials. Sarah, a 55-year-old woman with stage IV breast cancer, who has not responded to therapy, has been asked to participate in a study. She has been offered participation in an institutional review board (IRB)–approved phase one clinical trial to evaluate the safety of a new biological agent. Although new to the unit, Jeanie knows that phase one trials are conducted to evaluate the safety of investigational agents in terms of dosage and side effects. While participants in such trials may benefit from the intervention, that is not the primary goal of the research and many patients may receive minimal to no benefit. After reading the informed consent required for participation in the study, Sarah tells Jeanie, "I know this says that the treatment may not help me but I really think it will." Jeanie is concerned that Sarah does not seem to fully understand the clinical trial informed consent and believes that the intervention will help her although it may have no benefit. In addition, Sarah does not seem to be aware of possible alternatives to participation, however limited.

Question to Consider Before Reading On

1. How would you respond to Sarah's initial misunderstanding of the clinical trial intervention?

BRIEF HISTORY OF ETHICAL GUIDELINES

The Code of Ethics for Nurses (American Nurses Association [ANA], 2015) and other guidelines are vital to our understanding of ethical research and evidence-informed practice. This understanding encompasses more than one document or a set of regulations and depends on the attention, knowledge, integrity, and courage of the professionals involved.

Nursing regulatory boards such as ANA and those in other countries such as Australia and Great Britain (Australian Nursing Federation [ANF], 2009; Haigh & Williamson, 2009; Royal College of Nursing [RCN], 2009) have provided direction for nurses in various roles on the ethical conduct of research and measures required to protect those participating in the process. These directions and mandates have resulted from ethical breaches committed during human experimentation in the past.

After World War II, the Nuremberg trials were conducted to prosecute Nazi leaders and physicians for crimes against humanity including subjecting prisoners to appalling procedures done in the name of clinical research. At this time, there were no regulations, codes, or formal documents that contained standards for ethical research on human subjects so the trials resulted in development of the Nuremberg Code (1949). The three essential elements of the Nuremberg Code are voluntary and informed consent, a favorable risk–benefit ratio, and the right to withdraw from a study without repercussion. These elements form the basis of subsequent ethics codes and international research regulations including the Declaration of Helsinki (World Medical Association, 1964), which states that the interests of the subject should supersede those of society and every subject should receive the best-known treatment available (Layman, 2009; Rice, 2008).

Although the United States was involved in the creation of the Nuremberg Code, federal regulations regarding research and IRB approval were not developed until 1974 with the National Research Act followed by guidelines based on principles outlined in the Belmont Report (The National Commission for the Protection of Subjects of Biomedical and Behavioral Research, 1978). The Belmont Report serves as the basis for regulations affecting research sponsored by the U.S. government including studies supported by the National Institute for Nursing Research (NINR). This report identifies three major principles in evaluating research: respect for persons, beneficence, and justice. These principles maintain that an individual must understand what he or she is being asked to do, make a reasoned judgment about the effect(s) of his or her participation, and make a choice free of coercive influence. In addition, individuals incapable of making their own informed choices should be protected. The investigator is obligated to ensure that the research is based on a sound design and has undergone review, and that the obligation to maximize benefits and minimize risks is heeded (Horner & Minifie, 2011a; Layman, 2009; Polit & Beck, 2014).

The Belmont Report also delineates the difference between research and treatment, emphasizes the assessment of risks and benefits, and reiterates the importance of informed consent. In addition, several populations are identified as "vulnerable" or requiring additional protection including children, pregnant women and fetuses, neonates, prisoners, and the institutionalized mentally disabled. Following development of the Belmont Report, the Department of Health and Human Services (DHHS) issued the Federal Policy for the Protection of Human Subjects or the "Common Rule" in 1991 to provide a uniform approach to human research in the United States. This document has been revised and amended several times with the latest revision occurring in 2009 (DHHS). While these regulations and guidelines may seem excessive, several egregious, unethical research studies that occurred in the United States before, during, and even after their development indicate the ongoing need for awareness and monitoring of research practices. Table 7.1 describes

Table 7.1

Examples of Unethical Research in the United States

STUDY AND YEAR(S) CONDUCTED	PARTICIPANTS AND PURPOSE	ETHICS BREACHES
Tuskegee, Alabama Syphilis Study 1932–1973 Study was funded by the U.S. Public Health Service (USPHS)	Men with syphilis from a poor African American community. To investigate the natural history of untreated syphilis in humans. When penicillin treatment became available, it was withheld from participants.	Participants who consented had no meaningful understanding of the research or their condition and many believed they were receiving medical care. Study risks outweighed potential benefits and withholding of treatment violates protection from harm.
Jewish Chronic Disease Hospital Study 1963 Brooklyn, NY Study was funded by the USPHS and the American Cancer Society	Chronically ill, senile, elderly, hospitalized patients with compromised immune systems. Patients received bloodstream injections of live liver cancer cells to determine the influence of weakened immunity on the spread of cancer.	Vulnerable patients who could not give informed consent. Subjects received no benefit and investigators had no proof that they would not develop cancer.

(continued)

Table 7.1

Examples of Unethical Research in the United States *(continued)*

STUDY AND YEAR(S) CONDUCTED	PARTICIPANTS AND PURPOSE	ETHICS BREACHES
Willowbrook State School Hepatitis Study 1955–1970 Staten Island, NY	Mentally and physically disabled children were infected with viral hepatitis by feeding them an extract from the feces of other infected residents. The purpose was to discover a vaccine for viral hepatitis.	Parents were coerced to sign consent forms so their children would be admitted to a "newer" part of the facility. Parents and children were not informed of the risks.
San Antonio Contraceptive Study 1969	Indigent Mexican American women seeking contraceptives. One randomized half received oral contraceptives and the others a placebo. The purpose was to determine the side effects of contraceptives.	Participants were not informed that they might receive the placebo and many became pregnant.
UCLA Schizophrenia Medication Study 1983–1994	Patients with schizophrenia had their treatment medication withheld. The purpose was to determine if some patients might improve without such medication that had untoward side effects.	Participants signed consent forms but were not informed of potential acute relapse or possible worsening of symptoms.

Sources: Hardicre (2014); Horner and Minifie (2011a); Polit and Beck (2014); Wilson and Stanley (2006).

the purpose of these studies and the ethical breaches that occurred (Hardicre, 2014; Horner & Minifie, 2011a; Polit & Beck, 2014; Wilson & Stanley, 2006).

Question to Consider Before Reading On

1. What elements of the Nuremberg Code are included in the informed consent used in your workplace?

COMPONENTS OF ETHICAL RESEARCH

Ethical conduct of research includes, but is not limited to, the three basic ethical principles outlined in the Belmont Report. These principles were integrated and expanded upon by Emanuel et al. (2000, 2011) in their framework for evaluating the ethics of research studies and adapted for critical care nursing research by Richmond and Ulrich (2013). This framework extends from study development through dissemination of findings and addresses aspects of care and virtue ethics. Framework components include assessment of social value, scientific validity, fair subject selection, favorable risk–benefit ratio, independent review, informed consent, respect for potential and enrolled subjects, and research integrity. While nurses may not be called upon to evaluate all components of the framework, an understanding is necessary as identified in the ANA Code of Ethics (2015) interpretive statements and Quality and Safety Education for Nurses (QSEN; Cronenwett et al., 2007) competencies (Boxes 7.1 and 7.2).

Question to Consider Before Reading On

1. Choose two of the QSEN competencies from Box 7.2. How are they demonstrated in your current practice?

Social Value

A study that has social value must help the researcher determine how to improve people's health and/or well-being. This can be accomplished directly through findings that may lead to better tests or treatments for disease, such as in the Case Scenario, or by obtaining data that increases understanding or leads to future research. As noted, "If the research doesn't help in . . . these ways, it wastes money and resources" (Emanuel, Abdoler, & Grady, 2011, p. 4). Clinical trials are certainly not the only type of research and nurses may be engaged in additional studies that evolve from clinical experience, the literature, or priority areas such as those identified by specialty groups. The assessment of social value or significance remains the same for all research studies. Conducting a needlessly redundant investigation or one based on a trivial

Box 7.2

Ethics in Research and Evidence-Informed Practice: Relevant QSEN Competencies

Describe EBP to include the components of research evidence, clinical expertise, and patient/family values. (Knowledge)

Adhere to institutional review board (IRB) guidelines. (Skills)

Value the need for ethical conduct of research and quality improvement. (Attitudes)

Analyze ethical issues associated with continuous quality improvement. (Knowledge)

Value ethical conduct in quality improvement efforts. Value the roles of others, such as IRBs, in assessing ethical and patient rights/informed decision making. (Attitudes)

Maintain confidentiality of any patient information used in quality improvement efforts. (Skills)

Value working in an interactive manner with the institutional review board. (Attitudes)

Actively engage with the institutional review board to implement research strategies and protect human subjects. (Skills)

Source: QSEN Institute (2014).

research question does not meet the criterion of social value. It is also unethical to put potential participants at risk of harm or discomfort when no benefit may be realized (Gennaro, 2014). *In the Case Scenario, Jeanie realizes that the biological agent has potential social value for future breast cancer patients. However, she questions Sarah's understanding of the value of the intervention in her own treatment, potential risks, and side effects.*

Scientific Validity

To be scientifically valid and ethical, a research study should be conducted in a methodologically rigorous manner and be expected to have useful results and add to the body of scientific knowledge. Whether a clinical trial or other quantitative or qualitative study, it must be designed using accepted principles and methods, be feasible, and have an appropriate data analysis plan. Nurses may be involved in ensuring the scientific validity of a study as primary investigators or coinvestigators or as members of an IRB. As care providers, nurses contribute to the scientific validity of a study through evaluation of adherence with the protocol or requirements and monitoring participants for adverse events. They also assess the impact of participation on the patient's/subject's disease process and overall well-being (Grady & Edgerly, 2009; Richmond & Ulrich, 2013). *For example, in the Case Scenario, Jeanie is concerned about the potential effects of the biological agent on Sarah's quality of life.*

Fair Subject Selection

Nurses may be involved in recruiting and enrolling patients in a research study. Fair subject selection means that the scientific goals of the study, not convenience, vulnerability, or other factors form the basis for recruiting individuals or groups to participate. As seen in Table 7.1, in the past certain individuals became research subjects because they were easily accessible or compromised in their ability to understand and/or protect themselves. *This is also a consideration in the chapter Case Scenario as Jeanie is assessing Sarah's understanding of participating in the clinical trial and whether she may be vulnerable given her present condition.*

Question to Consider Before Reading On

1. Patients like Sarah, who are asked to be research participants, are often considered "vulnerable" because of their advanced illness. What additional safeguards can the nurse implement when recruiting such patients for research studies?

Since it is important that research results be useful to the population for whom the intervention is intended, certain groups or individuals should not be excluded without good reason. This requirement comes from past instances when women and children were excluded from research studies. If a potential intervention is likely to be used for women and/or children, then these groups should be included. The IRB review process requires investigators to identify inclusion/exclusion criteria and justify why certain individuals or groups may be excluded.

Favorable Risk–Benefit Ratio

To be ethical, the risks in participating in a research study must be balanced by benefits to the subjects and/or the importance of new knowledge to be gained. This comparison is called the *risk–benefit ratio.* "The riskier the research study, the more benefit it must offer to be considered ethical" (Emanuel et al., 2011, p. 5). *For example, in the Case Scenario, the potential risks of participating may be quite high for Sarah and could include accelerating disease progression and mortality. Therefore, the overall benefit of determining the safety and efficacy of the new investigational agent for treatment of breast cancer must be considered highly important to meet this ethical requirement.*

All research involves some degree of risk but in many studies, the risk is considered minimal or expected to be no more than is encountered in daily life or during routine physical care, procedures, or tests. When risks are more than minimal, they are considered burdensome and the researcher must ensure that steps are taken to reduce their occurrence. Potential risks for participants may be fatigue, emotional distress, loss of privacy, and loss of time, among others. Such risks must be weighed against possible benefits including satisfaction from participation, direct benefit from the intervention, or gains from incentives or stipends provided. Aspects of the risk–benefit ratio are addressed in IRB review process and throughout the course of the study. As a caregiver, the nurse is often in the best position to assess daily risks and possible burdens for the patient/participant and communicate these to the investigator and/or research team (Grady & Edgerly, 2009). *In the chapter Case Scenario, although Jeanie is new to the oncology unit, she has extensive experience in assessing the effects of various interventions and treatments on patients' physical condition and well-being. Her professional relationship with Sarah contributes to Jeanie's ability to determine Sarah's complete understanding of the proposed clinical trial.*

Independent Review

Designing a research study is extremely time consuming. Although investigators believe strongly in their work, they may experience various conflicts or distractions that result in overlooking ways to ensure adherence to ethical principles and other research requirements. Independent review by individuals not associated with the proposed research study helps ensure that the investigation is consistent with these requirements. Most hospitals, universities, and other institutions where research is conducted have established formal review committees called "human subjects committees" or IRBs. The United States requires that any research that receives federal funding must be approved by an IRB as do other granting organizations and editorial review boards that review manuscripts for professional scholarly journals (Barrett, 2010; Richmond & Ulrich, 2013).

The National Research Act of 1974 requires that the IRB must have at least five members who reflect professional, gender, racial, and cultural diversity. At least one member must have a nonscientific background and one must be unaffiliated with the institution. Primary responsibilities of the IRB are outlined in Box 7.3. Based on assessment of subject risk level, the IRB determines if the research proposal is exempt (minimal risk), is expedited (no greater than minimal risk), or requires full board review (Richmond & Ulrich, 2013; Sims, 2008). *In general, clinical trials such as presented in the Case Scenario require full board IRB approval (DHHS).*

Box 7.3

Responsibilities of Institutional Review Boards

1. Determine if the research is reasonable.

2. Ensure that risks are minimized and reasonable in relation to anticipated benefits.

3. Determine if subject selection is equitable.

4. Review informed consent procedures.

5. Monitor data collected to ensure subject safety and privacy.

6. Ensure that safeguards are in place for vulnerable participants.

Source: U.S. Food and Drug Administration (2016).

Question to Consider Before Reading On

1. Do you have a mechanism for independent review of research in your current practice setting? Compare its responsibilities with those in Box 7.3.

Informed Consent

Informed consent is the foundation of ethical research. Nurses participate in the process to ensure informed consent at many levels. The purpose of informed consent is to ensure that individuals control whether or not to participate in a research study and that they participate only "when the research is consistent with their values, interests, and preferences" (Emanuel, Wendler, & Grady, 2000, p. 2706). This process promotes the principle of respect for persons, their autonomous choices, and is a requirement of justice, understood in terms of participant empowerment. Informed consent also reflects the virtue of fidelity and care in the professional–patient/participant relationship (Messer, 2004).

Conditions of informed consent include competence, adequate information, and voluntariness. Competence can be both a medical and legal issue but essentially refers to the ability to perform a task, and in the research context, to make decisions about one's own health care and participation in the study. Competence is the ability to understand the proposed action or intervention, reason about it, and choose to express that choice. To make an informed choice, the participant must have adequate information about the proposed intervention, probable consequences and possible alternatives, and their consequences. More information is not necessarily better and a limited amount of accurate and relevant information may be considered sufficient. The decision to participate must also be voluntary and not the result of pressures such as undue inducement or coercion (Emanuel et al., 2011; Judkins-Cohn et al., 2014). *In the chapter Case Scenario, although Sarah may be competent, Jeanie questions whether she has adequate information to make an informed decision that is consistent with her values and preferences.*

In clinical trials and other types of research, the potential participant should be evaluated for therapeutic misconception or misestimation. The former refers to the erroneous belief that the research intervention is based on the individual participant's needs and is designed to benefit him or her personally. Therapeutic misestimation occurs when the participant does not fully understand the estimated risks or benefits or believes that a greater chance of personal benefit exists while failing to understand possible risks. To prevent therapeutic misconception and misestimation, the nurse may ask potential participants to repeat consent information using their own words in order to identify need for clarifications and further education (Scott, 2013).

Several elements of an informed consent document include explanation of the purpose of the research, expected duration, and a description of the procedures and foreseeable risks or discomforts, among other components. Additional information included in the consent may address termination of the subject's participation by the researcher and the sharing of findings with the subject. See the Code of Federal Regulations, Title 21, Part 50 (2CFR50.35), for a complete description of the elements of informed consent.

Question to Consider Before Reading On

1. In the Case Scenario, what are some questions Jeanie could ask Sarah to further assess her understanding of the clinical trial informed consent?

Variations to the signed informed consent process do occur. In studies employing a self-administered questionnaire, *implied consent* is assumed when the participant returns the completed questionnaire. Certain qualitative studies require repeated contact with subjects and continued participation may be renegotiated throughout the investigation (*process consent*). The rights of vulnerable subjects including children, pregnant women, and those who are mentally or physically disabled or severely ill must be protected through additional procedures. In research, *vulnerability* refers to the inability to provide informed consent because of incapacity, educational or emotional burdens. Participant safeguards may include obtaining *assent* to participate from children who are least 7 years of age or the use of surrogate or proxy decision makers for critically ill patients. Surrogates are generally asked to use the *substituted judgment standard* or consider what the patient would have wanted based on previously expressed wishes or other factors such as prognosis or religious/moral beliefs. In certain circumstances, such as emergency care research, a waiver of consent may be justified by the IRB if it meets specific criteria (Grove, Burns, & Gray, 2013; Polit & Beck, 2014). These criteria and additional information about IRBs and the informed consent process are available on the U.S. Department of Health and Human Services, Office of Human Research Protections website (2016a; 2016b).

CASE SCENARIO (*CONTINUED*)

Returning to the Case Scenario, Jeanie considers the ethical framework (see Chapter 2) for decision making and determines that Sarah's autonomy may be compromised. Jeanie also thinks that Sarah's ability to fully understand the consequences of participation may have been affected by recently administered pain medication. Although initially hesitant to speak up, Jeanie reflects on the virtue and caring components of the ethical framework and decides to call the primary investigator (PI).

In speaking with the PI about her concerns, he agrees with Jeanie that Sarah may not fully understand the difference between research and treatment or "therapeutic misconception." The primary purpose of the research trial is to evaluate the safety and efficacy of the intervention, not to provide specific treatment for Sarah's cancer. It is very difficult for patients/participants to understand this distinction, as they may inherently trust that the provider would not offer the treatment if he or she thought it would not provide benefit.

Following a multidisciplinary patient care conference, the PI, oncologist, and Jeanie speak with Sarah and her family. They clarify the intent of the research and discuss possible care alternatives, including hospice. After meeting with a member of the hospice care team, Sarah and her family decide that this is the best choice.

Respect for Potential and Enrolled Subjects

Respect for subjects is inherent in acknowledging their autonomy in the research process and extends from initial approach, throughout the project, and after the investigation ends. In addition to autonomy, patients/participants have identified respect to include empathy, care, and dignity, among other elements (Dickert & Kass, 2009). *For seriously ill or vulnerable patients like Sarah, this may require recognizing their right to choose whether to be approached by a research member or team. Nurses often have an integral role in this initial process, as they may be most knowledgeable about the patient's daily physical, mental, and emotional status. As a patient advocate, a nurse may express legitimate concern about the burden on the patient and question his or her ability to provide informed consent.*

Respect is also given to those individuals who choose not to participate in a study (Entwistle, Cater, Cribb, & McCaffery, 2010). Should an individual decide to participate in research, Emanuel et al. (2000) note that respect involves at least five activities: maintaining privacy and confidentiality, respecting a decision to withdraw from the study, sharing significant new information, monitoring the participant's status, and informing the participant of overall study findings. While privacy is about people, confidentiality is about data and maintaining both helps protect individuals from potential harm (beneficence). Private health information in medical records is protected both legally and ethically. Participants have the right to expect that any data they provide will be kept in strictest confidence. This includes assurance of privacy during interviews and ensuring or minimizing the collection of identifiable information, among other measures.

An individual's right to withdraw at any time during the course of the study is included in the informed consent document. This right encompasses freedom from coercion or threat to the care they would otherwise receive. Participants may not be able to evaluate the potential burdens or inconveniences of participation until they are enrolled in the study (Schafer & Wertheimer, 2010, 2011). In caring for and monitoring the patient/participant, the nurse may be the first to identify these unforeseen consequences. Any significant new information obtained during the study, whether of benefit or risk to the participant, should be shared with him or her in addition to knowledge regarding new available interventions.

Offering the results of completed research studies to participants recognizes their dignity and contribution to the investigation. Whether in summary or individual format, most participants indicate that they place a high value on the offer of results. The components of a process to return results may vary based on specific needs and context. This ethical obligation is reflected in several national and international regulatory requirements and is recognized by IRBs (Fernandez et al., 2012; Ferris & Sass-Kortsak, 2011).

In the chapter Case Scenario, had she agreed to participate in the clinical trial, the PI would be primarily responsible for ensuring that Sarah is afforded the five components of respect outlined by Emanuel et al. (2000). Nurses, however, may be in the best position to safeguard these aspects of patient care and dignity.

Research Integrity

As noted, nurses participate in research at many levels and in different roles. To meet IOM recommendations and Magnet requirements, nursing research is no longer limited to academic settings but is conducted in clinical areas by bedside nurse scientists. The pace of this overall growth may exceed understanding of the ethical components of research, presented in the section Components of Ethical Research. The clinical environment may also lack the support required to ensure research integrity, thus contributing to the possibility of research misconduct. *Research integrity* is defined as "active adherence to the ethical principles and professional standards essential for the responsible practice of research." In contrast, *research misconduct* means "fabrication, falsification, or plagiarism in proposing, performing, or reviewing research, or in reporting research results" (Korenman, 2006).

Fabrication involves making up data and reporting it while *falsification* is changing or omitting data or manipulating results such that the research is not accurately reported. For example, in the Case Scenario, falsification would occur if Sarah enrolled in the study and she and other participants experienced adverse events that were omitted from the final research report or publication. *Plagiarism* is, unfortunately, a well-known form of misconduct and involves using someone's (or one's own) words, ideas, or results without giving credit or citing (Fierz et al., 2014).

While these three forms of misconduct are considered the most egregious, others include, but are not limited to, bad data practices such as intentional protocol violations, failure to disclose conflicts of interest, and issues related to authorship and publication. Not reporting facts, including funding sources and other conflicts of interest that could affect the interpretation of published articles, is unethical. Repeated publication, use of ghostwriters, and the conferment of unmerited authorship are additional forms of research misconduct. In addition to the Office of Research Integrity (ORI), there are several useful websites and resources that provide guidance on these issues including the Committee on Publication Ethics, the International Committee of Medical Journal Editors (ICMJE), and the International Academy of Nurse Editors (INANE; Fierz et al., 2014; Horner & Minifie, 2011b).

The effects of scientific misconduct can impact patients, researchers, the institution, and the larger community. Patients may be harmed if providers rely on fabricated or falsified data and public trust in science may be damaged. Individual careers and the reputation of the research institution may also be discredited. It has been estimated that the cost of investigating incidents of scientific misconduct reported to the ORI exceeds $100 million each year (Horner & Minifie, 2011b).

Participation in and use of research is considered an essential component of professional nursing practice as stated in the Code of Ethics (2015) and other documents. An environment that supports research integrity is vital. Despite these mandates, most nurses in clinical practice may not have received information about their role in the research process or scientific integrity in their educational programs. Strategies to promote research integrity in the clinical setting identified by nurses overseeing the process at Magnet hospitals include basic and continuing education about the responsible conduct of research, nursing research councils, and the use of research mentors. The role of the mentor in providing ongoing support and guidance was deemed particularly important to cultivating research confidence and accountability. Mentoring differs from formal instruction as the mentor demonstrates how to be a competent, professional, and ethical researcher. This process is reflective of a virtue approach to research integrity as it focuses on the character traits of the ethical researcher (Barrett, 2010; Resnik, 2012).

Question to Consider Before Reading On

1. As part of a Magnet project in your unit, the primary investigator, an RN academic faculty member, asks that you identify potential research participants for a study exploring family caregiver stress. How would you evaluate the ethical components of this study?

ETHICS AND EVIDENCE-INFORMED PRACTICE

The systematic collation, synthesis, and application of high-quality evidence have improved the quality and safety of health care delivery. The EBP movement is not without critics, however, in nursing and other disciplines. These authors/providers suggest that the overwhelming emphasis on use of evidence to guide practice may devalue other knowledge, decrease patient safety, and damage the ethical foundation of the patient–provider relationship (Cody, 2013; Greenhalgh, Howick, & Maskrey, 2014; Upshur, 2013). When the nurse begins to practice, he or she may rely solely on guidelines, protocols, and evidence. With increasing experience, the nurse may internalize or refer to these strategies but develops a more nuanced, holistic practice that integrates additional forms of knowing such as aesthetics and ethics. Clinical expertise may evolve from mastery of these skills leading to an intuitive ability to efficiently make complex patient care decisions while grasping the entire nature of a situation. While some nurses become experts, others remain at the competent level and continue to capably apply rules and protocols to patient care. However, they may miss the subtle patient differences that represent exceptions to these protocols or lack the skills to practice in situations for which there are no guides or sufficient evidence. As a result, patient safety may be compromised, if it is dependent on the nurse's expert anticipation of potential problems and consequences. Indeed, in a clinical environment focused solely on efficiency and empirical evidence, an inexperienced clinician may engage mechanically and defensively. This reductionist approach may impede development of critical thinking and delivery of quality, patient/family-centered care (McHugh & Lake, 2010; Walker, 2015). *In the chapter Case Scenario, for example, a competent nurse may have overlooked Sarah's therapeutic misconception regarding the clinical trial in an endeavor to obtain her timely consent in accordance with the study protocol.*

Mitchell (2013) observes that, over the last decade, many nurses have been "indoctrinated with the mantra that research evidence is knowledge and individual nurses require evidence to be competent professionals." The EBP movement is so dominant in nursing and health care that we may not consider it with the same critical appraisal recommended for evaluating the ethical components of research. Critics of EBP question whether the findings from average results in clinical studies can inform decisions about real patients who may not resemble the textbook description of disease and differ from participants in clinical trials. They note that the evidence from large trials may be statistically but not clinically significant and often overestimates benefits while underestimating risks (social and scientific value and risk–benefit analysis; Greenhalgh et al., 2014; Miles & Loughlin, 2011).

Mitchell (2013) and Porter, O'Halloran, and Morrow (2013) question whether evidence actually exists to guide all nursing practice. Mitchell observes that evidence about clinical issues such as the effects of prolonged immobility in the ICU or prevention of infection is available. However, other questions relevant to nursing practice are often not addressed in systematic reviews or the results reported are deemed inconclusive. An example is cancer-related fatigue, the most common problem in patients with cancer. The only evidence-based nursing intervention recommended among the dozens listed for this pervasive symptom is exercise (Oncology Nursing Society, 2014).

The amount of relevant evidence available may also be unmanageable. One study of 18 patients with 44 diagnoses identified 3,679 pages of national guidelines relevant to their immediate care (Greenhalgh et al., 2014). In addition, there are important issues that cannot be studied completely by quantitative methods; ethical decision making is one of those areas. Rigid compliance with best evidence and guidelines can become an end in itself and may diminish patient-centered care and provider integrity (Benner, Hughes, & Sutphen, 2008; Miles & Mezzich, 2011).

Question to Consider Before Reading On

1. Do you have questions/issues in your current practice for which the evidence to support your nursing practice is unavailable, inconclusive, or not relevant?

Ethical, Evidence-*Informed* Practice

Ethical, evidence-*informed* practice builds on a strong relationship between the nurse and the patient/client/family. It acknowledges that there are factors other than empirical, quantifiable, evidence that influence clinical and ethical decision making in patient/family-centered care (Miles & Loughlin, 2011; Walton, 2017). Individualized, evidence-informed practice asks, What is the best course of action for *this* patient, in *this* circumstance, at *this* point? Being autonomous, the patient is free to make appropriate decisions that may not match current best evidence. This approach acknowledges the values and expertise of clinicians and the values and preferences of patients/clients who may be in a better position to guide respectful and ethical nursing practice (Benner, Sutphen, Leonard-Kahn, & Day, 2008; Greenhalgh et al., 2014). Walton provides an excellent Case Scenario example of this ethical, patient/family-centered approach in Chapter 6.

Cody (2013) acknowledges the important distinction between evidence-informed clinical care and values-based, ethical nursing practice. Ghinea and colleagues (2014) note that the use of evidence is itself a matter of values, stating, "What the evidence tells us to do tends to depend on what we see as important" (p. 38). The nurse chooses how to practice based on personal/professional values and provides care to address the patient's/client's needs that is informed by the best evidence available combined with other forms of knowledge such as personal, ethics, and aesthetics. While evidence may be important to a practice decision or intervention, it does not determine that decision or intervention. Nurses provide evidence-informed interventions, but they are also educated to make ethical judgments, provide care and comfort, and bear witness to suffering (Greenhalgh et al., 2014; O'Halloran, Porter, & Blackwood, 2010).

Case Scenario *(CONTINUED)*

Jeanie visits Sarah in the in-patient hospice unit and observes her interacting with the therapy dog, Ruby, a large golden retriever. Sarah is smiling and appears to be in less pain as she pats Ruby on the head. Jeanie speaks with one of the hospice nurses, who tells her that complementary alternative therapies (CAM) such as animal-assisted therapy and acupuncture seem to be providing symptom relief for Sarah and other hospice patients experiencing chronic pain from metastases. While definitive effectiveness of these therapies has not been established, offering and using such alternatives also enable Sarah to remain alert and interact with her family and friends.

Greenhalgh et al. (2014) suggest that ethical, evidence-informed health care may be characterized by:

- Making ethical care of the patient the top priority

- Demanding individualized evidence in a format that clinicians and patients can understand

- Using expert judgment rather than mechanical following of rules

- Sharing decisions with patients through meaningful conversations

Greenhalgh et al. (2014) state that these principles can also be applied at the community level for evidence-informed public health. This approach refuses to let process such as tests and procedures dominate the agreed-upon health care goal or outcome. It involves finding out what matters to the patient and family and incorporating evidence in a way that informs a conversation about what best to do, how, and why. Evidence-informed, individualized nursing care is not bound by rules but integrates clinical expertise, personal knowledge, ethics, and judiciously selected research evidence. Box 7.4 provides an example of this approach to ethical, individualized nursing care.

Box 7.4

Evidence, Ethics, and Individualized Care

As a recent BSN graduate, Samantha (Sam) is eager to begin her new position in the neurology unit in a large, academic medical center in the Midwest. Following orientation, Sam is assigned to care for Paul, a 32-year-old retired Marine. Paul completed two tours in Afghanistan and was medically retired after suffering a severe traumatic brain injury from an improvised explosive device (IED). Paul has been readmitted several times for treatment of debilitating migraines, persistent nausea, and seizures that have responded poorly to conventional medications. Paul tells Sam that he has been unable to work for several months because of his condition. He confides that he has been experiencing depression since he is unable to engage in the physical activities he used to enjoy with his two young sons.

After discussing the treatment plan with Paul, Dr. S, his neurologist, proposes use of medical marijuana which is legal in their state of California. Although initially reluctant, Paul agrees to try this option as it may enable him to participate in the everyday functions that he values. When he mentions Dr. S's suggestion of medical marijuana to Sam, she states, "But there is no real evidence that it works and you might get addicted!" Heather, who has been working on the unit for 2 years and has cared for Paul on previous admissions, overhears Sam's comment and approaches her in the break room. Heather reminds Sam of her role as a caring, patient advocate. She states that Paul and Dr. S. had a long, detailed conversation about the goals of treatment and what Paul valued in his life. Heather acknowledges that controversy surrounds beliefs, policies, and the efficacy of medical marijuana. While continued research is needed, several professional health care organizations including the American College of Physicians (ACP, 2008) and the ANA (2008), also support provider education and supervised access to use for identified patients. Sam agrees with Heather and shares that she might have a personal bias against the use of medical marijuana because of a relative with an addiction problem. Heather and Sam decide to speak with Dr. S regarding collaboration on presentation of an in-service on medical marijuana.

Sources: American College of Physicians (2008); American Nurses Association (2008).

CONCLUSION

This chapter provided an overview of the expanding role of the professional nurse in applying and evaluating the ethical components of research studies and evidence-based recommendations. The historical development of ethical guidelines in the context of ethical breaches was presented in addition to a framework for evaluating the ethics of research studies from initial development to dissemination of findings. The distinction between values-based nursing practice and evidence-informed, individualized nursing care was discussed.

Critical Thinking Questions and Activities

1. What have you learned from the chapter Case Scenario?

2. Describe a recent patient/family scenario in which you employed an evidence-based guideline or recommendation with other forms of nursing knowledge such as personal, ethics, and/or aesthetics.

3. Explore and discuss the information available on the IRB or human subjects committee website in your current practice setting or in the following link:

http://research.uthscsa.edu/irb/forms_NewResearch.shtml

4. Read and discuss *Ethical Issues in the Creation of Clinical Practice Guidelines* (Fulda, 2014). How do you see or could you see these guidelines applied in your current workplace setting?

http://www.sccm.org/Communications/Critical-Connections/Archives/Pages/
Ethical-Issues-in-the-Creation-of-Clinical-Practice-Guidelines.aspx

REFERENCES

American College of Physicians. (2008). Supporting research into the therapeutic role of marijuana: A position paper. Philadelphia, PA: Author. Retrieved from https://www.acponline.org/acp_policy/policies/supporting_medmarijuana_2008.pdf

American Nurses Association. (2008). Position statement: In support of patients' safe access to therapeutic marijuana. Silver Spring, MA: Author. Retrieved from http://www.nursingworld.org/MainMenuCategories/Policy-Advocacy/Positions-and-Resolutions/ANAPositionStatements/Position-Statements-Alphabetically/In-Support-of-Patients-Safe-Access-to-Therapeutic-Marijuana.pdf

American Nurses Association. (2015). *Code of ethics for nurses with interpretive statements.* Silver Spring, MA: Nursebooks.

American Nurses Credentialing Center. (2014). *Magnet application manual.* Silver Spring, MD: American Nurses Association.

Australian Nursing Federation. (2009). *Standards for research for the nursing profession.* Melbourne, Victoria, Australia: Australian Nursing Federation Publications Unit.

Barrett, R. (2010). Strategies for promoting the scientific integrity of nursing research in clinical settings. *Journal for Nurses in Staff Development, 26*(5), 200–205.

Benner, P., Hughes, R., & Sutphen, M. (2008). Clinical reasoning, decision-making, and action: Thinking critically and clinically. In R. G. Hughes (Ed.), *Patient safety and quality: An evidence based handbook for nurses* (pp. 1–23). AHRQ Publication No. 08-0043. Rockville, MD: Agency for Healthcare Research and Quality.

Benner, P., Sutphen, M., Leonard-Kahn, V., & Day, L. (2008b). Formation and everyday ethical comportment. *American Journal of Critical Care, 17*(5), 473–476.

Cody, W. (2013). Values-based practice and evidence-based care: Pursuing fundamental questions in nursing philosophy and theory. In W. Cody (Ed.). *Philosophical and Theoretical Perspectives for advanced nursing practice* (pp. 5–13). Burlington, MA: Jones & Bartlett.

Cronenwett, L., Sherwood, G., Barnsteiner, J., Disch, J., Johnson, J., Mitchell, P., . . . Warren, J. (2007). Quality and safety education for nurses. *Nursing Outlook, 55*(3), 122–131.

Dickert, N., & Kass, N. (2009). Understanding respect: Learning from patients. *Journal of Medical Ethics, 35*(7), 419–423.

Emanuel, E., Abdoler, E., & Grady, C. (2011). Research ethics: How to treat people who partici- pate in research. U.S. Department of Health and Human Services, National Institutes of Health Clinical Center. Retrieved from https://www.opt.uh.edu/onlinecoursematerials/PHOP 6275/2015_Materials/PHOP6275_Class3_1_Human_Subjects_NIH_Bioethics.pdf

Emanuel, E., Wendler, D., & Grady, C. (2000). What makes clinical research ethical? *Journal of the American Medical Association, 283*(20), 2701–2711. Retrieved from http://www.dartmouth.edu/ ~cphs/docs/jama-article.pdf

Entwistle, V., Cater, S., Cribb, A., & McCaffery, K. (2010). Supporting patient autonomy: The impor- tance of the clinician-patient relationship. *Journal of General Internal Medicine, 25*(7), 741–745.

Fernandez, C., Ruccione, K., Wells, R., Long, J., Pelletier, W., Hooke, M., . . . Joffee, S. (2012). Recommendations for the return of research results to study participants and guardians: A report from the children's oncology group. *Journal of Clinical Oncology, 30*(38), 4573–4579.

Ferris, L., & Sass-Kortsak, A. (2011). Sharing research findings with research participants and com- munities. *International Journal of Occupational and Environmental Medicine, 2*(3), 172–181.

Fierz, K., Gennaro, S., Dierickz, K., Achterberg, T., Morin, K., & DeGeest, S. (2014). Scientific mis- conduct: Also an issue in nursing science? *Journal of Nursing Scholarship, 46*(4), 271–280.

Fowler, M. (2015). *Guide to the code of ethics with interpretive statements: Development, interpretation, and application* (2nd ed.) Silver Spring, MD: Nursebooks.org.

Fulda, G. (2014). Ethical issues in the creation of clinical practice guidelines. *Society of Critical Care Medicine.* Mount Prospect, IL: Author.

Gennaro, S. (2014). Conducting important and ethical research. *Journal of Nursing Scholarship, 46*(2), 73.

Ghinea, N., Lipworth, W., Kerridge, I., Little, M., & Day, R. (2014). Evidence in medical debates: The case of recombinant activated factor VII. *Hastings Center Report, 44*(2), 38–45.

Grady, C., & Edgerly, M. (2009). Science, technology, and innovation: Nursing responsibilities in clinical research. *Nursing Clinics of North America, 44*(4), 471–481.

Greenhalgh, T., Howick, J., & Maskrey, N. (2014). Evidence-based medicine: A movement in crisis? *British Medical Journal, 348*, g3725. doi:10.1136/bmj.g3725

Grove, S., Burns, N., & Gray, J. (2013). Ethics in research. In S. Groves, N. Burns, & J. Gray (Eds.), *The practice of nursing research: Appraisal, synthesis, and generation of evidence* (pp. 159–190). St. Louis, MO: Elsevier.

Haigh, C., & Williamson, T. (2009). *Research ethics: RCN guidance for nurses.* London, UK: Royal Col- lege of Nursing. Retrieved from http://www.yorksj.ac.uk/pdf/RCN%20Research%20ethics.pdf

Hardicre, J. (2014). An overview of research ethics and learning from the past. *British Journal of Nursing, 23*(9), 483–486.

Horner, J., & Minifie, F. (2011a). Research ethics I: Responsible conduct of research (RCR): Histor- ical and contemporary issues pertaining to human and animal experimentation. *Journal of Speech, Language, and Hearing Research, 54*, S303–S329.

Horner, J., & Minifie, F. (2011b). Research ethics III: Publication practices and authorship, conflicts of interest, and research misconduct. *Journal of Speech, Language, and Hearing Research, 54*(2), S346–S362.

Institute of Medicine. (2011). *The future of nursing: Leading change, advancing health*. Washington, DC: National Academies Press.

Judkins-Cohn, T., Kielwasser-Withrow, K., Owen, M., & Ward, J. (2014). Ethical principles of informed consent: Exploring nurses' dual role of care provider and researcher. *Journal of Continuing Education, 45*(1), 35–42.

Korenman, S. (2006). Teaching the responsible conduct of research in humans (RCRH). Office of Research Integrity, U.S. Department of Health and Human Services, Rockville, MD. Retrieved from http://ori.hhs.gov/education/products/ucla/

Layman, E. (2009). Human experimentation: Historical perspective of breaches of ethics in U.S. health care. *The Health Care Manager, 28*(4), 354–374.

McHugh, M., & Lake, E. (2010). Understanding clinical expertise: Nurse education, experience, and the hospital context. *Research in Nursing and Health, 33*(4), 276–287.

Messer, N. (2004). Professional–patient relationships and informed consent. *Postgraduate Medicine, 80*, 277–283. doi:10.1136/pgmj.2003.012799

Miles, A., & Loughlin, M. (2011). Models in the balance: Evidence-based medicine versus evidence-informed individualized care. *Journal of Evaluation in Clinical Practice, 17*, 531–536.

Miles, A., & Mezzich, J. (2011). The care of the patient and the soul of the clinic: Person-centered medicine as an emergent model of modern clinical practice. *The International Journal of Person Centered Medicine, 1*(2), 207–222.

Mitchell, G. (2013). Implications of holding ideas of evidence-based practice in nursing. *Nursing Science Quarterly, 26*(2), 143–151.

The National Commission for the Protection of Human Subjects of Biomedical and Behavioral Research. (1978). *The Belmont report: Ethical principles and guidelines for the protection of humans subjects of research*. Bethesda, MD: The Commission.

O'Halloran, P., Porter, S., & Blackwood, B. (2010). Evidence-based practice and its critics: What is a nurse manager to do? *Journal of Nursing Management, 18*, 90–95.

Oncology Nursing Society. (2014). Putting evidence into practice (PEP): Fatigue. Retrieved from http://www.ons.org/practice-resources/pep/fatigue

Polit, D., & Beck, C. (2014). Ethics in research. In D. Polit & C. Beck (Eds.), *Essentials of nursing research: Appraising evidence for nursing practice* (pp. 80–99). Philadelphia, PA: Lippincott, Williams, & Wilkins.

Porter, S., O'Halloran, P., & Morrow, E. (2011). Bringing values back into evidence-based nursing: The role of patients in resisting empiricism. *Advances in Nursing Science, 34*(2), 106–118.

QSEN Institute. (2014). Competencies. Retrieved from http://www.qsen.org

Resnik, D. (2012). Ethical virtues in scientific research. *Accountability in Research, 19*(6), 329–343.

Rice, T. (2008). The historical, ethical, and legal background of human subjects research. *Respiratory Care, 53*(10), 1325–1329.

Richmond, T., & Ulrich, C. (2013). Ethical foundations of critical care nursing research. *American Association of Critical Care Nurses*. Retrieved from http://www.aacn.org/wd/practice/docs/research/ethical-foundations-critical-care-nursing-research.pdf

Royal College of Nursing (RCN). (2009). Research ethics: RCN guidance for nurses. London, UK: Royal College of Nursing.

Sackett, D., Rosenberg, W., Gray, J., Haynes, R., & Richardson, W. (1996). Evidence-based medicine: What it is and what it isn't. *British Medical Journal, 312*(7023), 71–72.

Schafer, O., & Wertheimer, A. (2010). The right to withdraw from research. *Kennedy Institute of Bioethics Journal, 20*(4), 329–352.

Schafer, O., & Wertheimer, A. (2011). Reevaluating the right to withdraw from research without penalty. *American Journal of Bioethics, 11*(4), 14–16.

Scott, J. (2013). Therapeutic misconceptions and misestimations in oncology: A clinical trial nurse's guide. *Clinical Journal of Oncology Nursing, 17*(5), 486–489. U.S. Department of Health and Human Services, Office for Human Research Protection. Retrieved from http://www.hhs.gov/ohrp

Sims, J. (2008). An introduction to institutional review boards. *Dimensions of Critical Care Nursing,* 27(5), 223–225.

Upshur, R. (2013). A call to integrate ethics and evidence-based medicine. *Virtual Mentor, American Medical Association Journal of Ethics,* 15(1), 86–89.

U.S Department of Health and Human Services. (2009). Federal policy for the protection of human subjects ("common rule"). Retrieved from http://www.hhs.gov/ohrp/humansubjects/common rule

U.S. Department of Health and Human Services. (2016a). Informed consent FAQs. Retrieved from http://www.hhs.gov/ohrp/regulations-and-policy/guidance/faq/informed-consent/#

U.S. Department of Health and Human Services. (2016b). IRB registration process FAQs. Retrieved from http://www.hhs.gov/ohrp/regulations-and-policy/guidance/faq/irb-registration-process /index.html

U.S. Food and Drug Administration. (2016). Institutional review boards frequently asked questions: Information sheet. Retrieved from http://www.fda.gov/RegulatoryInformation/Guidances/ ucm126420.htm

U.S. Government Printing Office. (1949). The Nuremberg Code. Trials of war criminals before the Nuremberg Military Tribunals under Control Council Law. 10(2), 181–182. Retrieved from http://www.history.nih.gov/research/downloads/nuremberg.pdf

Walton, M. (2017). Exploring ethical issues related to patient and family-centered care. In C. Robichaux (Ed.), *Ethical competence in nursing practice: Competencies, skills, decision-making* (pp. 137–154). New York, NY: Springer Publishing.

Wilson, S., & Stanley, B. (2006). Ethical concerns in schizophrenia research: Looking back and moving forward. *Schizophrenia Bulletin,* 32(1), 30–36.

World Medical Association. (1964). Declaration of Helsinki—Ethical principles for medical research involving human subjects. World Medical Association. Retrieved from http://www.wma.net/ en/20activities/10ethics/10helsinki

8

Applying Ethics to the Leadership Role

CATHERINE ROBICHAUX

Upon completion of this chapter, the reader will be able to:

- Identify prominent leadership theories in nursing
- Describe components of ethical leadership and their relation to leadership theories used in nursing
- Discuss the behaviors and responsibilities of ethical leaders at the micro-, meso-, and macro-levels
- Identify and apply strategies to develop ethical leadership

A ll nurses are leaders in their roles as health care providers and advocates, meeting the needs of patients and families directly or indirectly from the classroom to the bedside and boardroom, as managers, executives, educators, or researchers. At the bedside, nurses communicate and collaborate with the patient, family, and health care team regarding the provision of safe, quality care. At the department and unit levels, nurse leaders engage nurses in decision making about patient flow and staffing, quality improvement activities, and continuous learning opportunities to improve overall care delivery. Nurse managers strive to ensure that appropriate staffing and other resources are in place to achieve safe care and optimal patient outcomes (Thompson, Hoffman, & Sereika, 2011; Tregunno et al., 2009). At the organizational level, nurse executives contribute to strategic directions through their participation in senior level decision making and their ability to influence how nursing is practiced and valued (Marquis & Huston, 2014; Wong, Spence Laschinger, & Cziraki, 2014). Academic faculty, nurse educators, and researchers assist in guiding students and developing the discipline. At the national and international level, nurse leaders participate in health care reform and policy formation. So regardless of your nursing role as a formal or informal leader, you will encounter ethical issues and will have ethical responsibilities associated with your role.

CASE SCENARIO

Sandy has worked in the labor and delivery unit of a large, academic medical center for 5 years. Recently there has been increased staff turnover and several new graduates have been hired for the 7 a.m. to 7 p.m. shift. In postpartum care, the nurse to mother-baby couplet ratio has been one nurse to four stable couplets with alterations based on acuity. For the past 2 weeks, Sandy has had several assignments of five couplets in which mothers had been immediate postoperative cesarean section or the baby was late preterm and at risk for complications. In addition, Sandy is serving as preceptor for two of the new graduates who also have patient assignments. As an active member of Association of Women's Health, Obstetric, and Neonatal Nurses (AWHONN), Sandy is aware of the recommendations for staffing of perinatal units (AWHONN, 2010) and realizes that these assignments jeopardize patient care and nurse professional integrity and licensure. She also knows that in her state, Texas, the Board of Nursing has a safe harbor regulation that can be invoked without employer retaliation when a nurse believes an assignment is unsafe (Texas Board of Nursing, 2013).

At the end of the shift, she discusses her concerns with the charge nurse, Irene, who states, "You better get used to it because I don't think they will be hiring any experienced nurses soon." Sandy informs the charge nurse that she intends to invoke safe harbor on her next shift if such unsafe patient assignments continue.

Questions to Consider Before Reading On

1. How would you respond to a similar situation in your workplace if you were Sandy?

2. How would you respond as the charge nurse?

LEADERSHIP IN NURSING

There are many definitions, types, and theories of leadership. One definition states that leadership is "the process through which an individual attempts to intentionally influence another individual or a group in order to accomplish a goal" (Pointer, 2006, p. 125). A distinction is often made between leadership and management or administration. While the latter may be positional roles, "leadership" is a qualitative statement of personal or individual ability. This difference suggests that while management is about tasks, leadership is about perception, judgment, and philosophy. In nursing, however, the two may overlap and be similar in that they involve determining what has to be done, collaborating to attain the goal, and ensuring that it is accomplished. As leaders in diverse roles, nurses establish a direction and motivate others to achievement through trust, credibility, and relationships. Thus, leadership is a set of knowledge, skills, and attitudes that can be used by all nurses. Effective leadership at the management and administration levels is also associated with a healthy work environment, improved patient safety and satisfaction, and decreased nurse turnover rates, among other factors (Laschinger & Smith, 2013; Zook, 2014).

The American Association of Colleges of Nursing (AACN) documents on baccalaureate (2008) and master's essentials (2011) support the development of leadership competencies in all nurses. Scott and Miles (2013) state that "if nurses are to make an impact on the advancement of patient care and the promotion of patient safety, then leadership must be considered an integral dimension of nursing education across the continuum" (p. 78). In the baccalaureate document, essential II states that "knowledge and skills in leadership, quality improvement, and patient safety are necessary for the provision of high-quality health care" (p. 3). This document also states that "Leadership skills . . . that emphasize ethical and critical decision making, . . . effective working relationships, . . . , and developing conflict resolution strategies" are needed. In addition, "The baccalaureate program prepares the graduate to engage in ethical reasoning and actions to provide leadership in prompting advocacy, collaboration, and social justice as a socially responsible citizen" (p. 12). Of the nine essentials for master's-prepared nurses, two contain the word "lead" and most imply the use of leadership knowledge, skills, and attitudes.

The American Association of Colleges of Nursing (AACN) Quality and Safety Education in Nursing (QSEN) graduate competencies state that "graduate nurses will be the future *leaders* in practice, administration, education, and research. It is essential that these nurses understand, provide *leadership* by example, and promote the importance of providing quality health care and outcome measurement" (author's emphasis; AACN, 2012, p. 2). Those QSEN competencies relevant to leadership in nursing are presented in Box 8.1.

Question to Consider Before Reading On

1. How do you or other nursing leaders in your workplace demonstrate the QSEN competencies in Box 8.1?

Box 8.1	

Ethics in the Leadership Role—Relevant QSEN Competencies

Understand principles of change management (Knowledge)—Demonstrate leadership in affecting necessary change (Attitudes).

Analyze human factors safety design principles as well as commonly used unsafe practices (Knowledge)—Demonstrate leadership skills in creating a culture where safe design principles are developed and implemented (Skills).

Analyze the impact of team-based practice (Knowledge)—Be open to continually assessing and improving your skills as a team member and leader (Attitudes).

Source: American Association of Colleges of Nursing (2012); Cronenwett et al. (2007).

LEADERSHIP THEORIES

Although numerous leadership theories exist, transactional, transformational, and authentic leadership are popular models in nursing literature and education. These theories have several similar or overlapping components or behavioral attributes and it has been suggested that authentic leadership evolved from transformational leadership (Tonkin, 2013). An in-depth discussion of these theories is beyond the scope of this chapter; however, transactional leaders focus on achieving goals through clarifying expectations and, at times, offering recognition and rewards. In contrast, transformational nurse leaders stimulate and inspire others to achieve through charisma, and authentic leaders accomplish the same through honesty and consistency.

A transactional leader is focused on the maintenance and management of ongoing, day-to-day functions. She or he may work within the existing organizational culture as a direct care provider or charge nurse and demonstrate effective, stable leadership (Huber, 2014). The transformational nurse leader encourages others to collaborate rather than compete with each other, inspiring a sense of being connected to a higher purpose. Authentic nurse leaders endeavor to speak the truth, be transparent in their actions, and encourage and mentor others to achieve higher levels of performance. Transformational and authentic leadership may be necessary for organizational culture change in circumstances of growth, change, and crisis and is future oriented (Clark, 2009; Huber, 2014). These leadership approaches or styles are not mutually exclusive; behaviors or characteristics associated with one or more may be appropriate or used in another given situation.

While leadership has been explored extensively across disciplines, the role of ethics in leadership or ethical leadership has received focused attention only within the last 15 years and primarily in the business literature (Storch, Makaroff, Pauly, & Newton, 2013). This current interest is undoubtedly related to recent and ongoing scandals in business, government, sports, nonprofits, religious, and health care organizations (Dinh, Lord, Gardner, Meuser, & Hu, 2014; Sama & Schoaf, 2008). In nursing, Nightingale and other early nurse leaders gave specific attention to ethics, with chapters, articles, and books written about the ethical behavior and responsibilities of nurse leaders (Aikens, 1916/1935; Ulrich, 1992). Makaroff, Storch, Pauly, and Newton (2014) note, however, that attention to ethics and nursing leadership has waned over the last two decades perhaps contributing to a deficient ethical climate and pervasive moral distress among nurses. These authors (Makaroff et al., 2014) and others (Edmonson, 2015; Gallagher & Tschudin, 2010; Keselman, 2012) call for renewed attention to ethics in nursing education and leadership. This attention is especially significant in the current health care environment as ethical leaders may influence peer/employee ethical conduct in situations that may have great impact on patient outcomes, safety, and quality care (Keselman, 2012; Piper, 2011; Piper & Tallman, 2015).

Question to Consider Before Reading On

1. Identify a nurse leader in your current workplace. Does he or she demonstrate characteristics or behaviors associated with one or more leadership theories in Figure 8.1?

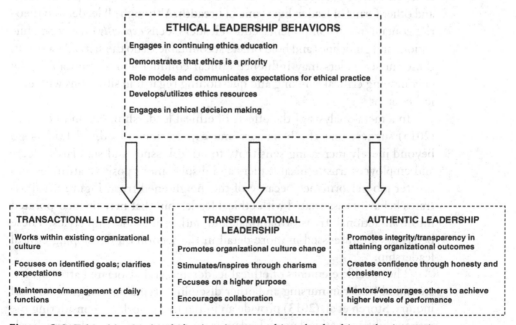

Figure 8.1 Ethical leadership behaviors integrated into leadership styles in nursing.
Sources: Fox, Crigger, Bottrell, and Bauck (2007); Huber (2014).

CASE SCENARIO *(CONTINUED)*

Returning to the Case Scenario, Sandy thinks about Irene's comment that she "better get used" to continued short staffing in the postpartum unit. She wonders if the charge nurse is aware of current research on the potential adverse outcomes for both mothers and infants that can occur from inadequate nurse staffing (Bingham & Rule, 2015). Sandy is certain that Irene realizes that providing safe care is the primary ethical and legal obligation of the hospital and all health care providers. She reviews the components of the ethical decision-making framework presented in Chapter 2. Sandy recognizes that the present staffing situation may both harm the patients, violating the principle of nonmaleficence, and is inconsistent with her perception of good nursing (virtue ethics). Sandy decides to bring copies of the Code of Ethics (2015) and AWHONN (2010) staffing guidelines to review with Irene before her shift begins in the morning.

ETHICAL LEADERSHIP

Ethical behavior is certainly a characteristic of transactional, transformational, and authentic leaders. These nurses are individuals of integrity who engage in ethical decision making and are role models for others. A distinction is made, however, in that in ethical leadership at all levels, nurses *proactively* influence others through personal conduct, communication, and expectations. As Zheng et al. (2015) note, the difference between ethical leadership and other forms of leadership is one of breadth. Although all leadership theories contain moral components, ethical leaders focus *explicitly* on ethical obligations and guidelines and hold others accountable to do the same. As a result, these nurse leaders may influence ethical conduct and accountability by encouraging critical thinking and questioning regarding situations with ethical content.

In a meta-analysis of the effects of ethical leadership, Ng and Feldman (2015) suggest that the behaviors and expectations of ethical leaders go beyond merely increasing sensitivity to ethical issues and standards. Peers and employees trust ethical leaders and display more positive attitudes and greater job performance because of this heightened trust. Figure 8.1 illustrates behaviors associated with ethical leadership that may be incorporated into transactional, transformational, and authentic leadership styles. These behaviors are discussed in more detail in the section on developing ethical leadership.

The specific elements of ethical leadership and associated attributes of an ethical leader in nursing and other disciplines remain an ongoing area of inquiry. Storch et al. (2013) provide an initial framework for considering the responsibilities of ethical nurse leaders at the macro-, meso-, and micro-levels both within and outside their organizations (Figure 8.2).

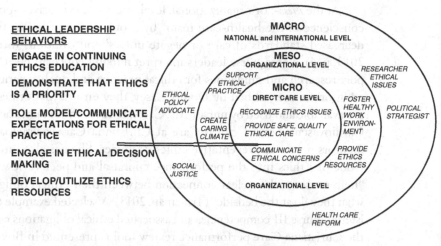

ETHICAL LEADERSHIP
BEHAVIORS

ENGAGE IN CONTINUING
ETHICS EDUCATION

DEMONSTRATE THAT ETHICS
IS A PRIORITY

ROLE MODEL/COMMUNICATE
EXPECTATIONS FOR ETHICAL
PRACTICE

ENGAGE IN ETHICAL DECISION
MAKING

DEVELOP/UTILIZE ETHICS
RESOURCES

Figure 8.2 Nursing ethical leadership responsibilities at micro-, meso-, and macro-levels. Ethical leadership behaviors cross all levels.

Questions to Consider Before Reading On

1. Figure 8.2 illustrates the responsibilities of ethical nurse leaders at three different levels. In addition, it depicts how ethical leadership behaviors cross all levels. How would you demonstrate these responsibilities and behaviors in your current workplace?

2. Can you identify a nurse leader with whom you have worked who demonstrates these behaviors and responsibilities at the macro-level?

The terms "macro," "meso," and "micro" reflect the environment of practice rather than the magnitude of influence of the ethical nurse leader. In addition, a nurse may be an ethical leader in several levels, for example, a staff nurse or nurse manager who is also a member of the institutional ethics committee or professional organization(s).

At the *macro-level*, ethical nursing leaders are spokespersons, political strategists, researchers, and advocates for social justice and health care reform. These leaders also ensure that nurses' views on and experiences of ethical issues are heard and represented in various national and international forums. For example, Marla Weston, Chief Executive Officer, American Nurses Association, has championed federal legislation regarding safe nurse staffing presently under review in the U. S. Senate, the Registered Nurse Safe Staffing Act of 2014 (ANA, 2014). Carol Pavlish, Associate Professor, UCLA School of Nursing, and colleagues have conducted extensive research on moral distress in nursing (2013, 2015a, 2015b), developed an early intervention tool to mitigate its deleterious effects (2014, 2015c), and an evidence-based action guide for nurse leaders (2016). Pavlish and her co-investigators have also explored gender-based violence in South Sudan and Rwanda and identified the global advocacy role of nursing in supporting these vulnerable populations (Pavlish, Ho, & Runkle, 2012).

At the *meso-*, or organizational, level, the nurse executive "serve(s) as the conscience of the health-care team" by avoiding compromises that lead to decreased standards of care or negate nurses' contributions (Storch et al., 2013, p. 4). These nurse leaders interpret nursing concerns clearly and support research and guidelines for ethical practice and quality patient care. In addition, as exemplified by Donna Casey, they ensure that ethics resources are available and used by nurses. Ms. Casey, Director of Patient Care Services, Cardiovascular and Critical Care at Christiana Care, participates in and mentors nurses in preventative ethics strategies. She has also integrated the Code of Ethics into the performance appraisal and peer review process to "help nurses make a clear connection between their ethical obligations and what they do at the bedside" (Trossman, 2013). A selected example of the Registered Nurse III competencies and associated ethical obligations contained in the Christiana Care performance review tool is presented in Box 8.2.

Nursing directors and nurse managers are leaders at both the organizational and unit levels. They are called on to foster healthy work environments and create a climate of caring and connectedness. These frontline leaders must also recognize the importance of meeting nurses' needs in order to meet client needs, and provide meaningful participation in decision making. The nurse director/manager position is critical to organizational success, patient outcomes, and nurse empowerment (Duffield, Roche, Blay, & Stasa, 2011; Lucas, Laschinger, & Wong, 2008; Wong et al., 2010). Over the past two decades, this role has become increasingly complex as these nurses may lead one or more units and have increased responsibility for budget, staffing, and regulatory compliance (Hewko, Brown, Fraser, Wong, & Cummings, 2014; Kath, Stichler, & Ehrhart, 2012; Shirey, McDaniel, Ebright, Fisher, & Doebbeling, 2010). These responsibilities and others may create tension between personal values, the ethical obligations of the profession, and working within the priorities and needs of the organization.

The challenging position of the frontline nurse manager or leader in ethical situations was explored by several researchers (Aitamaa, Leino-Kilpi, Puukka, & Suhonen, 2010; Pavlish et al., 2015b; Porter, 2010). Many issues identified by the nursing leaders in these studies are similar to those reported by direct care nurses. However, they occur at multiple levels as presented in Box 8.3, and reflect the nurse manager/leader's complex role in navigating diverse perspectives. Rather than taking a proactive stance or intervening early in these situations, Pavlish and colleagues (2015b) reported that the nurse leaders in their investigation often waited until the conflicts escalated. Reasons for the delay included perceptions that intervening could be risky, harm relationships, and/or jeopardize their ability to accomplish other initiatives. Although many participants believed that system-level issues contributed to ethical conflicts, few identified approaches to operate at the organizational level to change those contributing factors. Pavlish and colleagues concluded that the frontline nurse manager or leader may need to develop "more awareness, skill, and confidence in working with institutional level ethics" (p. 317).

Box 8.2

Registered Nurse III Performance Review Tool Selected Competencies

ADVOCACY/MORAL AGENCY
PATIENT ASSESSMENT/ETHICAL PLAN OF CARE
Works on another's behalf to help resolve ethical and clinical concerns within the clinical setting for patients and families when they cannot represent themselves.

Cultivates an environment that is supportive of colleagues' development in ethical reasoning and advocacy.

Represents the patient when the patient cannot represent self. Seeks available resources to help understand, formulate, and implement ethical decisions.

PATIENT/FAMILY SATISFACTION/ETHICAL INVOLVEMENT
Supports ongoing initiatives and implements new initiatives that improve patient satisfaction and foster ethical decision making.

Assumes a leadership role to provide support to other members of the team seeking resolution to patient satisfaction concerns or ethical solutions.

Empowers the patient and family; knows what rules or guidelines can be suspended or modified to allow patients and families to represent themselves or meet their moral needs.

Serves as a resource and a patient advocate. Is alert to and takes appropriate action regarding incompetent, unethical, illegal, or impaired practice by any member of the health care team.

PROFESSIONALISM IN NURSING—EXEMPLARY PROFESSIONAL PRACTICE
The nurse owes the same duties to self as to others, including the responsibility to preserve integrity and safety, to maintain competence, and to continue personal and professional growth (ANA Code of Ethics, 2015).

Attended a local or national nursing conference

Submitted an article for publication in a nursing or medical journal within the current review year

Active member of the unit or hospital nursing Quality and Safety Council

Adapted from Registered Nurse III Performance Review Tool (2012). Used with permission.

Question to Consider Before Reading On

1. Are the ethical issues identified by nurse managers in Box 8.3 similar to, or different from, those in your current workplace?

Recognizing that the frontline nurse manager role is crucial to sustaining a healthy, ethical work environment and optimal patient outcomes, the American Association of Critical-Care Nursing (AACN) and the American Organization of Nurse Executives (AONE) have collaborated to develop educational and certification programs to recognize and support the leadership role of nurse managers and directors. Several of the ethical leadership competencies identified by these organizations are consistent with Pavlish and colleagues' (2015b) recommendations:

- Engage in discussions with entity and system leaders that advance familiarity with ethical principles and incorporate values as guardrails for ethical decision making.

Box 8.3

Ethical Issues Identified by Frontline Nurse Managers

PATIENT CARE LEVEL

Development and maintenance of the quality of care

Disagreement between patients and/or families and health care professionals about treatment decisions

Ethical practices in end-of-life care

Patient suffering

STAFF LEVEL

Adequate staffing and competence

Professionalism in patient care

Provision of ethics resources

Respectful, collaborative, inter/intraprofessional relationships

ORGANIZATIONAL LEVEL

Ethical climate

Resource allocation

Conflict between nursing professional values and organizational goals

Respect and dignity for employees

Sources: Aitamaa et al. (2010); Pavlish, Brown-Saltzman, et al. (2015b); Porter (2010).

- Facilitate standardized approaches to competency development in ethics and monitor regularly for all members of the system.

- Role model principled, values-based, ethical thinking to the system.

- Develop moral courage in expressions of clinical priorities, values, and perspectives at all system levels effectively. (AONE, 2015, p. 12)

Box 8.4 presents an exemplar of ethical leadership in the nurse manager role.

Box 8.4

Exemplar—Ethical Leadership at the Meso-Level in the Nurse Manager Role

JL is a 44-year-old woman with a complicated medical history including hydrocephalus, asthma, and obesity. She has also been diagnosed with bipolar disease and has required frequent surgeries for foreign body ingestion to include pens, paper clips, and flash drives. As she is prone to agitation and physical aggression necessitating hospital security intervention and application of 4-point restraints, JL is usually assigned a 1:1 safety companion. Immediately following her last discharge, JL was readmitted for further ingestion of noxious objects requiring the extensive involvement of both trauma and thoracic surgery.

Nurse managers in the emergency department and unit to which JL had been admitted in the past became aware of the emotional and moral distress experienced by nurses and other providers caring for JL. They also recognized that this complex ethical situation included elements of futility, allocation of scarce resources, patient autonomy, and duty to treat. The nurse managers requested an ethics consultation, which was conducted in an open, interdisciplinary format to facilitate dialogue and problem solving.

Following the discussion, administrators, nurses, social workers, and physicians recognized that repeated foreign body ingestion may be considered an addiction and is resistant to treatment (Lytle, Stagno, & Daly, 2013). They acknowledged that progress for JL may be slow or she may eventually die from her addiction. A plan of care was developed that emphasized partnering with JL and understanding what triggers her ingestions. If readmission is absolutely necessary, all positive reinforcement such as a private room and access to snacks and movies is to be omitted. JL will continue to receive intensive psychotherapy in the community setting.

(continued)

Box 8.4

Exemplar—Ethical Leadership at the Meso-Level in the Nurse Manager Role *(continued)*

These nurse leaders at the meso-level demonstrated the ethical skill of relational involvement as they were engaged in this situation in an open and attentive manner that enabled them to collaborate and intervene (Cathcart, 2014). This relational skill, and moral courage, empowered them to participate in a discussion with health system administrators and members of the ethics committee to collectively develop a plan of care for JL.

Sources: Cathcart (2014); Lytle, Stagno, and Daly (2013).

In ethical nursing leadership at the *micro-*, or direct patient care, level, nurses such as Sandy in the Case Scenario recognize ethical issues and communicate their concerns:

CASE SCENARIO *(CONTINUED)*

Sandy approaches Irene the next morning to discuss the AWHONN (2010) staffing guidelines and relevant statements from Provision 4 of Code of Ethics (2015; Box 8.5). Although initially reluctant, stating, "I am too busy to sit down and read that," Sandy persists and Irene agrees to review the documents with her. Irene expresses surprise and concern after reading the AWHONN staffing guidelines related to immediate postpartum recovery and mother-baby care and how these recommendations are not currently known or followed in their unit. As the census is lower this morning, she and Sandy arrange a meeting with Kate, the nurse manager.

Kate has been in her position for 3 months, having worked as a staff nurse in the unit for several years. She is familiar with the staffing shortages but has been directed to cut her budget as the census has varied but is usually lower than in recent years. Kate is also a member of AWHONN and the hospital nursing ethics committee. She recognizes that, as a nurse manager, her primary obligation remains to the patient, as stated in the Code of Ethics (2015) and the Standards for Professional Nursing Practice in the Care of Women and Newborns (AWHONN, 2009). Kate has advocated for hiring additional experienced nurses and increasing the number of assistive staff. Kate meets with Sandy and Irene and together they develop a plan to present their documents and research to the chief nursing officer (CNO).

Question to Consider Before Reading On

1. As a nurse manager at the meso- or organizational level, what ethical behaviors and responsibilities (Figure 8.2) did Kate demonstrate?

Ethical issues identified by staff nurses are often similar to those described by nurse managers and directors and include concerns regarding protection of patient autonomy, staffing, and surrogate decision making (Ulrich et al., 2010). In addition, witnessing unnecessary patient suffering and differing perspectives on treatment goals are often associated with experiences of moral distress (Pavlish et al., 2015b; Varcoe, Pauly, Storch, Newton, & Makaroff, 2012).

The ability to initiate and engage in discussions such as withdrawal of aggressive treatment and transitioning to palliative care is a skill often demonstrated by experienced ethical leaders in the ICU. This is a complex and nuanced communication process in which the nurse (a) organizes and interprets knowledge from different sources, (b) learns who the patient is as a person, (c) helps the family see the deteriorating status of the patient, (d) reminds the family what the patient may have wanted, and (e) facilitates saying good-bye (Peden-McAlpine, Liaschenko, Traudt, & Gilmore-Szott, 2015). An example of this leadership skill is provided by Blas Villa, a clinical nurse at University Health System in San Antonio, Texas, who stated (personal communication Feb. 15, 2015):

> So often as a bedside nurse here in the Medical-Coronary Care Unit (MCCU), we encounter many patients that are in the end stages of a particular disease. It is a disheartening experience to hear those words "Am I going to die?" during patient encounter. I remember as a young inexperienced nurse, when faced with that question, often I would find myself answering jokingly "not on my watch" because I believed in my ability to care for them to at least get them through another day with their loved ones. But in the back of my mind I knew their time was limited but I never let that show in the way I delivered my care to them. But, in every sense as a nurse or even any member of the health care team, we want to give the patients hope. With all the technological advances in medicine and people living longer, I think we as nurses we don't ask enough of those tough questions. Such as: What is your understanding of the disease process? What are your priorities now that you are in the hospital? What are you willing to give up as a patient, mother, father, brother, husband or wife in order to gain something that may or may not help you get better? I think if we could tailor the care based on the patient's understanding of the disease process, we could see more of a meaningful quality of care that could potentially increase their quality of life. So now being more mature in my answers, I think being serious, more empathetic, and honest will show you on your patient's side. It certainly won't make miracles happen, but it's the best thing any nurse should do. As with my own patients,

when I am in charge, I make it a point to ask the nurses if the palliative care team should be consulted sooner rather than later.

DEVELOPING ETHICAL LEADERSHIP

Gallagher and Tschudin (2010) state that becoming an ethical leader in
nursing is "a complex and multifaceted process" (p. 226). Many nursing educational programs offer or require a basic ethics course or have content integrated throughout the curriculum. The competence necessary for ethical
leadership, however, requires additional knowledge and skills. Ethical competence includes, but is not limited to, self-understanding or awareness of
personal values, knowledge of diverse professional codes of ethics, ethical
principles and theories, and decision-making frameworks. As discussed in
Chapter 2, it also requires ethical sensitivity or the ability to recognize a
situation with ethical content and conflict resolution skills. Of course, ethical leadership is demonstrated not only by what leaders do, their conduct,
but also by their character. Thus, these nurses develop a range of moral virtues including courage and trustworthiness through practice and reflection
(Brown & Trevino, 2006; Fox et al., 2007; Gallagher & Tschudin, 2010).

As part of the integrated ethics program at the Veterans Health Administration, Fox et al. (2007) propose four components or behaviors of ethical
leaders that can be adapted and used by nurses at all levels: demonstrate
that ethics is a priority, role model and communicate expectations for ethical practice, engage in ethical decision making, and develop/utilize ethics
resources. In addition, this author has added a fifth component, engage in
continuing ethics education, discussed in the next section and in Chapter 2.
Many of these components or behaviors are demonstrated in the examples and Case Scenarios presented previously and illustrated in Figures 8.1
and 8.2.

ENGAGE IN CONTINUING ETHICS EDUCATION

If included in the curriculum, ethics courses have been shown to increase
students' ethical perceptions and reasoning processes. To be effective, teaching strategies should include both didactic content and carefully constructed
case studies. Case studies should be consistent with students' own clinical
practice, and be analyzed in a safe environment that encourages discussion
of conflicting viewpoints and self-examination (Cannaerts, Gastmans, &
Dierckx de Casterle, 2014; Park, Kjervik, & Crandall, 2012). Since ethics is
a collaborative endeavor, several educational institutions have developed
interprofessional ethics education courses in which students from nursing,
medical, dental, and other schools learn the skills necessary to respectfully

address ethical issues within the team (UT Houston, OHSU). This approach, while logistically challenging in terms of class scheduling, addresses the competency of "values and ethics for interprofessional practice" identified in the Core Competencies for Interprofessional Collaborative Practice (2011).

As with clinical competence, maintaining ethical competence is a continuous, ongoing process that is emphasized in Chapters 2 and 4 of this book. The responsibility to develop and maintain this competence is an individual professional obligation that should also be supported at the organizational level by formal nurse leaders (Poikkeus, Numminen, Suhonen, & Leino-Kilpi, 2013).

DEMONSTRATE THAT ETHICS IS A PRIORITY

In their research exploring ethical leadership among nurse managers and executives, Makaroff et al. (2014) discovered that many participants chose not to identify issues as "ethical" or use the language of ethics as they believed it was "too scientific" and/or created distance between themselves and others. The use of euphemisms that obscure ethical uncertainty or conflict diminishes the essential role of ethics in everyday nursing practice. Fox et al. (2007) suggest that to demonstrate that ethics is a priority, leaders identify and talk about ethical concerns using explicit language. For example, nurses should use words and phrases such as "ethical principles," "advocacy," "integrity," and "duty" and refer to illustrative provisions in the Code of Ethics (2015), when applicable. Box 8.5 illustrates several provisions and statements from the Code of Ethics relevant to the leadership role.

Question to Consider Before Reading On

1. As a nurse leader at the meso- or macro-level, how would you support one of the provisions/statements in Box 8.5?

Ethical leaders in nursing can create or take advantage of opportunities to discuss ethical issues with peers or staff members and use cases or narratives to illustrate the importance of ethics. Examples include initiating conversations about situations with ethical content such as saying, "The bullying on this unit is causing moral distress for many nurses and several are talking about leaving; let's discuss why this is happening" or "I believe an ethics consultation is needed because this patient's autonomy is being ignored. I would like to hear your opinion about this situation." As mentors, ethical nursing leaders use such conversations to encourage others to think about ethics in their own practices and professional relationships.

Box 8.5

Ethics in the Leadership Role—Relevant Provisions and Statements From the Code of Ethics

PROVISION 1

INTERPRETIVE STATEMENT 1.3

THE NATURE OF HEALTH

Nurses are leaders who actively participate in ensuring the responsible and appropriate use of interventions in order to optimize the health and well-being of those in their care. This includes acting to minimize unwarranted, unwanted, or unnecessary medical treatment and patient suffering.

PROVISION 4

INTERPRETIVE STATEMENT 4.3

RESPONSIBILITY FOR NURSING JUDGMENTS, DECISIONS, AND ACTIONS

The nurse acts to promote inclusion of appropriate individuals in all ethical deliberations. Nurse executives are responsible for ensuring that nurses have access to and inclusion on organizational committees and in decision-making processes that affect the ethics, quality, and safety of patient care.

INTERPRETIVE STATEMENT 4.4

ASSIGNMENT AND DELEGATION OF NURSING ACTIVITIES OR TASKS

Nurses in management and administration have a particular responsibility to provide a safe environment that supports and facilitates appropriate assignment and delegation. This includes orientation, skill development . . . and policies that protect both the patient and nurse from inappropriate assignment or delegation of nursing responsibilities, activities, or tasks.

PROVISION 5

INTERPRETIVE STATEMENT 5.2

PROMOTION OF PERSONAL HEALTH, SAFETY, AND WELL-BEING

These [health maintenance and promotion] activities and satisfying work must be held in balance to promote and maintain the health and well-being of the nurse. Nurses in all roles should seek this balance and it is the responsibility of nurse leaders to foster this balance within their organization.

(continued)

Box 8.5

Ethics in the Leadership Role—Relevant Provisions and Statements From the Code of Ethics *(continued)*

INTERPRETIVE STATEMENT 5.4
PRESERVATION OF INTEGRITY
Nurse executives should ensure policies addressing conscientious objection are available.

PROVISION 6
INTERPRETIVE STATEMENT 6.3
RESPONSIBILITY FOR THE HEALTH CARE ENVIRONMENT
Nurse executives have a particular responsibility to ensure that employees are treated fairly and justly, and that nurses are involved in decisions related to their practice and working conditions.

PROVISION 7
INTERPRETIVE STATEMENT 7.1
CONTRIBUTIONS THROUGH RESEARCH AND SCHOLARLY INQUIRY
Nurse executives and administrators should develop the structure and foster the processes that create an organizational climate and infrastructure conducive to scholarly inquiry.

Source: American Nurses Association (2015).

ROLE MODEL AND COMMUNICATE EXPECTATIONS FOR ETHICAL PRACTICE

To be effective, the nurse at any level must role model moral behavior before he or she is seen as an ethical leader by peers, staff, and others. In their extensive exploration of ethical leadership in business, Brown and Trevino (2005), Brown, Trevino, and Harrison (2006), and Jordan, Brown, Trevino, and Finklestein (2013) propose that this perception by others is based on the leader's consistent ethical conduct and actions with *everyone*. Thus, in ethical leadership, the principles of autonomy, beneficence, nonmaleficence, and justice, in conjunction with caring and virtue ethics, are applicable to patient/family care and interactions with peers/staff and others. While nurses are familiar with these principles in patient/family care, their relevance to all professional relationships may not be as well understood. As an example, autonomy in professional practice is defined as the ability to make autonomous decisions based on an extensive knowledge base, clinical expertise, and evidence (Papathanassoglou et al., 2012). The inability to exercise autonomy in nursing practice is directly related to job dissatisfaction and perceptions of poor quality care. Limited nurse autonomy may also be associated with lack of interprofessional collaboration and contribute to moral distress and turnover (Galletta, Portoghese, Battistelli, & Leiter, 2013). The nurse leader role models ethical behavior by supporting nurse autonomy through recognition and respect at the bedside, including staff nurses on practice and operation committees, and other actions. He or she also demonstrates the principle of justice and caring in treating everyone with fairness and dignity.

Role modeling ethical behavior and practice can positively influence and motivate others to do the same. However, it is often necessary for the nurse leader to explain the values and principles underlying his or her actions and expectations. We may erroneously assume that others are familiar with aspects of ethical practice when their knowledge may be limited to an abstract understanding rather than concrete, everyday application. For example, the nurse leader can describe how the virtue of courage and principle of nonmaleficence apply to advocating for a colleague who is being bullied: "To work together as a team for quality patient care, we have to actively support and speak up for one another; at times, this may take courage. Comments that belittle (name of nurse) or imply that his patient care is substandard is harmful to him and the team. If you have concerns about (name of nurse) patient care, it would be more constructive to discuss them with him personally."

ENGAGE IN ETHICAL DECISION MAKING

Through self-understanding and ethical sensitivity, leaders in all areas of nursing should be able to identify issues with ethical content and discuss their concerns using appropriate language, as noted previously. At times, this may require the skill of moral courage, addressed in Chapter 2. Once the nurse determines that the situation requires an ethical decision, he or she must address the decision in a systematic manner. Depending on the complexity of the situation, this process may include collecting relevant facts, identifying stakeholders, understanding differing values, analyzing potential benefits and burdens of possible courses of action, and reasoning in a coherent, logical manner. Using a systematic model such as the one in this text serves to improve the quality of ethical decisions (Grace, 2014). In addition, sharing the process by which one reaches and implements a decision serves to mentor and inform others.

DEVELOP AND/OR UTILIZE ETHICS RESOURCES

Ethical nursing leaders are aware of the ethics resources in their respective institutions. Nurse managers and executives are responsible for ensuring that such resources are available and communicating their expectations for access and use by staff members. All providers should be informed of the process for calling for an ethics consultation and what to expect. Chapter 3 and others discuss instances in which a formal ethics consultation might be indicated.

Chapter 5 presents the three roles of an ethics committee—education, policy review/creation, and consulting. In addition, the differences between an ethics committee and an ethics consultant, and the types of consultation that can occur are discussed.

While The Joint Commission (2016) and American Nurses Credentialing Center (ANCC) Magnet® (2014) program require that hospitals have such ethics resources, nurses may work in settings where they do not exist or where what is available is insufficient. Ethical nurse leaders in these institutions can collaborate to develop initial resources that include ethics education and nursing ethics groups or committees and ethics journal clubs as discussed in Chapter 2.

Questions to Consider Before Reading On

1. Choose one of the ethical leadership behaviors discussed previously and illustrated in Figure 8.1. Describe how you would demonstrate this behavior in a chosen leadership style.

2. How would a transformational or authentic leader at the meso- or organizational level integrate/demonstrate this behavior?

CONCLUSION

Recognizing that all nurses are leaders in their respective positions, the purpose of this chapter was to discuss the important role of ethical leadership. Relevant leadership theories used in nursing were briefly reviewed and their relationship to ethical leadership presented. The behaviors and responsibilities of ethical leaders at the micro-, meso-, and macro-levels of the nursing practice environment were described. Five strategies to develop and maintain ethical leadership in nursing were explored.

Critical Thinking Questions and Activities

1. Recall a recent ethical situation from your practice. Discuss the behaviors and responsibilities of an ethical nurse leader in this situation at the micro-, meso-, and macro-levels.

2. You are considering applying for the certified nurse manager and leader (AONE/AACN, 2016) credential. Review the candidate handbook available at http://www.aone.org/docs/certification/cnml-handbook.pdf

   Then describe how the role of the ethical nurse leader is integrated into the exam within the four practice areas of (a) financial management, (b) human resource management, (c) performance improvement, and (d) strategic management.

(continued)

Critical Thinking Questions and Activities *(continued)*

3. Nurse leaders are responsible for contributing to an ethical climate or moral environment. The Hospital Ethical Climate Survey (Olson, 1998) has been used extensively in studies conducted nationally (Sauerland, Marotta, Peinemann, Berndt, & Robichaux, 2014 and 2015; Whitehead, Herbertson, Hamric, Epstein, & Fisher, 2015) and internationally (Hwang & Park, 2014; Suhonen, Stolt, Gustafsson, Katajisto, Charalambous, 2014; Numinen, Leino-Kilpi, Isoaho, & Meretoja, 2015).

Review the items in the HECS (Box 8.6) and used in the study by Sauerland, Marotta, Peinemann, Berndt, and Robichaux (2014, p. 240) to assess the ethical climate in your workplace. Compare and contrast your answers and overall score with those of a class peer or colleague (score can range from a low of 26 to a high of 130).

http://journals.lww.com/dccnjournal/Fulltext/2014/07000/Assessing_and_Addressing_Moral_Distress_and.9.aspx

Box 8.6

Hospital Ethical Climate Survey

Directions: Here is a series of statements relating to various practices within your work setting. Please respond in terms of how it is in your current job on your current unit. As you read and respond to each statement, think of some difficult patient care issues you have faced. For those items that refer to your manager, think of your immediate manager (nurse manager, assistant nurse manager, shift supervisor). It is important that you respond in terms of how it really is on your unit, not how you would prefer it to be. It is essential to answer every item. There are no right or wrong answers, so please respond honestly. Remember, all your responses will remain anonymous.

Please read each of the following statements. Then, circle one of the numbers on each line to indicate your response.

	Almost Never True	Seldom True	Sometimes True	Often True	Almost Always True
1. My peers listen to my concerns about patient care	1	2	3	4	5
2. Patients know what to expect from their care	1	2	3	4	5

(continued)

Box 8.6

Hospital Ethical Climate Survey *(continued)*

	Almost Never True	Seldom True	Sometimes True	Often True	Almost Always True
3. When I'm unable to decide what's right or wrong in a patient care situation, my manager helps me............ 1		2	3	4	5
4. Hospital policies help me with difficult patient care issues/problems.................. 1		2	3	4	5
5. Nurses and physicians trust one another.................. 1		2	3	4	5
6. Nurses have access to the information necessary to solve a patient care issue/problem............... 1		2	3	4	5
7. My manager supports me in my decisions about patient care..... 1		2	3	4	5
8. A clear sense of the hospital's mission is shared with nurses.... 1		2	3	4	5
9. Physicians ask nurses for their opinions about treatment decisions.................. 1		2	3	4	5
10. My peers help me with difficult patient care issues/problems.............. 1		2	3	4	5
11. Nurses use the information necessary to solve a patient care issue/problem............ 1		2	3	4	5
12. My manager listens to me talk about patient care issues/problems 1		2	3	4	5

(continued)

Box 8.6

Hospital Ethical Climate Survey (continued)

	Almost Never True	Seldom True	Sometimes True	Often True	Almost Always True
13. The feelings and values of all parties involved in a patient care issue/problem are taken into account when choosing a course of actions	1	2	3	4	5
14. I participate in treatment decisions for my patients	1	2	3	4	5
15. My manager is someone I can trust	1	2	3	4	5
16. Conflict is openly dealt with, not avoided	1	2	3	4	5
17. Nurses and physicians here respect each others' opinions, even when they disagree about what is best for patients	1	2	3	4	5
18. I work with competent colleagues	1	2	3	4	5
19. The patient's wishes are respected	1	2	3	4	5
20. When my peers are unable to decide what's right or wrong in a particular patient care situation, I have observed that my manager helps them	1	2	3	4	5
21. There is a sense of questioning, learning, and seeking creative responses to patient care problems	1	2	3	4	5
22. Nurses and physicians respect one another	1	2	3	4	5

(continued)

Box 8.6				

Hospital Ethical Climate Survey (continued)

	Almost Never True	Seldom True	Sometimes True	Often True	Almost Always True
23. Safe patient care is given on my unit	1	2	3	4	5
24. My manager is someone I respect.	1	2	3	4	5
25. I am able to practice nursing on my unit as I believe it should be practiced.	1	2	3	4	5
26. Nurses are supported and respected in this hospital	1	2	3	4	5

© Copyright 1995 Linda Olson.

REFERENCES

Aikens, C. (1916/1935). *Studies in ethics for nurses*. Philadelphia, PA: W. B. Saunders.

Aitamaa, E., Leino-Kilpi, H., Puukka, P., & Suhonen, R. (2010). Ethical problems in nursing management: The role of codes of ethics. *Nursing Ethics, 17*(4), 469–482.

American Association of Colleges of Nursing. (2008). *The essentials of baccalaureate education for professional nursing practice*. Washington, DC: Author.

American Association of Colleges of Nursing. (2011). *The essentials of master's education in nursing*. Washington, DC: Author.

American Association of Colleges of Nursing. (2012). *Graduate level QSEN competencies: Knowledge, skills, and attitudes*. Washington, DC: Author. Retrieved from http://www.qsen.org

American Nurses Association (ANA). (2014). Nurse staffing legislation. Retrieved from http://nursingworld.org/FunctionalMenuCategories/MediaResources/PressReleases/2014-PR/RN-Safe-Staffing-Bill-Introduced-in-Senate.pdf

American Nurses Association. (2015). *Code of ethics for nurses with interpretive statements*. Silver Spring, MD: Author.

American Nurses Credentialing Center. (2014). *Magnet application manual*. Silver Spring, MD: Author.

American Organization of Nurse Executives and American Association of Critical Care Nurses. (2016). *Certified nurse manager/leader handbook*. Washington, DC: AONE. Retrieved from http://www.aone.org/docs/certification/cnml-handbook.pdf

American Organization of Nurse Executives (AONE). (2015). System CNE competencies. Retrieved from http://www.aone.org/resources/nec-system-cne.pdf

Association of Women's Health, Obstetric, and Neonatal Nurses. (2009). *Standards for professional nursing practice* (7th ed.). Washington, DC: Author.

Association of Women's Health, Obstetric, and Neonatal Nurses. (2010). *Guidelines for professional nurse staffing for perinatal units.* Washington, DC: Author. Retrieved from https://www.awhonn.org/store/ViewProduct.aspx?id=5152716

Bingham, D., & Ruhl, C. (2015). Planning and evaluating evidence-based perinatal nursing. *Journal of Obstetric, Gynecologic, and Neonatal Nursing, 44,* 290–308.

Brown, M., & Trevino, L. (2006). Ethical leadership: A review and future directions. *The Leadership Quarterly, 17,* 595–616.

Brown, M., Trevino, L., & Harrison, D. (2005). Ethical leadership: A social learning perspective for construct development and testing. *Organizational Behavior and Human Decision Processes, 97*(2), 117–134.

Cannaerts, N., Gastmans, C., & Dierckx de Casterle, B. (2014). Contribution of ethics education to the ethical competence of nursing students: Educators and students' perceptions. *Nursing Ethics, 21*(8), 861–878.

Cathcart, E. (2014). Relational work: At the core of leadership. *Nursing Management, 45*(3), 44–46.

Clark, C. (2009). Theories of leadership and management. In C. C. Clark (Ed.), *Creative leadership and management in nursing* (pp. 3–29). Sudbury, MA: Jones & Bartlett.

Cronenwett, L., Sherwood, G., Barnsteiner, J., Disch, J., Johnson, J., Mitchell, P., . . . Warre, J. (2007). Quality and safety education for nurses. *Nursing Outlook, 55*(3), 122–131. Retrieved from http://qsen.org/competencies/pre-licensure-ksas/

Dinh, J., Lord, R., Gardner, W., Meuser, J., & Hu, J. (2014). Leadership theory and research in the new millennium: Current trends and changing perspectives. *The Leadership Quarterly, 25,* 36–62.

Duffield, C., Roche, M., Blay, N., & Stasa. H. (2011). Nursing unit managers, staff retention, and the work environment. *Journal of Clinical Nursing, 20*(1–2), 23–33.

Edmonson, C. (2015). Moral courage and the nurse leader. *OJIN: The Online Journal of Issues in Nursing, 20*(2). Retrieved from http://www.nursingworld.org/MainMenuCategories/EthicsStandards/Courage-and-Distress/Moral-Courage-for-Nurse-Leaders.html

Fox, E., Crigger, B. J., Bottrell, M., & Bauck, P. (2007). Ethical leadership: Fostering an ethical environment and culture. Retrieved from http://www.ethics.va.gov/Elprimer.pdf

Gallagher, A., & Tschudin, V. (2010). Educating for ethical leadership. *Nurse Educator Today, 30*(3), 224–227.

Galletta, M., Portoghese, I., Battistelli, A., & Leiter, M. (2013). The roles of unit leadership and nurse-physician collaboration on nursing turnover intention. *The Journal of Advanced Nursing, 69*(8), 1771–1784.

Grace, P. (2014). *Nursing ethics and professional responsibility in advanced practice.* Burlington, VT: Jones & Bartlett Learning.

Hewko, S., Brown, P., Fraser, D., Wong, C., & Cummings, G. (2015). Factors influencing nurse managers' intent to stay or leave: A quantitative analysis. *Journal of Nursing Management, 23*(8), 1058–1066.

Huber, D. (2014). *Leadership and nursing care management.* St. Louis, MO: Elsevier.

Hwang, J., & Park, H. (2014). Nurses' perceptions of ethical climate, medical error experience, and intent-to-leave. *Nursing Ethics, 21*(1), 28–42.

Interprofessional Education Collaborative Expert Panel. (2011). *Core competencies for interprofessional collaborative practice: Report of an expert panel.* Washington, DC: Interprofessional Education Collaborative.

The Joint Commission. (2016). *Comprehensive accreditation manual, hospitals (CAMH).* Oakbrook Terrace, IL: Author.

Jordan, J., Brown, M., Trevino, L., & Finklestein, S. (2013). Someone to look up to: Executive-follower reasoning and perceptions of ethical leadership. *Journal of Management, 39*(3), 660–683.

Kath, L., Stichler, J., & Ehrhart, M. (2012). Moderators of the negative outcomes of nurse manager stress. *The Journal of Nursing Administration, 42*(4), 215–221.

Keselman, D. (2012). Ethical leadership. *Holistic Nursing Practice, 26*(5), 259–261.

Laschinger, H., & Smith, L. (2013). The influence of authentic leadership and empowerment on new graduate nurses' perceptions of interprofessional collaboration. *The Journal of Nursing Administration, 43*(1), 24–29.

Lucas, V., Laschinger, H., & Wong, C. (2008). The impact of emotional intelligent leadership on staff nurse empowerment: The moderating effect of span of control. *Journal of Nursing Management, 16*(8), 964–973.

Lytle, S., Stagno, S. J., & Daly, B. (2013). Repetitive foreign body ingestion: Ethical considerations. *Journal of Clinical Ethics, 24*(2), 91–97.

Makaroff, K., Storch, J., Pauly, B., & Newton, L. (2014). Searching for ethical leadership in nursing. *Nursing Ethics, 21*(6), 642–658.

Marquis, B., & Huston, C. (2014). *Leadership roles and management functions in nursing* (8th ed.). Philadelphia, PA: Wolters Kluwer, Lippincott, Williams, & Wilkins.

Ng, T., & Feldman, D. (2015). Ethical leadership: Meta-analytic evidence of criterion-related and incremental validity. *Journal of Applied Psychology, 100*(3), 948–965.

Numinen, O., Leino-Kilpi, H., Isoaho, H., & Meretoja, R. (2015). Newly graduated nurses' competence and individual and organizational factors: A multivariate analysis. *Journal of Nursing Scholarship, 47*(5), 446–457.

Olson, L. (1998). Hospital nurses' perceptions of the ethical climate of their work setting. *Journal of Nursing Scholarship, 30*(4), 345–349.

Papathanassoglou, E., Katanikola, E., & Kalafati, M. (2012). Professional autonomy, collaboration with physicians, and moral distress among European intensive care nurses. *American Journal of Critical Care, 21*(2), 41–52.

Park, M., Kjervik, D., & Crandall, J. (2012). The relationship of ethics education to moral sensitivity and moral reasoning skills of nursing students. *Nursing Ethics, 19*(4), 568–580.

Pavlish, C., Brown-Saltzman, K., Fine, A., & Jakel, P. (2015a). A culture of avoidance: Voices from inside ethically difficult clinical situations. *Clinical Journal of Oncology Nursing, 19*(2), 159–165.

Pavlish, C., Brown-Saltzman, K., Jakel, P., & Fine, A. (2014). The nature of ethical conflicts and the meaning of moral community in oncology practice. *Oncology Nursing Forum, 1*(41), 130–140.

Pavlish, C., Brown-Saltzman, K., So, L., Heers, A., & Iorillo, N. (2015b). Avenues of action in ethically complex situations: A critical incident study. *The Journal of Nursing Administration, 45*(6), 311–318.

Pavlish, C., Brown-Saltzman, K., So, L., & Wong, J. (2016). SUPPORT: An evidence-based model for leaders addressing moral distress. *Journal of Nursing Administration, 46*(3), 313–320.

Pavlish, C., Hellyer, J., Brown-Saltzman, K., Myers, A., & Squire, K. (2013). Barriers to innovation: Nurses' risk appraisal in using a new ethics screening and early intervention tool. *Advances in Nursing Science, 36*(4), 304–319.

Pavlish, C., Hellyer, J., Brown-Saltzman, K., Myers, A., & Squire, K. (2015c). Screening situations for risk of ethical conflicts: A pilot study. *American Journal of Critical Care, 24*(3), 248–256.

Pavlish, C., Ho, A., & Rounkle, A. (2012). Health and human rights advocacy: Perspectives from a Rwandan refugee camp. *Nursing Ethics, 19*(4), 538–549.

Peden-McAlpine, C., Liaschenko, J., Traudt, T., & Gilmore-Szott, E. (2015). Constructing the story: How nurses work with families regarding withdrawal of aggressive treatment in ICU: A narrative study. *International Journal of Nursing Studies, 52*(7), 1146–1156

Piper, L. (2011). The ethical leadership challenge: Creating a culture of patient- and family-centered care in the hospital setting. *Health Care Manager. 30*(2), 125–132.

Piper, L., & Tallman, E. (2015). The ethical leadership challenge for effective resolution of patient and family complaints and grievances: Proven methods and models. *Health Care Manager, 34*(1), 62–68.

Poikkeus, T., Numminen, O., Suhonen, R., & Leino-Kilpi, H. (2013). A mixed method systematic review: Support for ethical competence of nurses. *Journal of Advanced Nursing*, *70*(2), 256–271.

Pointer, D. (2006). Leadership: A framework for thinking and acting. In S. Shortell & A. Kaluzny (Eds.), *Health care management: Organization design and behavior* (5th ed.). Albany, NY: Delmar.

Porter, R. (2010). *Nurse managers' moral distress in the context of the hospital ethical climate.* (Unpublished doctoral dissertation). University of Iowa, Iowa City. Retrieved from http://ir.uiowa .edu/cgi/viewcontent.cgi?article=2738&context=etd

Registered Nurse III Performance Review Tool. (2012). *Christiana health care system*. Wilmington, DE.

Sama, L., & Schoaf, V. (2008). Ethical leadership for the professions: Fostering a moral community. *Journal of Business Ethics*, *78*(1–2), 39–46.

Sauerland, J., Marotta, K., Peinemann, M., Berndt, A., & Robichaux, C. (2014). Assessing and addressing moral distress and ethical climate. *Dimensions of Critical Care Nursing*, *33*(4), 234–245.

Sauerland, J., Marotta, K., Peinemann, M., Berndt, A., & Robichaux, C. (2015). Assessing and addressing moral distress and ethical climate, Part II: Neonatal and pediatric perspectives. *Dimensions in Critical Care Nursing*, *34*(1), 33–46.

Scott, E., & Miles, J. (2013). Advancing leadership capacity in nursing. *Nursing Administration Quarterly*, *37*(1), 77–82.

Shirey, M., McDaniel, A., Ebright, P., Fisher, M., & Doebbeling, B. (2010). Understanding nurse manager stress and work complexity: Factors that make a difference. *The Journal of Nursing Administration*, *40*(2), 82–91.

Storch, J., Makaroff, K., Pauly, B., & Newton, L. (2013). Take me to my leader: The importance of ethical leadership among formal nurse leaders. *Nursing Ethics*, *20*(2), 150–157.

Suhonen, R., Stolt, M., Gustafsson, M. L., Katajisto, J., & Charalambous, A. (2014). The associations among the ethical climate, the professional practice environment and individualized care in care settings for older people. *Journal of Advanced Nursing*, *70*(6), 1356–1368.

Texas Board of Nursing. (2013). Safe harbor forms—nursing peer review. Retrieved from https:// www.bon.texas.gov/forms_safe_harbor.asp

Thompson, D., Hoffman, L., & Sereika, S. (2011). A relational leadership perspective on unit level safety climate. *The Journal of Nursing Administration*, *41*(11), 479–487.

Tonkin, T. (2013). Authentic versus transformational leadership: Assessing their effectiveness on organizational citizenship behavior of followers. *International Journal of Business and Public Administration*, *10*(1), 40–61.

Tregunno, D., Jeffs, L., Hall, L., Baker, R., Doran, D., & Bassett, S. (2009). On the ball: Leadership for patient safety and learning in critical care. *The Journal of Nursing Administration*, *39*(7–8), 334–339.

Trossman, S. (2013). Code interwoven into job performance, peer review. *The American Nurse*. Retrieved from www.theamericannurse.org/index.php/2013/09/03/code-interwoven-in-job -performance-peer-review

Ulrich, B. (1992). *Leadership and management according to Florence Nightingale*. Norwalk, CT: Appleton & Lange.

Ulrich, C., Taylor, C., Soeken, K., O'Donnell, P., Farrar, A., Danis, M., & Grady, C. (2010). Everyday ethics: Ethical issues and stress in nursing practice. *Journal of Advanced Nursing*, *66*(11), 1365–1380.

Varcoe, C., Pauly, B., Storch, J., Newton, L., & Makaroff, K. (2012). Nurses' perceptions of and responses to morally distressing situations. *Nursing Ethics*, *19*(4), 488–500.

Whitehead, P., Herbertson, R., Hamric, A., Epstein, E., & Fisher, J. (2015). Moral distress among healthcare professionals: Report of an institution-wide survey. *Journal of Nursing Scholarship*, *47*(2), 117–125.

Wong, C., Spence Laschinger, H., & Cziraki, K. (2014). The role of incentives in nurses' aspirations to management roles. *The Journal of Nursing Administration, 44*(6), 362–367.

Zheng, D., Witt, L., Waite, E., David, E., van Driel, M., McDonald, D. P., . . . , Crepeau, L. J. (2015). Effects of ethical leadership on emotional exhaustion in high moral intensity situations. *The Leadership Quarterly, 26*(5), 732–748.

Zook, E. (2014). Effective leadership promotes perioperative success. *AORN Journal, 100*(1), 4–7.

9

Public Health Ethics and Social Justice in the Community

JOAN KUB

Upon completion of this chapter the student will be able to:

- Define public health and public health ethics
- Differentiate public health ethics from clinical ethics
- Describe the ethical tensions inherent in addressing public health problems
- Discuss different theoretical approaches and principles used in public health ethics
- Apply a public health framework in analyzing the development of a new program or policy
- Discuss ethical principles involved in implementing programs and designing policies in the community

As a practicing nurse, you more than likely have experienced situations that involve clinical ethics. In general, clinical ethics focuses on the nurse and other providers' roles in individual patient/family issues such as confidentiality, privacy, respect, and autonomy. In contrast, public health ethics is concerned with the overall health of communities and populations. Public health also seeks to better understand social inequities in health and to address them using a social justice lens, a responsibility of all nurses as identified in the Code of Ethics (2015). Since public health nursing is a specialty area you may or may not have experienced public health ethical situations.

This chapter discusses the development of the burgeoning field of public health ethics. In doing so it (a) differentiates clinical ethics from public/population health ethics; (b) discusses theoretical foundations and principles of public health ethics; (c) discusses the relevance of human rights and social justice as key to public health ethics; (d) presents one framework for analyzing public or population health decision making; and (e) uses selected public health issues to illustrate the application of theory and principles in the analysis and justification of public health decisions and actions.

CASE SCENARIO

On January 5, 2015, the California Department of Health was notified of a suspected case of measles. The 11-year-old unvaccinated child had visited one of two adjacent Disney theme parks located in Orange County, California. On that same day, six additional suspected measles cases, all of whom had visited the same theme parks from December 17 to 20, were also reported in California and Utah. By February 11, a total of 125 measles cases with a rash occurred from December 28, 2014 to February 8, 2015 (Zipprich et al., 2015). "Among the 110 California patients, 49 (45%) were unvaccinated; five (5%) had 1 dose of measles-containing vaccine, seven (6%) had 2 doses, one (1%) had 3 doses, 47 (43%) had unknown or undocumented vaccination status, and one (1%) had immunoglobulin G seropositivity documented, which indicates prior vaccination or measles infection at an undetermined time" (Zipprich et al., 2015, p. 153). From January 1 to August 21, 2015, 188 people from 24 states and the District of Columbia developed reportable measles. One hundred and seventeen cases (62%) were part of a large multistate outbreak linked to the amusement park in California (Centers for Disease Control and Prevention, 2015a).

This Case Scenario raises several ethical questions that have implications for the health of the public. The key question is whether compulsory mandated measles vaccination that impinges upon individual autonomy, privacy, and liberty is justifiable for reasons of protecting the health of the entire population and realizing public health goals?

Questions to Consider Before Reading On

1. Do you believe compulsory mandated measles vaccination that impinges upon individual autonomy, privacy, and liberty is justifiable for reasons of protecting the health of the entire population and realizing public health goals?

2. Are certain vaccinations mandatory for nurses where you currently work?

Measles is a serious illness with the potential of putting the health of the public at risk with devastating outcomes for individuals and populations. Controversies and tensions exist surrounding concerns about vaccine safety, mandatory school vaccination regulations, suboptimal vaccine coverage, the prevalence of preventable cases of disease, the fairness of exemptions to the law, and liberty/personal rights (Ransom, Swain, & Duchin, 2008). In 2013, the Institute of Medicine report *Childhood Immunization Schedule and Safety: Stakeholder Concerns, Scientific Evidence, and Future Studies* provided an update on the safety of immunizations for children (Chi, 2014; Institute of Medicine, 2013). Despite this report, it is clear that hesitancy about immunizing children and refusals to immunize children are growing problems, so much so that a study of families in California found that personal belief exemption rates rose by 9.2% from 0.6% in 1994 to 2.3% in 2009 (Richards et al., 2013). This Case Scenario illustrates concerns about individual rights/autonomy versus concern for the overall good of the public.

PUBLIC HEALTH AND PUBLIC HEALTH ETHICS

The field of public health ethics evolved in the early 1980s with the emergence of a number of infectious diseases such as AIDS and severe acute respiratory syndrome (SARS; Knight, 2015; Simón-Lorda, Barrio-Cantalejo, & Peinado-Gorlat, 2015). Debates concerning the relationship of ethics, public health, and human rights surfaced at this time. It became clear that actions required in public health practice are different from actions required in clinical ethics. These differences stem in large part because of the nature of public health.

In 1988, the Institute of Medicine (IOM) defined public health as what we, as a society, do collectively to ensure the conditions in which people can be healthy (Institute of Medicine, 1988). The IOM report went on to define the core functions of public health as assessment, assurance, and policy development (Figure 9.1). The American Public Health Association further defined public health by the 10 essential services that help define effective performance (American Public Health Association, n.d.; Table 9.1). Public health seeks to improve the health of communities and populations. It is concerned with not only understanding the causes of disease but first and foremost the prevention of disease. It is often focused on underlying social, economic, and environmental conditions and population-level health interventions, policies, or programs that shift the distribution of health risk.

A five-tier health impact pyramid illustrates the focus of interventions in public health. (Figure 9.2; Frieden, 2010). The broad base focuses on what has now been called social determinants of health (housing, sanitation, nutrition) followed by interventions that change the context for health (clean water, safe roads, eliminating trans fat in foods), followed by protective interventions such as immunizations, followed by direct clinical care and counseling and education. The two top tiers are focused more on individual care and are dependent on individuals changing their behavior. The lowest

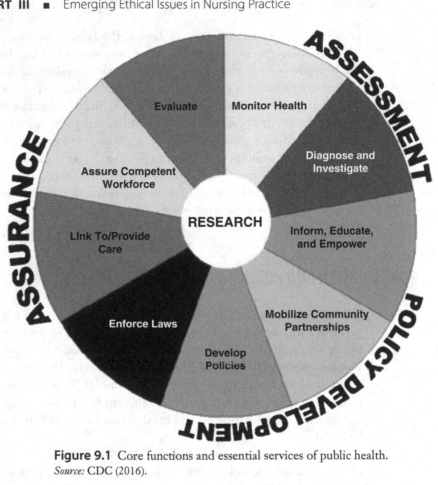

Figure 9.1 Core functions and essential services of public health.
Source: CDC (2016).

tier has the greatest potential to change population health, while tier 2 usually consists of the most effective public health actions (Frieden, 2010).

 Questions to Consider Before Reading On

1. What interventions could nurses implement at each tier in Figure 9.2?

2. What are the ethical implications of these interventions?

PUBLIC HEALTH ETHICS

In 2002, the American Public Health Association adopted a code of ethics for public health practice (Public Health Leadership Society, 2002; Thomas, Sage, Dillenberg, & Guillory, 2002; see Table 9.2). Until that time, public health was guided by medical ethics with the four principles of autonomy, beneficence, nonmaleficence, and justice (Thomas, 2008). Although these

Table 9.1

Ten Essential Public Health Services

1. **Monitor** health status to identify community health problems.

2. **Diagnose and investigate** health problems and health hazards in the community.

3. **Inform, educate, and empower** people about health issues.

4. **Mobilize** community partnerships to identify and solve health problems.

5. **Develop policies and plans** that support individual and community health efforts.

6. **Enforce** laws and regulations that protect health and ensure safety.

7. **Link** people to needed personal health services and ensure the provision of health care when otherwise unavailable.

8. **Ensure** a competent public health and personal health care workforce.

9. **Evaluate** effectiveness, accessibility, and quality of personal and population-based health services.

10. **Research** for new insights and innovative solutions to health problems.

Source: American Public Health Association (n.d.).

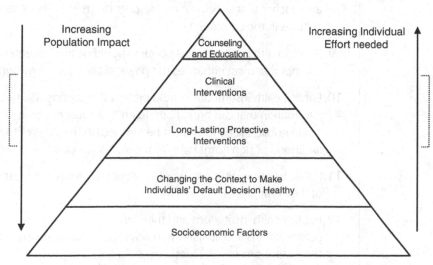

Figure 9.2 Five-tier health impact pyramid.
Source: Frieden (2010).

Table 9.2

Principles of Public Health

1. Public health should address principally the fundamental causes of disease and requirements for health, aiming to prevent adverse health outcomes.

2. Public health should achieve community health in a way that respects the rights of individuals in the community.

3. Public health policies, programs, and priorities should be developed and evaluated through processes that ensure an opportunity for input from community members.

4. Public health should advocate and work for the empowerment of disenfranchised community members, aiming to ensure that the basic resources and conditions necessary for health are accessible to all.

5. Public health should seek the information needed to implement effective policies and programs that protect and promote health.

6. Public health institutions should provide communities with the information they have that is needed for decisions on policies or programs and should obtain the community's consent for their implementation.

7. Public health institutions should act in a timely manner on the information they have within the resources and the mandate given to them by the public.

8. Public health programs and policies should incorporate a variety of approaches that anticipate and respect diverse values, beliefs, and cultures in the community.

9. Public health programs and policies should be implemented in a manner that most enhances the physical and social environment.

10. Public health institutions should protect the confidentiality of information that can bring harm to an individual or community if made public. Exceptions must be justified on the basis of the high likelihood of significant harm to the individual or others.

11. Public health institutions should ensure the professional competence of their employees.

12. Public health institutions and their employees should engage in collaborations and affiliations in ways that build the public's trust and the institution's effectiveness.

Source: Public Health Leadership Society (2002).

principles guide the interactions between individuals and their health care providers, ethical quandaries in public health are concerned with the needs of populations. The moral considerations generally include concerns with . . .

> producing benefits; avoiding, preventing, and removing harms; producing the maximal balance of benefits over harms and other costs (often called utility); distributing benefits and burdens fairly (distributive justice) and ensuring public participation including the participation of affected parties (procedural justice); respecting autonomous choices and actions, including liberty of action; protecting privacy and confidentiality; keeping promises and commitments; disclosing information as well as speaking honestly and truthfully (often grouped under transparency); and building and maintaining trust. (Childress et al., 2002, pp. 171–172)

Although some of these moral considerations apply to clinical ethics, there are distinct differences between public health ethics and clinical ethics. Clinical ethics is concerned with the individual patient and relationships with individual clinicians. Typical concerns include issues of confidentiality, privacy, respect, and autonomy (Carter, Kerridge, Sainsbury, & Letts, 2012). In contrast, public health ethics is focused on collective thinking and tradeoffs between the well-being of communities and the well-being of individuals (Carter et al., 2012). According to the Canadian Institutes of Health Research (2012), public health ethics differs from traditional bioethics because of its emphasis on moral evaluations related to populations, the realization that "upstream" interventions occur outside the health care system, and the focus on the prevention of illness and disease.

The prevention imperative is evident, for example, in current global HIV/AIDS policy discussions. Although the initial focus of HIV/AIDS policy was focused on individual behavior and ensuring access to biomedical treatment, public health efforts are now focused on a combination of behavioral, structural, and biomedical prevention strategies (Meier, Brugh, & Halima, 2012). The behavioral approaches include not only traditional educational and motivational approaches but also community normative approaches. The aim of structural approaches is to change the social, economic, political, and environmental factors that influence HIV risk and vulnerability. The biomedical approaches involve technological interventions not solely dependent on behavior change (Meir et al., 2012).

Question to Consider Before Reading On

1. What are some of the identified public health needs in your community?

THEORETICAL FOUNDATIONS AND PRINCIPLES OF PUBLIC HEALTH ETHICS

Within both clinical and public health ethics, it is important to examine the theory and principles guiding normative behavior. Theories that are particularly pertinent to public health ethics are utilitarianism, deontology, libertarian theories, and communitarianism. These theories have been described in earlier chapters but often have particular relevance to public health. Utilitarianism, for example, is often used to justify public health interventions supporting the belief that the most ethical course of action is the one that produces the greatest good for the greatest number (Buchanan, 2008). The moral worth of actions using utilitarianism is based on their contributions to overall "utility" (Mill & Bentham, 1987). Utilitarianism often utilizes economic approaches such as cost–benefit analyses or cost-effectiveness analyses to guide decision making in public health (Faden & Powers, 2008). Deontology is the theory proposed by Kant that begins with the premise that human beings have the capacity for reason and are worthy of respect and dignity. Therefore, human beings have a duty to respect the dignity of other human beings and humans should not be treated as a means to an end (Misselbrook, 2013). In public health, appeals to the avoidance of stigmatization of vulnerable groups such as individuals with HIV have been used to guide moral decision making within the public realm (Dean, 2014). Libertarian theory is concerned with ensuring that public policies do not violate human rights or rights to property influencing tax policies (Faden & Powers, 2008). Communitarianism is a social philosophy concerned with a collective reflection on shared values and what is good for society. Communitarians examine the ways shared good or values are formed, transmitted, justified, and enforced (Etzioni, 2006). Communitarian ethics can be used in examining the allocation of scarce resources and rationing of care or resources in time of need (Etzioni, 2011) or in the development of infectious disease policies (Cheyette, 2011).

PRINCIPLES OF PUBLIC HEALTH ETHICS

The principles that have particular relevance to our discussion of public health ethics are paternalism, human rights, and social justice.

Paternalism Versus Autonomy

Distinguishing clinical ethics from public health ethics is often concerned with identifying when paternalistic interventions that override individual autonomy are justified (Buchanan, 2008). Paternalism is described by Schickle as the interference with a person's autonomy by performing an act or agreeing to perform an act without the consent of that person with the intention of improving or preventing a decline in the welfare of that person (Schickle, 2009).

Discussions of paternalism often relate back to a 1905 single Supreme Court case, *Jacobson* v. *Massachusetts*. The court found:

> The liberty secured by the Constitution of the United States to every person within its jurisdiction does not impart an absolute right in each person to be, at all times and in all circumstances, wholly freed from restraint. There are manifold restraints to which every person is necessarily subject for the common good. (Supreme Court of the United States, decided February 20, 1905, cited by Buchanan, 2008)

In thinking about communicable diseases, overriding individual rights or autonomy for purposes of controlling infectious diseases is often justified. Tuberculosis, for example, is a classic example when individual patients have been "quarantined" in the past to ensure a cure and to protect others from the disease. This is an example of John Stuart Mill's theory of liberty and "harm principle" that is invoked to control risk and to control infectious diseases. This is justified since an individual poses a significant harm to others and therefore liberty-limiting interventions are supported (Gostin & Gostin, 2009).

In cases of infectious diseases, it is easier to justify what appear to be paternalistic public health interventions. Today we are not only concerned about infectious diseases, however, but also the growing public health emphasis on noncommunicable diseases. The key question is whether any public health intervention can rightfully infringe upon individual autonomy. Childress and colleagues defined five "justificatory conditions" when this could occur. These criteria include (a) effectiveness, (b) proportionality, (c) necessity, (d) least infringement, and (e) public justification. An intervention or policy must show evidence of realizing its goal, being necessary for the accomplishment of the goal, and justifiable by public health agents. In addition, it is essential to show that the public health benefits outweigh the infringed moral considerations (proportionality) and the public health agents seek to minimize and attain the least infringement of general moral considerations (Childress et al., 2002).

Question to Consider Before Reading On

1. Recall a recent incident of communicable or noncommunicable disease. Did the interventions proposed and/or implemented meet the criteria defined by Childress et al. (2002)?

CASE SCENARIO *(CONTINUED)*

Returning to our Case Scenario, mandating school vaccinations would be considered an example of overriding individual autonomy for the welfare of the entire community with the goal of achieving health for children. This case does raise other complex concerns. There are often differing opinions about not only

(continued)

CASE SCENARIO (*CONTINUED*)

the justification of mandating the vaccines, but also the legitimacy of allowing exceptions to the mandate. The arguments used against mandatory vaccination requirements are often based on autonomy and various beliefs that vaccinations cause more individual harm than benefit. The "vaccine hesitant" parents cite several reasons for their concerns including negative beliefs that children receive too many vaccines, the side effects outweigh the benefits, perceptions that vaccines may negatively impact their immune systems, there is an increased risk of autism, and fears about mercury or thimerosal in vaccines (Williams, 2014). Consequently parents sometimes seek exemptions to the policies.

These arguments illustrate the complexity involved with justifying public health interventions and the tensions between traditional principles of autonomy, beneficence, and nonmaleficence. In the case of mandatory vaccinations for children, the ultimate goal is the health of the community. At the end of this chapter, a framework applied to mandatory vaccination of health care workers (HCWs) is presented that can also be used in thinking about mandatory childhood vaccination (Kass, 2001). Ethical questions for consideration include:

- What are the public health goals of the mandatory vaccination program?

- How effective is mandatory vaccination in achieving its stated goals?

- What are the known or potential burdens of the program including considerations of the threat to individual liberty?

- Can burdens be minimized and are there alternative approaches?

In the case of mandatory childhood vaccinations, exemptions often include medical or personal beliefs. States are currently making exemption processes more restrictive in hopes of reducing the numbers of exemptions (Constable, Blank, & Caplan, 2013). Two additional questions for consideration are whether programs are implemented fairly and if benefits and burdens of a program such as mandatory vaccination can be fairly balanced. The ultimate concern, though, of mandatory childhood vaccination is the health of the community.

In other examples of public health interventions such as regulating seatbelt usage, wearing motorcycle helmets, or fluoridation of water at a community level, regulations are intended to safeguard the individual's own health and safety (Gostin & Gostin, 2009). Using Mill's concept of liberty, these public health efforts would not necessarily be justified since the intervention primarily affects the person concerned. Others would argue, however, that "hard paternalism" in which a person knows that his or her actions or inactions can be harmful is justified if the interventions do not pose a truly significant burden on individual liberty but safeguards the health and well-being of the population (Gostin & Gostin, 2009; Schickle, 2009).

These arguments for the justification of "hard paternalism" in public health are also evident in the most recent approaches in addressing noncommunicable diseases, especially with the rising rates of overweight and obesity in populations (Carter & Rychetnik, 2013). Hard paternalism is defined as an action that may be permissible when the individual knows that actions or inactions could be harmful (Shickle, 2009). Approximately one third of U.S. adults and 16% of children and adolescents aged 2 to18 years are obese (Flegal, Carroll, Kit, & Ogden, 2012; Ogden, Carroll, Kit, & Flegal, 2012).This growing concern about the negative effects of overeating and unhealthy eating has resulted in the development and implementation of policies that are meant to improve healthy eating. These policies include bans on trans fat in restaurants, nutritional requirements for fast-food meals, policies to limit unhealthy food from food assistance programs, taxes on sugary drinks, or policies to limit the sale of large sugary drinks (Barnhill & King, 2013; Resnik, 2015). The ethical concerns about such policies have focused on concepts such as "fairness, equality, respect, legitimacy, paternalism, infantization, as well as liberty and freedom" (Barnhill & King, 2013, p. 117). According to Barnwall and King (2013), concerns about obesity policies actually focus on three dimensions of autonomy—liberty, understanding of available options, and psychological capacity—to make choices and to act on them. Using the ban on the sale of sugary drinks as an example, one ethical criticism is that these policies limit individual liberty due to external restraint while a counter argument stresses that these policies actually promote autonomy since they increase an individual's psychological capacity to make good choices.

Questions to Consider Before Reading On

1. Do you agree or disagree with the ethical criticism of the ban on sugary drinks?

2. What is your opinion about the counter argument that the ban promotes autonomy?

Human Rights, Health, and Health Care

A human rights approach is used to think about public health problems (Easley & Allen, 2007; Ivanov & Oden, 2013). This approach strengthens public health ethics by defining health as a human right, protecting human rights as a determinant of health, and focusing on the duties of states to realize the health of citizens (Nixon & Forman, 2008). Human rights can be both negative rights (noninterference) and positive rights (receiving or possessing certain goods; Carter et al., 2012). In the case of paternalism, the concern is often with negative rights (noninterference). In contrast, positive rights are concerned with a right to health, privacy, and/or confidentiality.

The World Health Organization (WHO) first articulated health as a fundamental human right in the 1946 Constitution of the WHO. It defined health as a "state of complete physical, mental, and social well-being and not merely the absence of disease or infirmity" (WHO, n.d.). These ideas were further developed in 1948 with the Universal Declaration of Human Rights that also mentioned health as part of the right to an adequate standard of living (Article 25; Office of the United Nations High Commissioner for Human Rights, n.d.).

> Everyone has the right to a standard of living adequate for the health and well-bing of himself and of his family including food, clothing, housing, and medical care and necessary social services, and the right to security in the event of unemployment, sickness, disability, widowhood, old age, or other lack of livelihood in circumstances beyond his control. Motherhood and childhood are entitled to special care and assistance.

In 2000, the United Nations Committee on Economic, Social, and Cultural Rights further developed these ideas by specifying that the right to health extends to timely and appropriate health care as well as underlying determinants of health such as water, sanitation, an adequate supply of food, housing, health education including sexual and reproductive health, and healthy occupational and environmental conditions (World Health Organization, 2013).

Within clinical ethics, individual rights–based frameworks are often used to support the provision of medical treatment initiatives. The HIV/AIDS pandemic was an example of how human rights were initially operationalized for public health (Meier, Brugh, & Halima, 2012). Initially the pandemic in the early stages of the disease led to the development of HIV/AIDS policy with a focus on prevention in contrast to treatment and concerns about discrimination, privacy, confidentiality, equal access to care, and other human resources (Easley & Allen, 2007).

Social Justice

Despite the fact that international conventions and institutions emphatically say that health is a human right, health statistics do not substantiate this (Eleftheriadis, 2012). Whether health is viewed as a right or a value, the important point is that health inequalities or inequities exist and these are of concern to public health. In 2007, the Nuffield Council on Bioethics published a report, *Public Health: Ethical Issues*, that outlines a model of public health ethics called the *stewardship model* (Lee, 2012; Nuffield Council on Bioethics, 2007). The model is based on a liberal framework with the belief that liberal states have a duty to look after the important needs of people individually and collectively. Although a major focus of the report was on clarifying the issues of individual rights versus collective needs, one of the major points of discussion was concerned with inequalities in health. Questions focused on whether success was defined by health outcomes or access to resources and within which groups or subgroups should equality be sought. This report also emphasized the importance of "community" defined as a society in which each person's welfare mattered to everyone else (Lee, 2012).

Terms used to discuss disparities such as *inequalities* and *inequities* are sometimes confusing and not well defined. *Health disparities* was defined by Margaret Whitehead in the early 1990s as differences that are unfair and unjust in addition to being avoidable and unnecessary (Whitehead, 1992). Health equity was defined by Braveman as "providing all people with fair opportunities to attain their full health potential to the extent possible" (Braveman, 2006, p. 181). There are two different types of health equity— horizontal and vertical. Horizontal equity means equal treatment for equal needs while vertical equity refers to different levels of treatment for different needs. In the latter case, one would expect greater expenditures of resources to treat people most in need—poor individuals with more chronic conditions in comparison to wealthier individuals (Giles & Leburd, 2010).

The relevance of justice or fairness to public health ethics in addressing inequalities and inequities is founded on "a societal responsibility to protect and promote the health of the population as a whole" (Buchanan, 2008, p. 15). Justice is central to the mission of public health and it is considered a core value that guides public health practice (Gostin & Powers, 2006). It is focused on health improvement for the population and fair treatment of the disadvantaged. Its attributes have been defined by Buettner-Schmidt and Lobo (2011) as follows:

- Fairness
- Equity in the distribution of power, resources, and processes that affect social determinants of health
- Just institutions, systems, structures, policies, and processes
- Equity in human development, rights, and sustainability
- Sufficiency of well-being

Justice is usually defined in two major categories: procedural and distributive (Summers, 2014). Procedural is concerned with whether certain procedures were followed while distributive justice is concerned with the allocation of resources.

John Rawls (1971) is perhaps best known for his philosophical egalitarian theory of justice as fairness presented in his original 1971 work, *A Theory of Justice*. Rawls addresses distributive justice issues by using a social contract theory. His theory consists of two principles of justice. The first principle is one of liberty with each person having the most extensive basic liberty in line with the liberty of others and the second principle stating that social and economic positions are to everyone's advantage (Wenar, 2013). Objective decisions are to then be made under a veil of ignorance maximizing the minimum level of primary goods (Ruger, 2008). This theory was not directly applied to health care although Norman Daniels has used it to argue that health care is a right because it provides equality of opportunity (Daniels, 1985). Three exemplars that have particular relevance to a discussion of justice are access to health services, social determinants of health, and allocation of scare resources in time of emergencies.

Questions to Consider Before Reading On

1. Provision 8.1 of the Code of Ethics (2015) states that health is a universal right. What is your understanding of this assertion?

2. What is the nurse's role in meeting this obligation?

ACCESS TO HEALTH SERVICES: A SOCIAL JUSTICE CONCERN

The United States is one of the few industrial countries that does not guarantee ongoing access to health care for its citizens (Dalen, Waterbrook, & Alpert, 2015). Health care outcomes including measures such as infant mortality and life expectancy are worse than in other Western countries. The Patient Protection and Affordable Care Act (ACA) that passed in March 2010 seeks to improve these statistics and target major impediments in accessing health care for millions of Americans. Its goal is to improve the health of Americans by increasing the number of individuals covered by insurance. This act was the culmination of decades of political debate revolving around issues of health care access, quality of care, costs, and the role of government in health care (Gable, 2011). The focus of the ACA is on health insurance reform with prevention as a key theme in its initiatives. It also supports marked expansions in Medicaid coverage, thus decreasing the number of uninsured individuals.

The Patient Protection and ACA completed the second enrollment period in February 2015 (Dalen et al., 2015; Sommers, Gunja, Finegold, & Musco, 2015). The percentage of uninsured individuals decreased from 18% to 19% after the introduction of the ACA (Geyman, 2015; Hall & Lord, 2014). Despite these improvements, many uninsured individuals reside within states that have chosen not to expand Medicaid services to the poor, a benefit that is possible with ACA. As of January 2016, 17 states have chosen not to extend Medicaid services to individuals (The Advisory Board Company, 2015). A recent study of 156 clinics in nine states found that clinics in Medicaid expansion states had a 40% decrease in the rate of uninsured visits in the postexpansion period and a 36% increase in the rate of Medicaid-covered visits. Clinics in nonexpansion states had a significant 16% decline in the rate of uninsured visits but no change in the rate of Medicaid-covered visits. Sommers and colleagues found similar findings supporting the fact that Medicaid expansions are associated with significant benefits for low-income individuals (Sommers et al., 2015). Despite the significant improvements associated with the ACA, challenges remain including the expansion of Medicaid services. It is still predicted that 36 to 45 million individuals will be uninsured by 2019 (Geyman, 2015; Hall & Lord, 2014).

Questions to Consider Before Reading On

1. What are some problems associated with access to health care in the community in which you live?

2. What are the ethical implications of limited access to health care?

3. What is the nurse's ethical role in improving access to health care?

DISPARITIES AND SOCIAL DETERMINANTS OF HEALTH

Disparities in health are often driven by social determinants that include socioeconomic status, social structure, education, social position, racism, and discrimination (Trin-Shevrin, Islam, Nadkarni, Park, & Kwon, 2015). Other significant determinants include housing, transportation, and concerns about the built environment. These inequalities are seen across the life span and across the globe. Life expectancy differences that span sometimes 40 years between high- and low-income countries are issues of social justice. Chronic illnesses including heart disease, stroke, type 2 diabetes, and certain types of cancer disproportionally affect minority populations in the United States. American Indian or Alaska Natives (15.9%) and non-Hispanic Blacks (13.2%), for example, have higher prevalence of diabetes compared with non-Hispanic whites (7.1%; Centers for Disease Control and Prevention, 2015b). A recent study examined the interplay of race, poverty, and place (neighborhood) to estimate the impact of these variables on the odds of having diabetes (Gaskin et al., 2014). The odds of diabetes increased for Blacks and those living in poverty and in poor neighborhoods. These findings illustrate the need to address health from a broad perspective and in all policies. Examples of evidence-based approaches can be found in the Community Guide (The Community Guide to Preventive Services, n.d.). An example of addressing disparities in a North Carolina community can be seen in Box 9.1.

Box 9.1

Creating Walkable Communities in North Carolina

Problem: North Carolina tipped the scales when more than one in five of its residents were classified as obese in 2002.

Granville's Greenways Master Plan: Outlines the future of a county that embraces changing the built environment to promote active lifestyles.

(continued)

Box 9.1

Creating Walkable Communities in North Carolina (continued)

Approaches
- Creation of or enhanced access to places for physical activity combined with information about other activities
- Community-scale urban design and land use policies
- Street-scale urban design and land use policies
- Transportation and travel policies and practices

Granville's Greenways Master Plan initiative was entered into the Public Health Foundation's 2011 "I'm Your Community Guide!"

Source: Creating Walkable Communities (2012).

PUBLIC HEALTH EMERGENCIES

Public health emergencies or disasters are another example of a public health issue illustrating the junction between social justice and public health, especially as they relate to a scarcity of resources. In thinking about past diasters such as Hurricane Katrina, it is clear that disenfranchised communities can suffer excessive burdens and that planning must address what Swain and colleagues call public health principles including interdependence (individual rights versus health of others), community trust, fundamentality (concern about underlying diseases and the environment), and justice (Swain, Burns, & Etkind, 2008).

In addition to natural disasters, other disasters such as pandemic influenza have been of concern. Some important ethical considerations were outlined by a Subcommittee of the Advisory Committee for the Centers for Disease Control (Kinlaw, Barrett, & Levine, 2009). Ethical issues in emergencies often revolve around sound planning maximizing preparedness, transparency, and engagement with the community, sound science, concerns with justice, and balancing individual and liberty and community interests (Kinlaw et al., 2009). Rationing of resources in diasters of this magnitude would most likely include, for example, a limited number of mechanical ventilators to treat patients. The key question of course would be how providers would make difficult decisions as to who should be placed on a ventilator or who should remain on one (Lin & Anderson-Shaw, 2009). Lin and Anderson-Shaw present a useful algorithm based on utilitarian principles that is intended to serve as a guide in the allocation of scarce resources in a just way (Lin & Anderson-Shaw, 2009).

Another infectious disease disaster is that of Ebola, also illustrating the importance of examining these situations with a public health ethical lens.

Questions to Consider Before Reading On

1. What factors should be considered in the use of scarce resources such as mechanical ventilators in a public health emergency?

2. What are the ethical implications of these factors?

Ebola and Social Justice–QSEN–Quality and Safety–Ebola

In August, 2014, the WHO declared Ebola a public health threat to the global community. At that time the primary ethical focus was whether it was permissible to use experimental drugs in the treatment of a few individuals. There was little focus on public health issues of establishing trust and a fair distribution of resources in the face of scarcity (Dawson, 2015). Dawson points out in her ethical analysis that this public health disaster resulted in many unanswered issues about global health inequities which were relevant to issues of quality and safety. By the end of the epidemic, many health care providers had lost their lives. A few of the questions that were not initially addressed related to an inadequate public health infrastructure in the countries affected including the capacity for surveillance, security, quarantine, and protection of health workers (Dawson, 2015).

FRAMEWORKS FOR PUBLIC HEALTH ETHICS

Frameworks can guide decision making in the development of public health programs and policies. Although public health ethics is a relatively new field, there are more than 13 frameworks that have been presented with an awareness that public health raises ethical issues that require a different approach than traditional bioethics (Lee, 2012; Marckmann, Schmidt, Sofaer, & Strech, 2015). One model that can then be used in discussing public health decision making related to program or policy development is a six-step framework proposed by Nancy Kass (Kass, 2001). This model serves as an analytic tool to help consider the implications of proposed interventions, policy proposals, research initiatives, and programs (Kass, 2001). The framework raises six important questions for consideration in making decisions (Table 9.3). Important points to consider under each question are also listed. The Case Scenario on mandatory HCW vaccination presents an opportunity to apply these questions within this framework to developing either a program or policy related to this health issue.

Table 9.3

Kass's Public Health Ethics Framework

STEPS	CONSIDERATIONS
What are the public health goals of the proposed program?	Should be expressed in terms of public health improvement Epidemiologic data can provide descriptive data Ultimate concern with morbidity/mortality Other benefits could be included (e.g., social benefits)
How effective is the program in achieving its stated goals?	What data exist to substantiate assumptions of program? Does program change not only knowledge but also behavior? Implement data-based policies and programs
What are the known or potential burdens of the program?	Consider risks to privacy and confidentiality; risks to liberty and self-determination; risks to justice
Can burdens be minimized? Are there alternative approaches?	If any risks exist, can the program or policy be modified to minimize burdens without effecting the efficacy?
Is the program implemented fairly?	This refers to the ethics principle of distributive justice—fair distribution of benefits and burdens
How can the benefits and burden of a program be fairly balanced?	Most burdensome programs/policies should be implemented in context of extensive and important benefits

Source: Kass (2001).

CONCLUSION

Public health ethics has been growing over the past decade as a distinct discipline that differs from the traditional theories of clinical and bioethics (Carter et al., 2012; Lee, 2012). This chapter briefly presented the traditional ethical frameworks that have been used to think about ethics as well as the principles important in any discussion of public health. Public health ethics is concerned with the moral questions that relate to the mission of public health—ensuring the conditions in which people can be healthy. The concern is with making the right decisions related to programs and policy development to achieve health for often the most vulnerable populations in our communities. Over the past decade there are many newer frameworks that provide some guidance in this decision-making process. We started this chapter with a public health issue, the increasing number of cases of measles in our country. While the issues are different, the one public health framework by Kass provides us with the tools to examine this issue as well as other issues such as that of examining mandatory influenza vaccinations for HCWs.

The field of public health ethics will continue to evolve as the health issues and technology become increasingly complex. The benefits and burdens of public health actions will need to be distributed equitably across our society requiring tools and analytics to address the public health and ethical issues that are likely to arise. Issues that are currently and likely to raise ethical issues in the future include public health genetics, public health access to personal health information, and public health lifestyle with the prevalence of chronic illness and behavioral health issues (Rothstein, 2012).

Critical Thinking Questions and Activities

Case Example

Similar to the measles vaccination, mandatory vaccination for HCWs is another public health issue that has raised many ethical controversies. Despite recommendations from the Centers of Disease Control (CDC) on influenza vaccination since the 1980s, the rates of vaccinations among HCWs are usually around 40% to 50% (Galanakis, Jansen, Lopalco, & Giesecke, 2013). The belief that mandatory vaccination for seasonal influenza is necessary stems from the need to reduce nosocomial transmission of influenza. Some questions to think about in the development of a policy for mandatory vaccination of HCWs relate to how HCW vaccination contributes to patients' health. We can use Kass's framework to think through mandatory vaccination programs for HCWs.

1. What are the public health goals of the proposed program?

   What questions would you want to consider? What is the primary goal of your program? Do patients and HCWs benefit as a result of the HCW vaccination?

2. How effective is the program in achieving its stated goals?

   How effective is the vaccine? What is the efficacy of immunizing HCWs in preventing nosocomial transmission in health care facilities? How are various beliefs about the disease or about the vaccines handled? Is the vaccine cost-effective?

3. What are the known or potential burdens of the program?

   Can burdens be minimized? Are there alternative approaches?

(continued)

Critical Thinking Questions and Activities *(continued)*

Can burdens including the restriction on individual liberty be minimized? Are there alternative approaches to the vaccination program addressing individual objections (i.e., alternative to thimerosal)? What are the penalties for nonparticipation? How safe is the vaccine? What are the side effects?

4. Is the program implemented fairly?

How can this program be fairly implemented? How does one evaluate the sincerity of beliefs for medical or nonmedical exemptions? How does one consider conscientious exemption? Do all HCWs have to be vaccinated or would it depend on their level of patient contact? Are different forms of exemptions treated equitably? Is the review process fair?

5. How can the benefits and burden of a program be fairly balanced?

Do the health benefits to patients outweigh the health risks to the HCWs? Do the health benefits outweigh the burdens on liberty? At what level is herd immunity achieved? Are the policies within the institution outlined explicitly? What is the scope of acceptable exemptions?

6. How would you frame justice issues in this discussion of mandatory seasonal influenza immunization for HCWs?

7. Choose a relevant topic from The Guide to Community Preventive Services in the following link. How are (or could) nurses be involved in implementing the recommendations and findings?
http://www.thecommunityguide.org

(Refer Antommaria [2013], Galanakis [2013], and Omer [2013])

REFERENCES

The Advisory Board Company. (2015). Where the states stand on Medicaid expansion. Retrieved from https://www.advisory.com/daily-briefing/resources/primers/medicaidmap

American Nurses Association. (2015). *Code of ethics for nurses with interpretive statements.* Washington, DC: Author.

American Public Health Association. (n.d.). 10 essential public health services. Retrieved from https://www.apha.org/about-apha/centers-and-programs/quality-improvement-initiatives/national-public-health-performance-standards-program/10-essential-public-health-services

Antommaria, A. H. M. (2013). An ethical analysis of mandatory influenza vaccination of health care personnel: Implementing fairly and balancing benefits and burdens. *The American Journal of Bioethics, 13*(9), 30–37.

Barnhill, A., & King, K. F. (2013). Ethical agreement and disagreement about obesity prevention policy in the United States. *International Journal of Health Policy and Management, 1*(2), 117–120.

Braveman, P. (2006). Health disparities and health equity: Concepts and measurement. *Annual Review of Public Health, 27,* 167–194.

Buchanan, D. (2008). Autonomy, paternalism, and justice: Ethical priorities in public health. *American Journal of Public Health, 98*(1), 15–21.

Buettner-Schmidt, K., & Lobo, M. L. (2011). Social justice: A concept analysis. *Journal of Advanced Nursing, 68*(4), 948–958.

Canadian Institutes of Health Research. (2012). Population health ethics: Annotated bibliography. Retrieved from http://www.cihr-irsc.gc.ca/e/40740.html

Carter, S. M., Kerridge, I., Sainsbury, P., & Letts, J. K. (2012). Public health ethics: Informing better public health practice. *New South Wales Public Health Bulletin, 23*(5–6), 101–6. doi:10.1071/NB12066

Carter, S. M., & Rychetnik, L. (2013). A public health ethic approach to non-communicable diseases. *Bioethical Inquiry, 10*, 17–18.

Centers for Disease Control and Prevention. (2015a). Measles cases and outbreaks. Retrieved from http://www.cdc.gov/measles/cases-outbreaks.html

Centers for Disease Control and Prevention. (2015b). Diabetes report card 2014. Atlanta, GA: Centers for Disease Control and Prevention, U.S. Department of Health and Human Services. Retrieved from http://www.cdc.gov/diabetes/pdfs/library/diabetesreportcard2014.pdf

Centers for Disease Control and Prevention (2016). Core functions of public health and how they relate to the 10 essential services. (2016). Retrieved from http://www.cdc.gov/nceh/ehs/ephli/core_ess.htm

Cheyette, C. M. (2011). Communitarianism and the ethics of communicable disease: Some preliminary thoughts. *Journal of Law, Medicine, and Ethics, 39*(4), 678–689.

Chi, D. (2014). Caregivers who refuse preventive care for their children: The relationship between immunization and topical fluoride refusal. *American Journal of Public Health, 104*(7), 1327–1333.

Childress, J. F., Faden, R. R., Gaare, R. D., Gostin, L. O., Kahn, J., Bonnie, R. J., . . . Nieburg, P. (2002). Public health ethics: Mapping the terrain. *Journal of Law, Medicine & Ethics, 30*(2), 170–178.

The Community Guide to Preventive Services. (n.d.). Retrieved from http://www.thecommunityguide.org

Constable, C., Blank, N. R., & Caplan, A. L. (2014). Rising rates of vaccine exemptions: Problems with current policy and more promising remedies. *Vaccine, 32*(16), 1793–1797.

Creating Walkable Communities. (2012). Retrieved from http://www.thecommunityguide.org/CG-in-Action/PhysicalActivity-NC.pdf

Dalen J. E., Waterbrook, K., & Alpert, J. S. (2015). Why do so many Americans oppose the Affordable Care Act? *The American Journal of Medicine, 128*(8), 807–10. doi:10.1016/j.amjmed.2015.01.032

Daniels, N. (1985). *Just health care*. Cambridge, UK: Cambridge University Press.

Dawson, A. J. (2015). Ebola: What it tells us about medical ethics. *Journal of Medical Ethics, 41*, 107–110.

Dean, R. (2014). Stigmatization and denormalization as public health policies: Some Kantian thoughts. *Bioethics, 28*(8), 414–9. doi:10.1111/bioe.12019

Easley, C. E., & Allen, C. E. (2007). A critical intersection: Human rights, public health nursing, and nursing ethics. *Advances in Nursing Science, 30*(4), 367–382.

Eleftheriadis, P. (2012). A right to health care. *Journal of Law, Medicine, and Ethics, 40*(2), 268–285. doi:10.1111/j.1748-720X.2012.00663.x

Etzioni, A. (2006). A communitarian approach: A viewpoint on the study of legal, ethical, and policy considerations raised by DNA tests and databases. *Journal of Law, Medicine & Ethics, 34*(2), 214–222.

Etzioni, A. (2011). On a communitarian approach to bioethics. *Theoretical Medicine and Bioethics, 32*, 363–374.

Faden, R. R., & Powers, M. (2008). Health inequities and social justice. The moral foundations of public health. *BundesgesundheitsblattGesundheitsforschungGesundheitsschutz, 51*(2), 151–157. doi:10.1007/s00103-008-0443-7

Flegal, K. M., Carroll M. D., Kit, B. K., & Ogden, C. L. (2012). Prevalence of obesity and trends in the distribution of body mass index among U.S. adults, 1999–2010. *The Journal of the American Medical Association, 307*(5), 491–497.

Frieden, T. R. (2010). A framework for public health action: The health impact pyramid. *American Journal of Public Health, 100*(4), 590–595.

Gable, L. (2011). The Patient Protection and Affordable Care Act, public health, and the elusive target of human rights. *The Journal of Law Medicine & Ethics, 39*(3), 340–354.

Galanakis, E., Jansen, A., Lopalco, P. L., & Giesecke, J. (2013). Ethics of mandatory vaccination for healthcare workers. *Euro Surveillance, 18*(45), 20627.

Gaskin D. J., Thorpe R. J, McGinty, E. E., Bower, K., Rohde, C., Young, J. H., . . . Dubay, L. (2014). Disparities in diabetes: The nexus of race, poverty, and place. *The American Journal of Public Health, 104*(11), 2147–2155. doi:10.2105/AJPH.2013.301420

Geyman, J. P. (2015). A five-year assessment of the affordable care act: Market forces still trump the common good in U.S. health care. *The International Journal of Health Services, 45*(2), 209–225. doi:10.1177/0020731414568505

Giles, W. H., & Liburd, L. C. (2010). Achieving health equity and social justice. In L. Cohen, V. Chavez, & S. Chehimi (Eds.), *Prevention is primary: Strategies for community well-being* (pp. 33–53). Oakland, CA: Prevention Institute.

Gostin, L. O., & Gostin, K. G. (2009). A broader liberty: J.S. Mill, paternalism and the public's health. *Public Health, 123,* 214–221. doi:10.1016/j.puhe.2008.12.024

Gostin, L. O., & Powers, M. (2006). What does social justice require for the public's health? Public health ethics and policy imperatives. *Health Affairs, 25*(4), 1053–1060.

Hall, M. A., & Lord, R. (2014). Obamacare: What the Affordable Care Act means for patients and physicians. *British Medical Association, 349,* g5376. doi:10.1136/bmj.g5376

Institute of Medicine. (1988). *The future of public health.* Washington, DC: National Academies Press.

Institute of Medicine. (2013). *Childhood immunization schedule and safety: Stakeholders concerns, scientific evidence, and future studies.* Washington, DC: National Academies Press.

Ivanov, L. L., & Oden, T. L. (2013). Public health nursing, ethics, and human rights. *Public Health Nursing, 30*(3), 231–238.

Kass, N. (2001). An ethics framework for public health. *American Journal of Public Health, 91*(11), 1776–1782.

Kinlaw, K., Barrett, D. H., & Levine, R. J. (2009). Ethical guidelines in pandemic influenza: Recommendations of the ethics subcommittee of the advisory committee of the director, Centers for Disease Control and Prevention. *Disaster Medicine and Public Health Preparedness,* Dec; 3 Suppl 2: S185–192. doi:10.1097/DMP.0b013e3181ac194f.

Knight, R. (2015). Empirical population and public health ethics: A review and critical analysis to advance robust empirical–normative inquiry. *Health, 20*(3), 274–290. doi:10.1177/13634593 15583156

Lee, L. M. (2012). Public health ethics theory: Review and path to convergence. *Journal of Law, Medicine, and Ethics, 40*(1), 85–98.

Lin, J. Y., & Anderson-Shaw, L. (2009). Rationing of resources: Ethical issues in disasters and epidemic situations. *Prehospital and Disaster Medicine, 24*(3), 215–221.

Marckmann, G., Schmidt, H., Sofaer, N., & Strech, D. (2015). Putting public health ethics into practice: A systematic framework. *Front Public Health, 3,* 23. doi:10.3389/fpubh.2015.00023 .eCollection 2015

Meier, B. M., Brugh, K. N., & Halima, Y. (2012). Conceptualizing a human right to prevention in global HIV/AID policy. *Public Health Ethics, 5*(3), 263–282.

Mill, J. S., & Bentham, J. (1987). *Utilitarianism and other essays.* London, UK: Penguin Classics.

Misselbrook, D. (2013). An A-Z of medical philosophy: Duty, Kant, and Deontology. *British Journal of General Practice, 63*(609), 211. doi:10.3399/bjgp13X665422

Nixon, S., & Forman, L. (2008). Exploring synergies between human rights and public health ethics: A whole greater than the sum of its parts. *BMC International Health and Human Rights, 8*, 2.

Nuffield Council on Bioethics. (2007). Public health: Ethical issues. Nuffield Council on Bioethics, London. Retrieved from http://nuffieldbioethics.org/wp-content/uploads/2014/07/Public-health-ethical-issues.pdf

Office of the United Nations High Commissioner for Human Rights. (n.d.). The right to health. Fact Sheet No. 31. Retrieved from http://www.who.int/hhr/activities/Right_to_Health_factsheet31.pdf?ua=1

Ogden, C. I., Carroll, M. D., Kit, B. K., & Flegal, K. M. (2012). Prevalence of obesity and trends in body mass index among U.S. children and adolescents, 1999–2010. *The Journal of the American Medical Association, 307*(5), 483–490.

Omer, S. B. (2013). Applying Kass's public health ethics framework to mandatory health care worker immunization: The devil is in the details. *The American Journal of Bioethics, 13*(9), 55–57.

Public Health Leadership Society. (2002). Principles of the ethical practice of public health. Retrieved from https://www.apha.org/~/media/files/pdf/membergroups/ethics_brochure.ashx

Ransom, J., Swain, G. R., & Duchin, J. S. (2008). Ethics, public health, and immunization mandates. *Journal of Public Health Management and Practice, 14*(4), 410–412.

Rawls, J. (1971). *A theory of justice.* Cambridge, MA: Harvard Press.

Resnik, D. B. (2015). Food and beverage policies and public health ethics. *Health Care Analysis, 23*, 122–133.

Richards, J. L., Wagenaar, B. H., Van Otterloo, J., Gondalia, R., Atwell, J. E., Kleinbaum, D. G., . . . Omer, S. B. (2013). Nonmedical exemptions to immunization requirements in California: A 16-year longitudinal analysis of trends and associated community factors. *Vaccine, 31*(29), 3009–3013. doi:10.1016/j.vaccine.2013.04.053

Rothstein, M. A. (2012). The future of public health ethics. *American Journal of Public Health, 102*(1), 9.

Ruger, J. P. (2008). Ethics in American health 1: Ethical approaches to health policy. *American Journal of Public Health, 98*(10), 1751–1756.

Shickle, D. (2009). The ethics of public health practice: Balancing private and public interest within tobacco policy. *British Medical Bulletin, 91*, 7–22.

Simón-Lorda, P., Barrio-Cantalejo I. M., & Peinado-Gorlat, P. (2015). Content of public health ethics postgraduate courses in the United States. *Journal of Bioethical Inquiry, 12*(3), 409–417. doi:10.1007/s11673-015-9608-x

Sommers, B. D., Gunja, M. Z., Finegold, K., & Musco, T. (2015). Changes in self-reported insurance coverage, access to care, and health under the Affordable Care Act. *The Journal of the American Medical Association, 314*(4), 366–74. doi:10.1001/jama.2015.8421

Summers, J. (2014). Principles of healthcare ethics. In E. Morreson & B. Furlong (Eds.), *Healthcare ethics critical issues for the 21st century* (pp. 47–64). Burlington, MA: Jones & Bartlett.

Swain, G. R., Burns, K. A., & Etkind, P. (2008). Preparedness: Medical ethics versus public health ethics. *Journal of Public Health Management and Practice, 14*(4), 354–357.

Thomas, J. C. (2008). An agenda for public health ethics. *Journal of Public Health Management and Practice, 14*(4), 329–331.

Thomas, J. C., Sage, M., Dillenberg, J., & Guillory, V. J. (2002). A code of ethics for public health. *American Journal of Public Health, 92*, 1057–1059.

Trin-Shevrin, C., Islam, N. S., Nadkarni, S., Park, R., & Kwon, S. C. (2015). Defining an integrative approach for health promotion and disease prevention: A population health equity framework. *Journal of Health Care for the Poor and Underserved, 26*(2), 146–163.

Wenar, Leif. (2003, Winter Edition). John Rawls. In Edward N. Zalta (Ed.), *The Stanford encyclopedia of philosophy*. Retrieved from http://plato.stanford.edu/archives/win2013/entries/rawls

Whitehead, M. (1992). The concepts and principles of equity and health. *International Journal of Health Services, 22*(3), 429–445.

Williams, S. E. (2014). What are the factors that contribute to parental vaccine-hesitancy and what can we do about it? *Human Vaccines & Immunotherapeutics, 10*(9), 2584–2596. doi:10.4161/hv.28596

World Health Organization. (n.d.). Definition of health. Retrieved from http://www.who.int/about/definition/en/print.html

World Health Organization. (2013). Health and human rights. Fact Sheet No. 323. Retrieved from http://www.who.int/mediacentre/factsheets/fs323/en

Zipprich, J., Winter, K., Hacker, J., Xia, D., Watt, J., & Harriman, K. (2015). Measles outbreak—California, December 2014–February 2015. *Morbidity and Mortality Weekly Report, 64*(6), 153–154.

10

Exploring Ethical Issues Encountered With the Older Adult

Maryanne M. Giuliante

Upon completion of this chapter, the reader will be able to:

- Discuss why nurses, regardless of the setting, frequently encounter older adults in the current health care system
- Describe why there is a current shortage of workers able to care for older adults
- Discuss how nurses can effectively advocate for the desires and preferences of older adult patients
- Discuss why cognitively impaired patients are at higher risk for encountering ethical dilemmas
- Describe how the nurse can advocate for patients who are older or those who have cognitive impairment in situations of medical futility
- Apply relevant provisions from the Code of Ethics to ethical issues encountered with the older adult
- Identify signs and symptoms of elder abuse
- Discuss risk factors that predispose one for elder abuse

C aring for older adults is not a specialty area that nurses frequently choose after graduating from nursing school. More popular specialties include critical care, medical–surgical, or oncology nursing. However, as a practicing RN, you have probably cared for many older adults regardless of your specialty, unless you are a pediatric or obstetrical nurse. In addition, you may have realized that ethical quandaries arise with a greater degree of frequency when working with the older adult population. Their medical, physical, economic, and social issues are often age specific. How medical issues manifest in older adults can differ greatly from the presentation of a younger individual. Ethical situations that arise in this population are often complex, leaving nurses to wonder about their role, and if they should voice their concerns to the rest of the health care team or remain silent. Consider the following Case Scenario.

CASE SCENARIO

Angel works in a medical–surgical unit of a large urban hospital. Although this unit has patients with mixed diagnoses and ages, he often finds himself caring for older adults with cancer. Angel works overnight, and often does not have a great deal of interaction with family members. Today, he has agreed to help out during the day and has found himself in the middle of an emotional family discussion. The topic of discussion was his patient, Mrs. Smith. Angel has taken care of her for several days, and has found her to be cognitively intact. She is 83, and has just been diagnosed with end-stage anaplastic thyroid cancer. Angel remembers that this cancer is one of the deadliest, and often patients with anaplastic thyroid cancer do not live past a few months following the diagnosis. Mrs. Smith is somewhat frail already, and has a history of emphysema, heart failure, osteoporosis, and type II diabetes. With his experience and education, Angel realizes that this diagnosis is terminal. She has recently been told by the oncologist working with her that she is unsuitable for chemotherapy, surgery, and radiation (the three forms of treatment for cancer). Her interprofessional team consisting of an oncologist, geriatrician, oncology nurse, oncology social worker, and palliative care specialist is recommending only palliative (comfort) care. Though saddened, Mrs. Smith seems accepting of this news and verbalizes her agreement to focus on her comfort. However, Mrs. Smith's daughter, her health care proxy (HCP), is visibly upset and agitated and tries to convince her to go to another hospital for a second opinion. Although Angel thinks that this request is reasonable, Mrs. Smith does not want to go, and is asking for him to convince her daughter that she should stay in this hospital. Mrs. Smith states, "I have had a long life, and I am ready to die." Angel is uncomfortable with this discussion, and believes that Mrs. Smith's wishes should be respected.

Question to Consider Before Reading On

1. How would you respond to Mrs. Smith's family if it asks why a geriatrician is needed on her medical team?

It is imperative that we make a clear distinction that older adults are not the same as middle-aged adults. They have different issues, by virtue of their age, that should cause us to evaluate what makes them unique. Age *does* become an important factor when we consider certain aspects of care (such as social support, physiologic functioning, and diseases that typically affect this population). However, we need to consider much more than *only* the chronological age of the patient. Functional, cognitive, and social issues must be taken in consideration to allow us to provide the most holistic care possible. Older adults should not be judged solely by their chronological age, as their age is just one of a variety of factors that informs us about their health status. An *unfit* 56-year-old is unlikely to have the same issues as a *fit* 76-year-old. This understanding will be the foundation of how we analyze our patients as it relates to questions surrounding ethics and other aspects of age-appropriate care.

GROWING POPULATION OF OLDER ADULTS

Question to Consider Before Reading On

1. Why are nurses more likely to care for older patients in the current health care environment?

It is important to recognize that there has been tremendous growth among the older population in the past decade. In addition, we should be aware of the data regarding anticipated growth in coming years. Evaluating these statistics can help properly frame this group's overrepresentation in health care markets, understand their unique needs, and anticipate the ethical quandaries that may arise. According to the U.S. Department of Health and Human Services, Administration for Community Living, the adult population over the age of 65 has increased from 35.9 million in 2003 to 44.7 million in 2013 (a 24.7% increase) and is projected to more than double to 98 million in 2060 (Administration on Aging, 2014). In addition to the growth of this segment of population, the subsegment considered "older-old" is expected to surge. This population of 85+ is projected to increase from 6 million in 2013 to 14.6 million in 2040 (Administration on Aging, 2014; see Figure 10.1).

CAUSES OF MORBIDITY AMONG OLDER ADULTS

These statistics may help us understand the proportion of the population that older adults represent; however, there is still more to know. To appreciate the entire picture, we must evaluate the most common patients that nurses are likely to encounter in their practice. Not only do older adults represent a fair percentage of the population as a whole, but they are frequent utilizers of health care. According to the National Council on Aging, "approximately 92% of older adults have at least one chronic disease, and 77% have two.

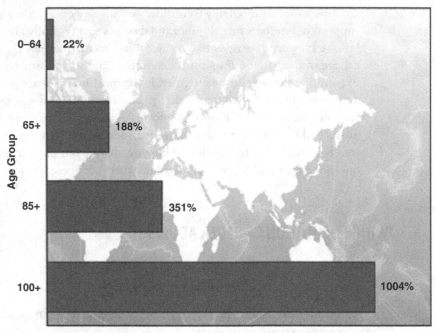

Figure 10.1 Percentage change in the world's population by age: 2010 to 2050.
Source: United Nations (2013).

Four chronic diseases—heart disease, cancer, stroke, and diabetes—cause almost two-thirds of all deaths each year" (NCA, 2016). This data may provide insight into the kind of ethical quandaries that older adults and their caregivers are likely to encounter.

Older adults frequently experience multiple chronic conditions (otherwise known as "multimorbidity"), making them potentially more frail and vulnerable. The degree of frailty and chronicity of illness that older adults experience can predispose them to ethical quandaries. According to *Journal of the American Geriatrics Society*, "Multi-morbidity is associated with higher rates of death, disability, adverse effects, institutionalization, use of healthcare resources, and poorer quality of life" (American Geriatrics Society [AGS], 2012). These data illustrate why nurses caring for older adults may encounter more ethical challenges than those caring for a younger population. Because their care can be more complex, nurses and other providers must understand the needs of the older adult and advocate for them using ethical competence and judgment.

Never before has the cost of health care been scrutinized as much as it is today. With the implementation of the Patient Protection and Affordable Care Act, commonly called the Affordable Care Act (ACA), cost has become a major influencing factor in health care decisions. The quality of care is also constantly evaluated. As a result, the provision of ethically competent care that is appropriate and cost-effective has become more important than ever before. As an example of this paradigm shift, we can return to the chapter Case Scenario and identify relevant issues that may arise in the era of the ACA.

CASE SCENARIO *(CONTINUED)*

As has already been established, Mrs. Smith is 83, and has recently been diagnosed with a terminal disease. She appears cognitively intact, accepting of the disease and its anticipated trajectory. However, her family seems unwilling to share this acceptance. If we examine this case through the lens of a provider who is conscious of current trends and limitations in health care, it may seem reasonable to forgo curative therapy and focus on keeping Mrs. Smith comfortable (especially given the fact that her medical team does not recommend any anticancer treatment). Interventions such as additional blood tests or scans and providing an anticancer therapy drug may be costly, burdensome, potentially uncomfortable, and likely result in poor clinical outcomes. Mrs. Smith may already be somewhat frail given her age and presence of multiple comorbid medical conditions, which will further undermine the medical team's ability to achieve a favorable outcome.

Question to Consider Before Reading On

1. How would you respond if Mrs. Smith's daughter asked, "If my mom is going to die anyway, why not try a little chemo on her. . . . what's the difference"?

Ageism

What is "ageism"? According to Ageismhurts.org, ageism is, "The stereotyping or discrimination of a person or group of people because of their age" (Ageism Hurts, n.d.). This stereotype suggests that people are treated differently based on their age, and not their functional ability. Generally speaking, employing stereotypes is frowned upon. However, ageism seems to have endured, while other prejudices such as racism and sexism are not socially acceptable. We often crack a smile when comedians joke about somebody with gray hair who drives too slowly. However, these insensitive comments can have long-lasting effects on older adults and those who care for them. We may be quick to react negatively to comments such as these when *we* become the subject of the jest. Remarks highlighting the noteworthy value of youth in our Western society seem to undermine our inability to appreciate and respect our older adults.

As nurses, we should support a paradigm shift that does not evaluate a person based on their chronological age, but on their functional status. Return to the chapter Case Scenario to explore how ageism could play an unintended role in Mrs. Smith's care. If she were not a frail 83-year-old with multiple comorbid medical conditions, but a *fit* 83-year-old who was healthy and jogged 2 miles a day, we may consider her ability to withstand the rigors of anticancer therapy differently. Although the medical team may persist in recommending a focus on palliation, this fit 83-year-old may have a different disease and life trajectory. Functional status and anticipated disease trajectory should be determining factors in the care provided, not merely how long Mrs. Smith has been alive.

To emphasize this point further, let us consider Mrs. Smith to be 53, not 83. At first glance, we might assume that this individual will be healthy and vibrant. However, as we learn about the functional status of *this* 53-year-old, we are surprised that she is bedbound and frail, resulting from double below-the-knee amputations secondary to uncontrolled diabetes. In addition, she is completely blind. This is not the image that we generally have of a 53-year-old, right? We should apply this insight to older adults as well. There are many 66-year-olds who are frailer, sicker, and less functional than 83-year-old adults. In summary, age is just a number!

Respecting Autonomy and Beneficence

Many older adults struggle with maintaining independence, often their most important goal. Multiple chronic conditions and frailty may affect their functional status. Care providers are sometimes met with resistance from older adults when we advocate for "safety over independence." This becomes a very difficult situation, especially when family members diminish in number or in their ability to participate in care of the older adult. How can we effectively advocate for the safety and health maintenance of the older adult when their care may exceed the ability of family members and/or their financial resources? These difficult questions become the basis for further discussion, and are rarely easy.

As nurses, we recognize our obligation to advocate for our patients. This role seems easier to enact at certain times than in others. For example, this professional responsibility may feel quite easy when we share a critical aspect of our patient's care that has been overlooked. Perhaps we think that integration of this key information will support a favorable clinical outcome. We may feel relatively comfortable providing the necessary information to clarify what our patient needs, and see ourselves as our older adult patient's strongest ally. We may feel satisfied when we witness our patient receiving more comprehensive, *patient-centered care* because of our efforts (Box 10.1). These successful advocacy experiences reinforce this aspect of nursing care in a positive way, and our patients and their caregivers may be overtly grateful for our efforts. The lines may become somewhat blurred, however, when we are advocating for the health care team's recommendation and it runs counter to the wishes of our older adult patient. It may be *then* that we question how to fulfill our responsibilities, without disrespecting our older adult patient. Providers are challenged when they perceive a dichotomy between what is deemed right and what the patient wants. How can we as nurses walk this "tight rope?"

Box 10.1

QSEN Box Example: Patient-Centered Care

Providing patient-centered care to the older adult population is critical. In the case of Mrs. Smith, Angel is mindful of this QSEN competency when he considers the best care that can be rendered to his patient with terminal cancer. He explores ways to deliver care in a safe, comprehensive manner while keeping her wishes at the forefront of his mind. Angel may be somewhat conflicted regarding his ability to successfully navigate this clinical situation. Requesting his colleagues in the medical team to help him tackle this situation is the best way to deliver high-quality, patient-centered care for this older adult patient.

Question to Consider Before Reading On

1. Your older adult patient refuses transfer to a facility to maintain safety following an acute care episode, stating, "I want to go home, even if it means I fall and break a hip, or die!" How would you respond?

CASE SCENARIO *(CONTINUED)*

Returning to the Case Scenario, let us reflect back to the clinical care of Mrs. Smith. We are going to modify the case a bit to illustrate the points discussed previously. Instead of agreeing with the team of health care providers and advocating for palliation (comfort), let us say instead that Mrs. Smith wanted to take the more aggressive approach, despite professional opinion that does not support anti-cancer treatment. Let us further imagine that her family was taking a spirited position of encouraging her to choose the less aggressive approach, and they are leaning toward seeing this difficult situation in the same way as her medical team: focusing on palliation. Additionally, let us say that Mrs. Smith reports having heard of an international clinic that reports great success with treating patients with her type of cancer. She reports all related expenses (including travel, hotel accommodations, and treatment costs) would total $1M, and she is willing to spend all of her life savings on this last-ditch effort. She reports being able to physically "make the trip." You disagree, and believe that she is so severely physically limited that you as her nurse believe that her safety would be at risk by taking such a trip. She may even die in transit.

Question to Consider Before Reading On

1. How can you apply Provision 3 of the Code of Ethics to promote, advocate for, and protect the rights, health, and safety of Mrs. Smith in the Case Scenario?

Box 10.2

Evidence-Based Practice Box: Decision Making in the Absence of Capacity

Determining who will make health care decisions when the patient cannot may be confusing for nurses and other health care professionals. There are two approaches that can be employed in the situation where your patient has lost the capacity to make decisions on his or her own. The first is looking for "advance directives," such as a "living will," which will guide health care teams regarding major medical interventions, procedures, and end-of-life care. The second is "surrogate decision making," such as health care proxy or other surrogate decision maker. This person has the same decision-making authority as the patient himself or herself. A health care surrogate may be any competent adult over the age of 18. Formal surrogates may be specified by state law in a hierarchy, typically in descending order of relation to the patient. Informal decision makers are other family members or close friends who are asked by the health care team to help make decisions on the patient's behalf. When a patient has not made his or her wishes clear, substituted judgements assess what the patient *would have wanted* based on prior statements and patterns of decision making.

Adapted from Boltz (2012).

It is important to restate that Mrs. Smith has no cognitive impairment, and does not seem to be confused. This situation is perplexing to us as nurses, and there is often not a "right" or "wrong" decision. To revisit what has already been stated in previous chapters, autonomy is the patient's right to make decisions about his or her health care (Box 10.2). Beneficence is the act of health care providers "doing good." It is clear that to support this patient in autonomous decision making, we may have to forgo our usual conception of "doing good," since we believe that by supporting her, she would be jeopardizing her safety. In this instance, however, we are abiding by Provision 3 of the Code of Ethics. Requesting an ethics consultation may also be indicated as they can provide recommendations to both the patient/family and medical team. This interprofessional approach may result in a reasonable and acceptable outcome for all involved.

DEMENTIA: ETHICAL IMPLICATIONS

The number of patients with dementia is on the increase. According to The Elder Workforce Alliance, "7.7 million people will have Alzheimer's disease in 2030, up from 4.9 million in 2007" (Figure 10.2; EWA, 2016). This growing segment of the population forces us to evaluate how to best care for

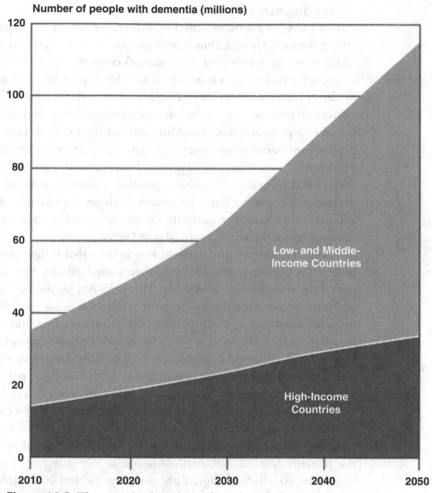

Number of people with dementia (millions)

Figure 10.2 The growth of numbers of people with dementia in high-income countries and low- and middle-income countries: 2010 to 2050.
Source: Alzheimer's Disease International (2010).

dementia patients and the frequent ethical issues that arise. The degree of the patient's memory/cognitive impairment increases the complexity of these issues and must be addressed by the health care team.

According to the Alzheimer's Association, "Concern for the autonomy of a person with dementia requires an assessment of an individual's capacity to understand the relevant options and consequences of a particular task or decision in light of one's own values" (2016). This recommendation allows us a basis for understanding the scope of our responsibilities as nurses. It also "keeps the door open" for the possibility that even those with dementia may be cognitively intact *enough* to make their own health care decisions. As we know, cognitive function can vary over the course of time, making ongoing assessments an important intervention. Factors such as certain medicines, time of day, and sleep patterns can influence cognitive function, so these factors must be considered when making an assessment.

It is imperative that the interprofessional team correctly interprets the patient's level of cognitive function. Misinterpretation can negatively influence a patient's choices, thus health care outcomes. There are two ways in which teams can falsely interpret a patient's cognitive status. The first involves caring for a patient who is impaired, but the impairment is not recognized by the health care team (Mitty, 2012). The second is the patient who *is* cognitively intact enough to make informed decisions, but the health care team is unable to recognize this state (Mitty, 2012). Either of these cases could result in poor patient/caregiver-centered outcomes. As nurses, we are often the ones who spend the most amount of time with our patients. This supports the idea that we may be in the most suitable position to alert the rest of the team that the patient's cognitive status has changed (either improved or devolved). In addition, nurses need to advocate for ongoing reassessments so that these changes are identified, and care adjusted accordingly.

Some health care professionals may believe that if their patients do not possess the cognitive ability to make their own decisions, they should be left out of the conversation altogether. This may not be the best approach. In addition, we need *not* think of cognitive function as an "on/off" switch. As previously mentioned, cognitive function is quite variable, and must be reassessed frequently. To do so, we need to include our patients in the conversation as often as possible. Although it is difficult to know exactly how much information is understood and retained by each individual patient, ongoing engagement remains an important aspect of patient-centered care. However, an important caveat exists. Some conversations may cause a patient with dementia to become agitated, and even more confused. Health care providers must constantly reassess as conversations unfold to determine if the patient's level of agitation/confusion is increasing. The conversation should be concluded if agitation/confusion occurs and reinitiated when appropriate.

To ensure understanding during these conversations, we must avoid using jargon and speak slowly to allow processing of information. However, speaking too slowly can insult patients. Too much or too little information can also undermine the ability of the health care team to paint a clear picture for the patient and their loved ones. Conversations with cognitively impaired patients may require additional planning. We must carve out as much time as possible, so that the information delivered to the patient and their loved ones is accomplished in a calm manner. The room should be free from extraneous noise, and the environment should be comfortable. Anticipating the needs of your patient with dementia, such as toileting them prior to the conversation, can help support success.

Questions to Consider Before Reading On

1. What are some strategies that interprofessional health care teams can use to improve the chances of a successful conversation with an older adult that has some degree of cognitive impairment?

2. How often should the health care team assess for cognitive impairment and why?

INTEGRATING THE INTERPROFESSIONAL TEAM INTO DEMENTIA CARE

According to the Robert Wood Johnson Foundation, "Research has long suggested that collaboration improves coordination, communication, and, ultimately, the quality and safety of patient care" (2011, p. 1). Social workers, psychologists, psychiatrists, neurologists, and geriatricians can add great value to clinical cases involving patients with dementia. These professionals may view difficult situations through a different lens, and add perspective to the situation at hand.

MEDICALLY FUTILE CARE AMONG OLDER ADULTS

Advances in technology and medical science have led to unimaginable breakthroughs. This progress has allowed life to be supported during acute episodes when the body cannot function independently. Life-sustaining measures such as ventilators, feeding tubes, critical care medicine, and other modalities were developed primarily as a bridge to eventual recovery. However, these measures are often employed to deter certain death among older adults and their younger counterparts. No one would argue that there are clinical cases in which the use of these life-sustaining measures is appropriate. Conversely, it is also true that there are cases where positive outcomes are unlikely—either with or without the use of these interventions. Moreover, the employment of life-sustaining treatments may only prolong suffering. These costly measures are also financially burdensome for family members.

When are life-sustaining therapies potentially "less appropriate" for older adults? First, we need to lay the groundwork for the discussion by stating the obvious; death is certain. It is not a failure of our medical system, but a known inevitability. All of us, on some level, understand this fact to be a reality, although many cultures consider the subject to be taboo. Many of us recognize the signs and symptoms of death as it draws near. Even before death is imminent, we may recognize that "things are not going well" with our patients. As nurses, we may be frustrated when our patient's condition becomes increasingly dire yet important conversations do not take place. And sadly, we may shake our heads when the health care team responds to a clinical crisis that *we* knew was looming for days or even weeks as if they were caught off guard. Perhaps the inappropriate use of life-sustaining interventions could be avoided by encouraging a conversation to take place earlier.

There are patients/family members who demand life-sustaining interventions despite all signs indicating a negative clinical outcome. Nurses and other providers may believe that these interventions are not appropriate, given the patient's clinical situation, age, and preexisting comorbidities . . . and we may be right! Inappropriate use of the interventions may be avoided by providing full disclosure regarding the patient's clinical condition. As professionals, we have a moral obligation to share our recommendations with patients and family members. Some providers avoid fully disclosing their opinion in the spirit of supporting patient/caregiver autonomy. They may argue that they do not want to "interfere" with what the patient wants at the end of his or her life. Perhaps they believe that their opinion will sway the patient/family in one direction or another. Well, it should! Patients and their caregivers *need to know* what our opinion is so they are able to formulate a plan based on the most recent information.

It is an unfortunate reality that discussing death and dying in our culture is not widely accepted. This resistance is not only among patients and their caregivers, but also among doctors, nurses, and other health care professionals. When opportunities for discussing end-of-life wishes are lost, patients may receive care that they would not have elected had the conversation taken place.

Question to Consider Before Reading On

1. How can you apply Provision 2 of the Code of Ethics to a situation such as the one stated previously, in which the nurse's commitment is to the patient, whether an individual, family, group, community, or population?

Not only is this care futile (in many cases), but is also costly, costly on many levels. We may first think of *monetary costs;* the actual cost of performing the intervention rather than not performing it. There is also a "time cost" associated with these interventions that may leave the patient unable to engage in meaningful dialogue with his or her family due to side effects, recovery times, or necessary sedation. Absent these interventions, our patients may have had more quality time to spend with loved ones.

LACK OF CAREGIVER SUPPORT FOR OLDER ADULTS—HOW CAN THIS INFLUENCE ETHICAL ISSUES?

Questions to Consider Before Reading On

1. How can you apply the Code of Nursing Ethics Provision 7: The nurse in all roles and settings advances the profession through research and scholarly inquiry, professional standards development, and the generation of both nursing and health policy to begin to improve the care of older patients in health care settings today?

2. How can you apply the Code of Nursing Ethics Provision 4: The nurse has authority, accountability, and responsibility for nursing practice, makes

decisions, and takes action consistent with the obligation to promote health and to provide optimal care to make sure the older patient receives optimal care to assist older patients and their families to seek the care they need?

3. What actions can you take to assist families with planning for the long-term care often needed by older patients?

4. Have you ever witnessed signs of elder abuse or risk factors associated with elder abuse? What are your responsibilities as an RN in such situations?

Have you heard of the "Silver Tsunami?" Well, we would better prepare like we would for any other storm! The Silver Tsunami describes the massive "wave" of patients over the age of 65 that will require care in the coming years. Even though we know this, we continue to have significantly less caregivers (both paid and unpaid) than we need. Paid caregivers, such as nurses, nurses' aides, and other allied support are the backbone of health care today. It is these (paid) caregivers upon whom we rely so heavily, the same people who often get the brunt of work when patient acuity increases. In this section, we will discuss the relationship that both paid and unpaid caregivers may have on ethical issues among older adults.

How influential are unpaid (family) caregivers to the care needed by our older adults? It may be shocking to discover just how many unpaid (family) caregivers there are providing care to our older adult patients. According to the Family Caregiver Alliance (2016), "65.7 million caregivers make up 29% of the U.S. adult population providing care to someone who is ill, disabled or aged." It is not difficult to imagine that having family caregivers can be a double-edged sword as it relates to ethical issues in this population. On one hand, it may seem like a significant advantage to be cared for by a person who has a familial relationship. It may seem safe to assume that the care provided is superior to that of paid caregivers. Unlike the paid caregiver, however, family members may experience undue stress in this role. Caring for a loved one can create personal and financial burdens. Because of personal feelings of attachment, family caregivers may also not be able to see what is in the best interest of the older adult.

According to AARP, "In 2009, about 42.1 million family caregivers in the United States provided care to an adult with limitations in daily activities at any given point in time, and about 61.6 million provided care at some time during the year. The estimated economic value of their unpaid contributions was approximately $450 billion in 2009, up from an estimated $375 billion in 2007" (AARP, n.d., p. 1). This caregiver involvement is imperative and heavily relied upon in today's health care climate. However, this reliance comes with a significant (and costly) disadvantage. One can anticipate that a *lack of* family caregivers will result in greater cost, the need to hire/train paid caregivers, or unfortunately, the need to institutionalize our older adults who lack home-based caregiver involvement. It is not difficult to predict that this increased demand on institutionalization will (and already does) stretch the paid/unrelated workforce beyond its current capabilities, creating an environment where ethical dilemmas can flourish.

There are certainly many challenges that are experienced by paid/unrelated caregivers, and these challenges likely differ from those experienced by family caregivers. The paid caregiver workforce is currently stretched thin, and it will only get worse as the number of baby boomers reach and exceed 65 years of age. Moreover, the number of caregivers who are adequately trained to deal with this population, their common health challenges, and potential ethical issues is grossly inadequate. According to the Eldercare Workforce Alliance, "It is estimated that by 2030, 3.5 million additional health care professionals and direct-care workers will be needed" (2015). This shortage of adequately prepared caregivers can have devastating, unintended, and costly consequences. How can we make a difference? We must recognize that the care of the older adult is a specialty. Formalized and ongoing education can help strengthen the nurse's understanding about the unique and challenging situations that can be encountered with this population. This understanding may serve to enhance care and communication among patients and the health care team and decrease the incidence of ethical issues.

The number of caregivers available to work with this population *within* these institutions is also shrinking, increasing the burden on the workforce as a whole. These workforce stresses may create environments where ethical issues abound. Institutionalized older adult patients may also lack a family member who can serve as their advocate. Often, institutions default to "life-sustaining treatment," unless they are directed otherwise. This may strike some as being odd, especially when the medical team has already determined that the patient's situation is dire, and there is no known cure for the disease. Yet, life-sustaining care is often provided. Aside from the costly nature of these (potentially inappropriate) interventions, the absence of a family advocate can create an environment in which the patient's best interest becomes entangled in strategies aimed at preserving life, even when death is near.

ELDER ABUSE AND NEGLECT

"Elder mistreatment (i.e. abuse and neglect) is defined as intentional actions that cause harm or create a serious risk of harm (whether or not harm is intended) to a vulnerable elder by a caregiver or other person who stands in a trust relationship to the elder" (NCEA, 2016). Types and examples of older adult abuse are presented in Box 10.3.

Unfortunately, elder abuse is quite common. According to the Centers for Disease Control, "Elder abuse, including neglect and exploitation, is experienced by 1 out of every 10 people ages 60 and older who live at home" (CDC, 2016). The nurse should be aware of risk factors associated with mistreatment of the older adult as described by Terry Fulmer, an expert in geriatric nursing:

A number of risk factors for elder mistreatment and its subsequent health outcomes create opportunities for prevention or intervention. These include: increased physical dependency of frail elders on care-givers; fewer family members living in the same geographic region or caregivers being elderly or impaired themselves; substance abuse, cognitive impairment and mental illness among caregivers and/or the mistreated as well as poverty, age, race, functional disability, frailty, loneliness and low education. (Fulmer, 2013)

Abuse or mistreatment of older adults can be inflicted by anyone: a rela-tive, friend, spouse, or unrelated (paid) caregiver. There are inherent barriers in the identification of such abuse, which are sometimes created by the victims themselves. There may be shame, denial, fear of reprisal, and other concerns

---

Box 10.3
_____

Types of Elder Abuse

Type of Elder Abuse	Definition
Physical abuse	Inflicting physical pain or injury on a senior, for example, slapping, bruising, or restraining by physical or chemical means
Sexual abuse	Nonconsensual sexual contact of any kind
Neglect	The failure by those responsible to provide food, shelter, health care, or protection for a vulnerable elder
Exploitation	The illegal taking, misuse, or concealment of funds, property, or assets of a senior for someone else's benefit
Emotional abuse	Inflicting mental pain, anguish, or distress on an elder person through verbal or nonverbal acts, for example, humiliating, intimidating, or threatening
Abandonment	Desertion of a vulnerable elder by anyone who has assumed the responsibility for care or custody of that person
Self-neglect	Characterized as the failure of a person to perform essential, self-care tasks and that such failure threatens his or her own health or safety

Source: National Institute on Aging (2016).

Box 10.4

Signs and Symptoms of Elder Abuse

- Trouble sleeping
- Seems depressed or confused
- Loses weight for no reason
- Displays signs of trauma, like rocking back and forth
- Acts agitated or violent
- Becomes withdrawn
- Stops taking part in activities he or she enjoys
- Has unexplained bruises, burns, or scars
- Looks messy, with unwashed hair or dirty clothes
- Develops bed sores or other preventable conditions

Source: National Institute on Aging (2016).

that may prevent older adults from reporting such abuse. For example, some victims may find it difficult to understand how their adult child could hurt them. There may be ashamed or embarrassed that the one inflicting such violence is the person whom the victim has raised. These difficult feelings can make reporting such behavior even more challenging.

As nurses, we must have a clear understanding of the "red flags" indicative of elder abuse. Often, nurses and other professionals miss key signs and symptoms because we have not had the proper training to identify abuse or because we do not want to be accusatory. Signs and symptoms of elder abuse/neglect are presented in Box 10.4.

Advocacy for older adults means asking the difficult questions, the ones that we typically avoid. It is imperative that we understand the risk factors, signs and symptoms, and the best way to proceed once abuse/neglect is suspected. This improved understanding can serve to minimize subsequent risk to the older adult victims, and protect their rights. It is of particular importance to underscore the added complexity when working with patients experiencing some type of cognitive impairment, such as dementia. For this group in particular, helping discover elder mistreatment and advocating for their rights may be even more difficult.

ADVANCE CARE PLANNING FOR THE OLDER ADULT

What prevents older adults from telling their loved ones what they would want, in the event that they become unable to do so? Perhaps it is the fear of poor treatment, neglect, or lack of available treatment options that cause some to not want to discuss this sensitive topic. As a nurse practitioner in an oncology practice, I often spend a great deal of time talking to older adults about advance care planning. In attempting to have meaningful dialogue with my patients and their loved ones, I often encounter barriers. The one that appears to be most frequent is wanting to "avoid" such discussions. Some say, "I don't want to talk about that right now" or "I am not prepared to make a decision." Although having these discussions are sure to bring up uncomfortable topics, the need to do so with our patients is imperative. Never before have we seen such technological advances leading to more opportunities to support life. With these advances comes an obligation to engage in meaningful dialogue with our patients about the ramifications of proceeding with this level of care, and the ramifications of not doing so.

How can we emotionally support our patients during these difficult discussions, while imparting to them the critical nature of such a decision? Nurses can encourage the medical team to engage in such discussions *before* the patient is critically ill. The irony is that we (both medical and nonmedical professionals alike) may choose to delay such conversations until they are absolutely necessary. Postponing such discussions serves only to illicit fear, as our patients may suspect that the "end is near." Instead, we can choose to engage in such discussions *before* the patient is critical/unstable, thereby decreasing the time-sensitive nature of such conversations and emotions that may arise. We can even portray such discussions as "standard," which may decrease the chances of patients thinking, "Why is he or she having this conversation with me *now*?" For example, you may say, "We have this conversation with all of our patients, to make sure that we don't do anything to you that you don't want. It's a way of making sure you are in the driver's seat when it comes to your care." You may want to follow this statement with one stating (if this is true) that the medical team does not expect anything critical to happen imminently, but that diseases tend to be unpredictable. It may be a helpful tactic to reveal to those patients that report that they "are not ready" to make such decisions, that they *are*, in fact, making a decision by *not* making one. Patients are often surprised to know that the default action when advance directives have not been discussed is the "do-everything" approach (in most cases); therefore, not making a decision can be viewed as indeed having made one.

So what is "right" in cases of older adults as it relates to end-of-life care? Well, it is a good start to establish that they need to be active participants in their care, whenever possible. It is essential that we as nurses provide them and their caregivers with all of the information that is needed to make an informed decision. Even more important may be to ensure (to the extent this is even possible) that they and their health care providers *understand* the information being provided to them, in clear, non-medical jargon. They should be given the opportunities to think about their choices, and we should spend some time with them trying to clear up any misconceptions. The time that we dedicate to these important tasks could mean the difference between patients dying peacefully, or spending their last days connected to equipment and medications that they never really wanted.

CASE SCENARIO (*CONTINUED*)

Returning to the chapter Case Scenario, as you may recall, Mrs. Smith has just been given a terminal diagnosis. When the diagnosis was initially discussed, her daughter seems resistant to the idea that her care will focus on palliation, forgoing anticancer treatment. Her daughter continues to ask Angel, the nurse, questions that he is unable to answer. Therefore, he asks the medical team to return to Mrs. Smith's room. The medical team returns and reiterates her diagnosis and treatment options. They also discuss the feasibility of leaving the hospital to get another medical opinion. Her daughter was provided adequate time to ask all of the questions that she had. Though disappointed, Mrs. Smith's daughter appears satisfied that all of her questions had been fully answered and that her mom seems to have peacefully come to terms with the possibility of dying from this disease. Mrs. Smith's daughter reports that her mom's choice to elect for comfort measures exclusively does not surprise her—she never wanted to be "hooked up to machines," so this decision seems consistent with that philosophy. Her daughter becomes supportive of the medical plan to focus on palliation. The next week, she is transferred to a hospice setting to live her remaining days, per her own wishes.

CONCLUSION

This chapter presented some of the unique challenges that may be encountered when working with the older adult patient. A background on geriatrics was provided, which gave the reader a better understanding of the distinctive needs of this population. We explored chronological age and how it may influence health care decisions. The causes of mortality among older adults were discussed and ethical issues associated with ageism, dementia, and elder abuse were explored. The need for advance care planning among the older adult population was explored, and the role of the nurse in this aspect of care was discussed. Throughout this chapter, a Case Scenario unfolded, and concepts outlined were applied to this Case Scenario, to help the nurse have a better understanding of how these issues can influence care and decision making.

Critical Thinking Questions and Activities

Case Study on Dementia Care

Mr. Alex Jones is a 92-year-old patient with a history of metastatic melanoma from a skin nodule to his brain, spinal cord, and liver. He also has a history of hypertension, osteoarthritis, diabetes (diet controlled), and advanced Alzheimer's dementia. Mr. Jones is an

(continued)

Critical Thinking Questions and Activities *(continued)*

inpatient on your medical unit, after falling in his home. He sustained a fracture to his humorous, and has multiple bruises. His primary caretaker is his daughter, who lives with him. Although she seems fairly active in Mr. Jones's care, the daughter claims that the care needed to keep her dad at home and safe has become "too much" for her, and she is advocating for institutional placement. Further, the daughter claims that her dad often wanders, and she is frightened that he will get lost. You are sitting at the nurse's station one Monday afternoon charting, when you are approached by the oncology attending physician. Dr. Ariano tells you that Mr. Jones is no longer a candidate for any additional anticancer therapies, as his cancer has progressed through all forms of therapy. He is too weak to withstand any additional treatment. Dr. Ariano reports to you that it is the oncology team's recommendation that he focus on palliation and be transferred to an inpatient hospice setting. Based on your interaction with him, you cannot imagine that Mr. Jones could meaningfully participate in his health care decisions. You remember reading that his HCP is his daughter. You walk into Mr. Jones's room, and find his daughter speaking with Dr. Ariano about Mr. Jones's condition. She seems distraught because she understands that her dad can no longer make decisions now, but sometimes she thinks he is "there." Mr. Jones's daughter asks you to revisit this conversation with her dad when he is more "with it."

1. How would you apply the Code of Nursing Ethics Provision 1 to practice with compassion and respect for the inherent dignity, worth, and unique attributes of Mr. Jones?

2. How would you apply the Code of Nursing Ethics Provision 2: The nurse's primary commitment is to the patient, whether an individual, family, group, community, or population to explain how you would respond to Mr. Jones's daughter. What is your rationale?

3. How would you apply Code of Nursing Ethics Provision 8 to collaborate with other health professionals and the public to protect human rights, promote health diplomacy, and reduce health disparities in the care of Mr. Jones?

4. What did you learn from the case studies of Mrs. Smith and Mr. Jones?

5. Have you ever had a similar situation occur in your workplace? If so, please provide details regarding similarities and differences you observed and experienced in your situation as compared to the chapter Case Scenario.

6. What would you do differently in your workplace, based on the principles and content presented in this chapter?

7. Using the website www.cdc.gov explain how a patient would properly communicate and document his or her wishes regarding advance directives.

8. Using the website http://www.rwjf.org/content/dam/farm/reports/issue_briefs/2011/rwjf72058 identify three strategies you can use to collaborate with other health care professionals when caring for older adults. Explain how these strategies may prevent the emergence of ethical issues.

REFERENCES

Administration on Aging. (2014). Administrative for Community Living. Retrieved from http://www.aoa.acl.gov/Aging_Statistics/Profile/2014/2.aspx

Ageism Hurts. (n.d.). What is ageism? Retrieved from http://ageismhurts.org/what-is-ageism

Alzheimer's Association. (2016). Respect for automony. Retrieved from http://www.alz.org/documents_custom/statements/Respect_for_Autonomy.pdf

Alzheimer's Disease International. (2010). World Alzheimer Report 2010. Retrieved from http://www.alz.co.uk/research/files/WorldAlzheimerReport2010.pdf

American Association of Retired Persons. (n.d.). Public Policy Institute 2011 Brief. Retrieved from https://assets.aarp.org/rgcenter/ppi/ltc/i51-caregiving.pdf

American Geriatrics Society Expert Panel on the Care of Older Adults with Multimorbidity. (2012). Patient-centered care for older adults with multiple chronic conditions: A stepwise approach from the American Geriatrics Society. *Journal of the American Geriatrics Society, 60*(10), 1957–1968. Retrieved from http://dx.doi.org/10.1111/j.1532-5415.2012.04187

Boltz, M. (2012). *Evidence-based geriatric nursing protocols for best practice*. New York, NY: Springer.

Centers for Disease Control. (2016). Elder abuse prevention. Retrieved from http://www.cdc.gov/features/elderabuse

Elder Workforce Alliance. (2016). 3.5 million workers needed by 2030 to care for older adults, current levels of workforce already stretched. Retrieved from http://www.eldercareworkforce.org/newsroom/press-releases/article:3-5-million-workers-needed-by-2030-to-care-for-older-adults-current-levels-of-workforce-already-stretched

Family Caregiver Alliance. (2016). Retrieved from https://www.caregiver.org/selected-caregiver-statistics

Fulmer, T. (2013). Mistreatment of older adults. In S. Durso & G. Sullivan (Eds.), *Geriatric review syllabus: A core curriculum in geriatric medicine* (8th ed., pp. 104–108). New York, NY: American Geriatrics Society.

Hartford Institute for Geriatric Nursing. (2016). Decision making in older adults with dementia. Retrieved from http://consultgeri.org/try-this/dementia/issue-d9

Mitty, E. (2012). Advance directives. In M. Boltz, E. Capezuti, T. Fulmer, & D. Zwicker (Eds.), A. O'Meara (Managing Ed.), *Evidence-based geriatric nursing protocols for best practice* (4th ed., pp. 579–599). New York, NY: Springer Publishing.

National Council on Aging. (2016). Healthy aging facts. Retrieved from https://www.ncoa.org/news/resources-for-reporters/get-the-facts/healthy-aging-facts

National Institute on Aging. (2016). Retrieved from https://www.nia.nih.gov/health/publication/elder-abuse#signs

Robert Wood Johnson Foundation. (2011). What can be done to encourage more interprofessional collaboration in health care? Retrieved from http://www.rwjf.org/content/dam/farm/reports/issue_briefs/2011/rwjf72058

United Nations. (2013). Department of Economic and Social Affairs. *World Population Prospects: 2012 Revision*. Retrieved from http://esa.un.org/unpd/wpp/index.htm

The U.S. Department of Health and Human Services. (2014). Administration for Community Living. Administration on aging (AoA). Retrieved from http://www.aoa.acl.gov/Aging_Statistics/Profile/2014/2.aspx

11

Exploring Ethical Issues Related to Emerging Technology in Health Care

Carol Jorgensen Huston

Upon the completion of this chapter, the reader will be able to:

- Discuss how the ethical principles of dignity and autonomy are challenged by technology
- Identify strategies to optimally integrate the use of technology with the human element or art of nursing
- Analyze difficulties in weighing the costs and benefits of technology use in health care
- Explain the challenges to ensuring ongoing, technological competence in nursing
- Identify the nurse's role in contributing to the ethical use of technology

As an RN you most likely have been able to see how technology is dramatically changing the world around us and this is especially evident in health care settings. Electronic health care records, smart devices, robotics, clinical decision support, and genetics are just a few of the technologies changing the health care landscape. In fact, one could argue that nothing has changed or will change the way nursing is practiced more than advances in technology. Indeed, the current rate of technology development and implementation is staggering. Andersen and Rasmussen (2015) suggest that society is transformed whenever new technologies emerge that change our means of production and ability to communicate and that the rapid technological development of the past century—in biotechnology, information technology, nanotechnology, and artificial intelligence—holds promise to do the same for our current, postindustrial world. As all of this occurs, it is good to reflect upon the statement made by Elvin Charles Stakman (1949): "Science cannot stop while ethics catches up. . . . And nobody should expect scientists to do all the thinking for the country."

CASE SCENARIO

As the "nurse" in the family, relatives often call to solicit health care advice. Julie, your sister-in-law, called this morning and shared that her 40-year-old sister was recently diagnosed with ovarian cancer. Because of a fairly strong family history of ovarian and breast cancers in her family, she is considering genetic testing (BRCA) to better assess her own risk, but is concerned about the confidentiality of these data.

When she discussed it with her husband, he discouraged her, suggesting that she was overreacting, that they could not afford it, and that having the genetic marker could increase the cost of life insurance or have other negative financial repercussions down the road. Julie feels she could keep the costs lower and control the confidentiality of results better if she did her testing privately through a low-cost commercial vendor online but knows that the results may have less reliability/validity and be less comprehensive than if it was ordered by her physician (subtyping could be included). She also mentions, however, that insurance might cover the cost of the testing if it was ordered by her physician, but the results then would be a part of her permanent medical record.

In addition, when she mentioned the possibility of genetic testing to her two daughters, one daughter said, "Do it if you must, but I do not want to know the results as it could influence my decision to marry and have children." The other daughter encouraged her to have the testing, suggesting that she would want to know the results right away so that she could do whatever necessary to mitigate her own risk.

Ethical issues contained in the case: confidentiality, autonomy, paternalism, beneficence, truth telling, duty-based ethics, nonmaleficence, justice

It is disconcerting that in many cases, technology mania has occurred without the much needed, prior critical analysis of the ethical questions surrounding its development and use. Certainly the old adage "If we build it, they will come" is at least somewhat true when discussing technology advances in health care. One must at least question whether some new technologies should be built at all, who should come, and what the unintended consequences might be once these technologies are created.

Pickersgill (2013) agrees, suggesting that as new health technologies are introduced, transformations in the meanings of care occur. For example, as patients gain new choices in care options as a result of emerging technologies, new questions arise as to how to mandate and monitor "good care." Thus, care becomes more mutable and context-specific; furthermore, risk increases

Table 11.1

Four Leadership Challenges Nurses Face in Integrating Technology and Health Care

Balancing the human element with technology
Balancing cost and benefits
Training a technology-enabled nursing workforce and ensuring
    ongoing competency
Ensuring that technology use is ethical

that "good" care may entail practices of coercion. Gabr (n.d.) concurs, suggesting that vigilance systems are needed to ensure that rapid advances in science and technology will not result in uncontrollable evolution or unacceptable deviation or harm.

Questions to Consider Before Reading On

Returning to the Case Scenario, Julie asks you to help her think through what decision she could make and asks you what other issues she should consider.

1. Can Julie make a decision that is truly unencumbered by the wishes of others?

2. Can Julie actually "control" confidentiality in this case?

3. Can Julie protect her "right to know her genetic data" and also protect her daughter's "right not to know"?

This chapter addresses some of the ethical considerations associated with emerging technologies in health care including how the basic ethical principles of dignity and autonomy are challenged by technology; the need to balance technology and the human element; the difficulty in weighing the costs and benefits of technology in health care; the challenges inherent in ensuring ongoing technological competence in the workforce; and the ongoing struggle by to ensure that technology use is ethical (Table 11.1). In addition, the chapter suggests strategies nurses might use to lessen the potential ethical dissonance between increasingly technologically driven practice and ethical practice.

DIGNITY AND AUTONOMY

A problem noted by Daniel Dennett ("Ethical Quotes," 2001–2015) was "that no ethical system has ever achieved consensus. Ethical systems are completely unlike mathematics or science. This is a source of concern." Multiple ethical principles are relevant when looking at the potential impacts of emerging technology: justice, autonomy, fidelity, paternalism, fairness, beneficence, confidentiality, dignity, autonomy, and agency, to name just a few. Given space constraints, however, only two are discussed in this chapter: dignity and autonomy.

Question to Consider Before Reading On

1. Do new discoveries related to human enhancement pose ethical threats to human dignity or are they supported by beneficence?

Dignity

Merriam-Webster defines *dignity* simply as "the quality or state of being worthy, honored, or esteemed" ("Dignity," 2016). The International Federation of Social Workers (2012), however, suggests a greater complexity to the definition of dignity, noting that dignity entails respecting the right to self-determination, promoting the right to participation, treating each person as a whole, and identifying and developing strengths in others.

The right to self-determination is discussed with autonomy in this chapter. It is the subdefinition of "treating each person as a whole" that may be most threatened by emerging health care technologies since technology-enhanced diagnosis and treatment are frequently directed at specific body parts rather than a more holistic approach.

For example, Chan (2015) suggests that dignity may be threatened by technology advances such as genetics since genetic research tends to reduce individuals to their genetic endowment. Wadhwa (2014) agrees, noting that, while access to and use of genetic information may promote better diagnosis and treatment, such information can also be used to restrict an individual's freedoms and right to participation by care as a sole result of his or her genetic structure. For example, Wadhwa notes that the Genetic Information Nondiscrimination Act of 2008 prohibits the use of genetic information in health insurance and employment, but provides no protection from discrimination in long-term care, disability, and life insurance. And, it places few limits on commercial use. There are no laws to stop companies from using aggregated genomic data in the same way that lending companies and employers use social-media data, or to prevent marketers from targeting ads at people with genetic defects.

Similarly, the John J. Reilly Center (2015a) suggests that new discoveries related to human enhancements pose ethical dilemmas to dignity since magnifying some aspect of human biological function beyond the social norms violates the treatment of the individual as a whole. It also results in physical risk and creates an unlevel playing field (some individuals are artificially enhanced). For example, drugs designed to treat attention deficit hyperactivity disorder can also be used to enhance the alertness and cognition of those without the disorder. While using performance-enhancing drugs such as stimulants, blood-boosters, and synthetic growth hormone is generally considered unethical by bodies that govern academics and athletics since they violate expectations of fairness and equity, the John J. Reilly Center (2015a) questions whether such enhancements are really unethical if they can be justified on utilitarian grounds. They also promote self-determination and promote strengths in individuals (part of the definition of dignity).

Allhoff, Lin, Moor, and Weckert (2009) suggest, however, that human enhancement technologies directly impact "human dignity" (p. 7); what it means to be human. For instance, they question whether the desire for enhancement shows ingratitude for what we have and (further) enables an attitude of unquenchable dissatisfaction with one's life. Would human enhancement technologies hinder moral development since many believe that "soul-making" is impossible without struggle? Is the frailty of the human condition necessary to best appreciate life? Can or should children be enhanced to give them an edge in society? Allhoff and colleagues (2009) conclude that a sensible middle path may be the best choice at this point in time and encourage individuals to use their own moral compass to find answers to these difficult questions.

 ### Questions to Consider Before Reading On

1. In reflecting on the Case Scenario, should Julie's desire to protect her daughter's "right not to know" change if she actually develops genetically susceptible cancer?

2. Should Julie's decision to be tested be influenced by her daughter's wish to not know the results?

3. Does the duty to warn outweigh the need to promote autonomy?

Autonomy

Merriam-Webster defines "autonomy" as "the quality or state of being self-governing" or having "self-directing freedom and especially moral independence" ("Autonomy," 2016). Rhodes (2013) agrees, suggesting that the ethical principle of autonomy represents a demanding standard for the self-regulation of one's actions since it gives beings moral worth and holds people responsible for their actions. With autonomy, individuals are viewed as having a distinctive self-legislating ability (assumes decisional capacity) and this requires others to respect their choices.

In health care, however, patients do not always have the capacity or the desire to make autonomous health care decisions. Indeed, the health care system historically has been paternalistic and the ethical principle of agency has been used to justify decision making based on what the provider considered the most appropriate course of action. Merriam-Webster defines *agency* as "the capacity, condition, or state of acting or of exerting power" to achieve an end ("Agency," 2016). Agency, however, should also be viewed as a moral directive as most individuals have notions of right and wrong and are held accountable to take actions that are beneficent.

The Internet is one example of an emerging technology that has significant potential to impact patient autonomy. Historically, providers were recognized as the keepers of medical information. This allowed them to be the primary health care decision maker, often relegating patients to a somewhat passive and dependent role (Huston, 2013). The Internet changed these dynamics because it expanded the power and control of health information from providers alone to patients themselves. Indeed, the Internet, which is growing faster than any other medium in the world, has great potential to improve health by enhancing communications and improving access to information for care providers, patients, health plan administrators, public health officials, biomedical researchers, and other health professionals.

Indeed, thousands of health information websites currently exist for consumers to explore in attempting to answer their health-related questions and more are launched daily. "Indeed, when it comes to health-related mobile technology, patients may be more frequent users than health care professionals. Thousands of software applications are developed each year just for personal health issues and medical conditions, and they are easily accessible from smartphones and tablets."

The end result is that patients have electronic access to medical information on virtually any topic, any time. This suggests that many consumers have at least the opportunity to be better informed about their health care problems and needs than in the past. In fact, this increased opportunity for consumers to access information has resulted in the creation of what is known as the *expert patient*—a patient who has the confidence, skills, information, and knowledge to participate in his or her health care.

Theoretically, expert patients are better informed and thus better able to be active participants in decision making. Although most providers appreciate well-informed patients who have demonstrated the initiative to learn more about their health care needs and problems, there are concerns regarding the accuracy and currency of information patients find on the Internet. In addition, many patients do not fully understand the information that is available to them, even when it is accurate. Some providers are concerned that patients will inappropriately self-diagnose, leading them to seek inappropriate treatment or no treatment at all.

In addition, little research has been done to validate the currency or accuracy of the information on health care Internet sites. Krotoski (2011), citing a recent study or more than 12,000 people across 12 different countries, noted that more people than ever are using the web to find out more about an ailment before or instead of visiting the doctor. Alarmingly, only a quarter of the people surveyed checked the reliability of health information they found online by looking at the credibility of the source. In addition, Krotoski suggests that "a typical medical consultation follows this trajectory:

1) you discover a growth, 2) do a Google search, 3) believe the first result that confirms your expectations" (para 6).

Krotoski concludes then, that while the wealth of health information online has contributed to a more informed public, the expertise of the professional should not be undermined by the leveling power of the web. Clearly, patients need to become experts at retrieving health care information and deciphering it to better empower themselves in health care decision making and to promote autonomy.

Question to Consider Before Reading On

1. What safeguards exist or could be created to better ensure accuracy and currency of layman health care information posted on the Internet?

BALANCING THE HUMAN ELEMENT AND TECHNOLOGY

Munro (2012) states:

> For each of us there is a moment of discovery. In the flash of a synapse we learn that life is elemental. This knowledge changes everything. We see all things connected. The element not listed on the chart— is the missing element—the human element. And when we add it to the equation—the chemistry changes. Every reaction is different. The human element is the element of change. Nothing is more fundamental. Nothing more elemental.

The human element is the art of nursing and nurses need to be actively involved in determining how best to use technology to supplement, not eliminate, human resources (Huston, 2013). One of the most significant challenges nurse leaders face in using technology is to find that balance between maximizing the benefits of using that technology, while not devaluing the human element. Nurses need to make sure that the human element is not lost in the race to expand technology. Pols (2015) agrees, suggesting that nurses, patients, and ethicists have expressed concern that "care through technology can become a cold and dehumanizing affair." This is certainly a potential concern with the use of robots as caregivers, with the Internet as a health care tool, and with some new technological devices.

Questions to Consider Before Reading On

1. What aspects of physical and mental nursing care do you believe could or should be replaced by robotics in the coming decade?

2. Are the elderly at greater risk of technology-related harm and ethics violations than other age groups?

Robots as Caregivers

Robotics provides a clear example of how the human element is being replaced by or supplemented with technology. Indeed, in some parts of the world, robots are being developed to provide direct patient care, particularly for the elderly. This is especially true in Japan, known as the "Robot Kingdom," as a result of a burgeoning elderly population and a low birth rate, which has resulted in a severe shortage of caregivers (Huston, 2013).

For example, physical service robots have been created to help with tasks such as washing or carrying elderly people, and mental service robots provide emotional support through therapeutic listening and feedback (robots use vision systems to monitor human expressions, gestures; use body language and voice sensors to pick up on intonation and individual words and sentences; and sense human emotion through wearable sensors that monitor pulse rate and perspiration). In addition, robotic walkers now exist that can obtain information about the environment through sensors, cameras, obstacle recognition systems and software. These walkers can guide elderly users to paths that minimize the chances of stumbling and falls (European Commission, 2015).

Sharkey and Sharkey (2012) suggest, however, that the increased use of robots in elder care raises a number of ethical concerns, including the potential reduction in the amount of human contact (opportunities for human social contact can be reduced); an increase in the feelings of objectification and loss of control (robots lack sensitivity to people's feelings and provide care at the convenience of caregivers); a loss of privacy; the loss of personal liberty; deception and infantilization (robots may restrict the behavior of humans); and a lack of clarity regarding the circumstances in which elderly people are allowed to control the robots (who is responsible if things go wrong?).

Sharkey and Sharkey suggest that at present:

> Apart from fundamental human rights legislation, there is little protection for elderly people against the potential downsides of robot care. In particular, there are no obvious restrictions on the amount of time that elderly people could be left in the care of robots, nor on the amount of human contact that they should experience. Like children, the very old and infirmed can be seen as being in need of special protection. (p. 33)

Huston (2013) notes that many consumers and health care providers negate these ethical concerns arguing that the lack of emotion in patient care robots is the element of human caregivers that can never be replaced. However, as technology continues to advance, the ability to distinguish robot from human caregiver is declining. The appearance of robot caregivers is increasingly lifelike, and Sharkey and Sharkey (2012) note that this physical embodiment means that they can be used to perform tasks in the world to a greater extent than purely computational devices. Their often personable appearance may lead them to be welcomed in the home and other locations, (where for instance a surveillance camera would not be accepted) and their personable, or animal-like, appearance can encourage and mislead people into thinking that robots are capable of more social understanding than is actually the case.

In addition, although machines have historically been unable to demonstrate caring, the development of new robotic devices is beginning to challenge this long-held belief. Researchers at the Georgia Institute of Technology have developed "Cody," a robotic nurse the university says is "gentle enough to bathe elderly patients" (Bilton, 2013). "Hector," a robot developed by the University of Reading in England, can remind patients to take their medicine, keep track of their eyeglasses, and assist in the event of a fall (Bilton, 2013).

Some robots are even being created with the purpose of therapeutic communication or interaction. Crisotomo (2015) and Bilton (2013) note that "Paro," a therapeutic robot that looks like a baby harp seal, is meant to have a calming effect on patients with dementia and Alzheimer's in health care facilities. First introduced last 2010, Paro was developed by Fujisoft to literally talk with its users and is currently used in nursing homes worldwide. More recently, Softbank's "Pepper" robot was designed not only to chat, but also to alter its reactions and speech by sensing and "feeling" the emotion of its users (Crisotomo, 2015).

Similarly, a laboratory at Carnegie Mellon has designed a robot to work with therapists and people with autism (Bilton, 2013). The machine can develop a personality and blinks and giggles as people interact with it. Jim Osborn, a roboticist and executive director of the Robotics Institute's Quality of Life Technology Center at the university, noted that those who tested it loved it and hugged it, and began to think of it as something more than a machine with a computer.

Indeed, Cynthia Breazeal, founder of the world's first social robot for the home called "Jibo," suggests that technology and humans can and should work hand in hand. She argues that what is being created are robots that are really teammates and that these robots should complement the services that human professionals can provide (Fox, 2015).

Sharkey and Sharkey (2012) agree in that they suggest that while all of us should be concerned about the use of robots for elder care, it is not the use of robots in elder care per se that should be of concern; it is the ways in which they are used. Sharkey and Sharkey suggest positive contributions by robotics including the following:

> Assistive robots and robotic technology could help to overcome problems of mobility, and reduce elderly people's dependence on busy, and sometimes inattentive, care staff. The use of remote controlled robots to monitor, and virtually visit elderly people could enable the elderly to live independently for longer. Robots could remind them

what medicines to take, watch out for health problems and safety risks. Companion robots could facilitate the social lives of elderly people, by giving them an interesting gadget to talk to other people about. Social interaction could also be facilitated by monitoring robots that enabled virtual visits from friends and family. (p. 30)

Bilton (2013) expresses concern, however, in his warning that given the increasing number of elderly people and the decline in the number of people to take care of them, it is likely that robots will start to fill in the care gaps. Sherry Turkle, a professor of science, technology, and society at the Massachusetts Institute of Technology and author of the book *Alone Together: Why We Expect More From Technology and Less From Each Other*, voiced her concerns as well in sharing that she was troubled when she saw a 76-year-old woman share stories about her life with Paro, the robotic seal. Turkle suggests, "We have been reduced to spectators of a conversation that has no meaning," and since robots do not have a true capacity to listen or understand something personal, tricking patients to think they can is unethical (Bilton, 2013). Debates, then, about how best to merge the human element of care (caring) and emerging robotic technology will undoubtedly continue.

The Internet

The Internet is another example of a technology that may significantly impact or interfere with the relationship between the caregiver and the patient, with Bajarin (2015) identifying the Internet as the most disruptive innovation of our time. For example, Dombo, Kay, and Weller (2014) suggest that maintaining professional boundaries becomes more challenging and critical for health care providers when online treatment or forms of communication are involved. The online setting may give the impression that the health care provider is always available, which can create unintentional opportunities for a client to feel rejected or for boundary violations on the part of the professional, particularly if she or he is immediately responsive on weekends and evenings through a variety of messaging mediums.

In addition, Harris and Robinson Kurpius (2014) report that mental health graduate students often engage in ethically questionable behavior as part of social networking, including such activities as conducting online searches for client information without informed consent. More than half of these students they studied did not believe their graduate programs adequately addressed professional social networking guidelines and slightly less than half did not believe their professional organization adequately addressed professional social networking guidelines. Students noted they needed additional guidance on how to navigate ethical dilemmas created by social networking.

Privacy concerns related to Internet use also pose ethical considerations. Walcerz (1999–2015) notes that many websites collect user data, from user-names and passwords to personal information such as addresses and phone numbers, without the explicit permission of users. Selling this information is widely considered unethical, but is often in a legal gray area because the user provides the data in the first place. Similarly, copyright and intellectual property rights are continually threatened by the Internet as a publishing medium with the end result being a host of ethical concerns related to plagiarism and piracy.

Technological Devices

Da Silva and Ferreira (2013) note that two forms of nursing action exist in the field of intensive care: caring and technological action. "Caring requires a greater application of knowledge, which directs the attention of nurses in search of the client's objective and subjective data, as well as data from the devices. The technological action is mostly sustained by information from the technological device, leading professionals to perform actions based on data supplied solely by the device" (p. 1324).

Da Silva and Ferriera (2013, p. 1324) suggest these two forms of nursing action lead to conflict with some suggesting that more attention to objectivity involved in care occurs with the technological actions and that this occurs at the expense of expressiveness or caring. Others, however, believe that "the fact that the nurse concentrate his observation more on certain critical situations that require technology for care does not presuppose a notion primarily of devaluation of subjectivity, indicating a mechanistic view, or lack of patient care, seen as inhumane conditions."

Van Manen (2015) suggests that even routine, noninvasive technologies, however, may impact the patient–provider or patient–family relationship and that these technologies are often a taken-for-granted part of the medical lifeworld. For example, van Manen suggests that while providers may view the neonatal cardiorespiratory monitor as a relatively simple technology to assist with vital signs and patient monitoring, it also may be a barrier to parent–child interaction. Van Manen concludes that, as the monitor is woven into human relationships, the monitor may carry more ethical significance than other seemingly ordinary things since the monitor penetrates the ethical moment, the ethicity of ethics, as it weaves into the relation of self and other, parent and child.

Dombo et al. (2014) also suggest that technology may promote a lack of face-to-face interactions between the patient and the provider. Practitioners may struggle with communication dynamics that inhibit building rapport and engagement when they are unable to read nonverbal cues when using e-mail or messaging. Additionally, there appears to be a distinct lack of regulation of what care should and should not be provided virtually.

Pols (2015), in detailing several case studies involving telecare, agrees, noting that "noisy technology" must be turned off since people and devices direct each other and each tries to "act back" at the other in order to establish a workable, livable, or even a good situation. In her case studies, telepatients . . .

> did not check their figures on the television, but trusted their nurses to call them if something was wrong. Webcams seduced people to contact each other about disease in daily life, but people used them to discuss many other things as well. Hard working nurses and frail elderly are notoriously difficult to organize "around the table." Attending to what they *do*, and how this expresses their practical knowledge and normative solutions is a way of making them heard. Not as autonomous spokespersons, but as the relational beings an empirical ethics wants to articulate. (p. 90)

Another ethical consideration associated with the use of medical devices includes whether adequate safeguards are in place for the patients who use them. For example, the John C. Reilly Center (2012) notes that implanted medical devices, such as pacemakers, are susceptible to hackers who can breach the security of the wireless device from a laptop and reprogram it to deliver an 830-volt shock. How do we make sure these devices are secure?

Similarly, Dodds (2015) notes that unlike the case of developing a new drug, stem cell therapy (e.g., that used in 3D printing) cannot be tested on a sizable number of healthy people prior to being tested on patients and then, finally, being made available as a standard treatment. The point of using a patient's own stem cells is to tailor the treatment quite specifically to that patient, and not to develop a treatment that can be tested on anybody else. She concludes that researchers must continue to develop new models for testing technological discoveries and treatments for safety and effectiveness before their implementation to overcome this ethical concern.

BALANCING COSTS AND BENEFITS

Questions to Consider Before Reading On

1. In reflecting on the Case Scenario, does potential socioeconomic discrimination discourage individuals from testing for genetically susceptible cancers?

2. What safeguards could be put in place to reduce this risk?

The United States is home to numerous technology developments that have led to health care advances and improved quality of life. Huston (2013) notes, however, that the U.S. health care system is already the most expensive health care system in the world and technology is one of the leading cost drivers. Sivy (2012) agrees, suggesting that while new technology sometimes reduces health care costs, mostly it drives spending higher.

In addition, since access to technology is often dependent on a person's ability to pay for that technology, many health care disparities still exist in this regard. Dodds (2015) asks, "Should these treatments only be available to those who can pay the additional cost? If so, then those patients who lack financial resources may not receive effective treatments that others can access for a range of serious conditions."

The reality is that emerging diagnostic and treatment technologies are expensive and thus may need to be used selectively. Decisions about who should have access to them and at what cost are at the heart of many ethical debates.

The Markkula Center for Applied Ethics (n.d.) suggests that the same technologies that offer hope for ever-increasing life expectancy (e.g., promising cancer treatments, surgical procedure and pharmacological break-throughs, and advanced genetic research) are also leading to increased demands on the health care system from a growing population of senior citizens. "Ethicists and health professionals alike are now raising questions about when and from whom treatments should be withheld, as competition for the scarce medical resources of the health care system grows beyond the system's capacity to provide care for everyone. Already, some forms of rationing have been implemented, and more rationing of health care resources may be inevitable" (Markkula Center, n.d., para 2). Should health care technology be rationed by age? By ability to pay? By perceived potential contributions to society at large?

Sivy (2012, para 4) agrees, suggesting that as health care spending soars, thorny ethical questions will become more urgent. When should aggressive treatment be limited for someone who is terminally ill? More than 30% of the Medicare budget is now spent on patients in their last year of life, and the benefits of that treatment vary enormously. Who decides how much to do?

Similarly, Dodds (2015) notes that while the introduction of 3D printing has offered great benefits in medicine, it also raises a number of ethical questions as the technology develops. For example, she notes that if the technology can be used to develop replacement organs and bones, could it not also be used to develop human capacities beyond what is normal for human beings? Should existing bones be replaced with artificial ones that are stronger and more flexible, less likely to break; or muscle tissue be improved so that it is more resilient and less likely to become fatigued, or new lungs be implanted that oxygenate blood more efficiently, even in a more polluted environment?

Dodds (2015) goes on to caution that 3D printing could be associated with military use with the idea that it could provide an advantage if our soldiers were less susceptible to being wounded, fatigued, or harmed in battle. She notes that "while it is clear that it would be preferable for military personnel to be less vulnerable to physical harm, the history of military technology suggests that 3D printing could lead to a new kind of arms race. Increasing the defenses that soldiers have in the face of battle would then lead to increasing the destructive power of weapons to overcome those defenses. And in so doing, increasing the harm to which civilians are exposed."

In addition, questions have been raised about whether need drives technology or whether technology is driving need. For example, a 2011 study showed that after Wisconsin hospitals acquired robotic surgery technology, the number of prostate removals they performed doubled within 3 months. In contrast, the number of prostate surgeries stayed the same at hospitals that did not purchase the new $2 million technology ("Do Robots Drive Up Prostate Surgeries?," 2011). One must question whether surgeons at hospitals with robots are recommending surgery for men with prostate cancer because the outcomes (potential reductions in incontinence and impotence) are better or whether the new technology is simply more exciting than alternative treatments like radiation or "watchful waiting" ("Do Robots Drive Up Prostate Surgeries?" 2011).

Furthermore, Hansen and Gee (2014) suggest that "scientific inertia" exists regarding new technology due to the scientific requirement for high levels of proof via well-replicated studies; the need to publish quickly; the use of existing intellectual and technological resources; and the conservative approach of many reviewers and research funders. Indeed, since 1996, the funding of environmental, health, and safety (EHS) research represented just 0.6% of the overall funding of research and technological development (RTD).

Compared with RTD funding, EHS research funding for information and communication technologies, nanotechnology, and biotechnology was 0.09%, 2.3%, and 4% of total research, respectively. The low EHS research ratio seems to be an unintended consequence of disparate funding decisions; technological optimism; a priori assertions of safety; collective hubris; and myopia. Clearly then, more EHS research is needed to anticipate and minimize potential hazards while maximizing the commercial longevity of emerging technologies (Hansen & Gee, 2014). Without such research, accurately balancing cost and benefits is almost impossible.

This is especially the case when emerging technologies may provide the only hope for patients. Sivy (2012) notes that newspapers feature on a regular basis, stories about patients being denied access to new high-tech treatments. Often, these treatments are outrageously expensive with only a small chance of extending life for a relatively short period. A public outcry ensues, debates continue about whether the treatment should be funded, and patients often die in the meantime. Whatever the outcome is, no one is ever really satisfied.

Sivy (2012, para 10) goes on to suggest that when it comes to controlling technology, directing medical research is a monumental task. "Some discovery that affects only an obscure disease might be the key to unlocking something much more important. And having made such a discovery, is it ethical to refuse to make it available to someone whose life might be saved, even if the odds are low? Similarly, should a hospital not buy and use some exotic scanning machine if that might be the only way to diagnose certain rare diseases? Should progress be limited simply because it might lead to higher costs?"

Sivy (2012, para 1) concludes then that:

> While policy experts complain that America has been slow to address its long-term economic problems—and unrealistic when such issues are actually discussed, there has been even greater evasion and denial when it comes to the ethical dilemmas that will accompany those economic problems, especially where healthcare is concerned. Politicians talk as though relatively painless solutions can be found. But in reality there is no magical escape from difficult choices—they can only be dealt with by facing up to them squarely.

ENSURING TECHNOLOGY COMPETENCE IN THE WORKFORCE

It has been said, "Technology is dominated by two types of people: those who understand what they do not manage, and those who manage what they do not understand" ("Technology," 1977–2001).

Technology is not only expensive (both initially and in terms of maintenance and technical support), but also needs constant upgrades, and the education needed to truly be competent in the use of all this technology is never ending. This is certainly the case in newer "smart" technologies such as infusion pumps, beds, bedside medication verification systems, drug dispensing machines, and other clinical tools in use today.

Perhaps though, one of the best current examples of where technology introduction has preceded workforce competence is the use of genetic testing. The John J. Reilly Center (2015b) notes that within the last 10 years, the creation of fast, low-cost genetic sequencing has given the public direct access to genome sequencing and analysis, with little or no guidance from physicians or genetic counselors on how to process the information.

Calzone and colleagues (2010) agree that despite a burgeoning body of evidence regarding the contribution of genetics and genomics to health or illness, there is little evidence of a genomically competent nursing workforce. They suggest that "in order for people to benefit from widespread genetic/genomic discoveries, nurses must be competent to obtain comprehensive family histories, identify family members at risk for developing a genomic influenced condition and for genomic influenced drug reactions, help people make informed decisions about and understand the results of their genetic/genomic tests and therapies, and refer at-risk people to appropriate health care professionals and agencies for specialized care."

Indeed, Calzone and colleagues (2010) argue that bringing all 2.9 million nurses in the U.S. workforce to the forefront of genetics/genomic health care practice is appropriate, as nurses must elicit health-related information, recognize what is important, and subsequently act upon that information in caring for the patients they serve. Calzone and colleagues suggest that public policies that affect heath care practice in the area of genetics/genomics will be stronger with inclusion of nurses and professional nursing organization representation in the policy-making process.

Similarly, Kamei (2013) suggests that telenursing requires advanced abilities and specialized knowledge since telenurses must have a deep understanding of the latest knowledge in the areas in which they conduct telenursing as well as highly developed critical thinking skills, the provision of information based on evidence, excellent patient teaching, counseling, and communication skills, and expertise in the use of telecommunication devices.

Huston (2013), however, asks:

> Who is going to train all the healthcare professionals who will work with new emerging technologies? More importantly, who will need to be responsible for assuring *ongoing competency* in a digital era where half of what someone knows is obsolete in three years?

There are no national standards for defining, measuring, or requiring continuing competence in nursing. In addition, specialty nursing organizations, state nurses associations, state boards of nursing, and professional nursing organizations have not reached consensus about what continuing competence is and how to measure it, although there is little debate that it is needed. Huston (2014a) suggests the reality is that given the multiplicity and variations of the definition of continuing competence and the number of stakeholders affected by its promulgation, identifying and mandating strategies that ensure the continuing competence of health care providers will be very difficult.

The responsibility, then, for initial as well as continued competence then in the use of emerging technologies really falls to the license holder. Ward (2012) iterates that patients trust that their nurses are competent in their practice. This means that nurses must be compliant with Board of Nursing standards and they must complete necessary continuing education or whatever is necessary to demonstrate their competency.

Questions to Consider Before Reading On

1. How much input do nurses have at your place of practice in terms of the selection and use of new technology? Are ethical considerations included in these acquisition decisions?

2. What can or should a nurse do when his or her personal values appear in conflict with the organizational values regarding the ethical use of technology?

ENSURING THAT TECHNOLOGY USE IS ETHICAL: NURSING'S ROLE

Wood (2013) suggests that when nurses encounter ethical dilemmas in situations in which they cannot do what they consider to be "the right thing," they experience moral distress. Indeed, the problems faced by health care leaders regarding technology will increasingly be what is called *wicked*—meaning that they have many causes, they are tough to describe, and there is no right answer.

To counter this moral distress in technology-related ethical dilemmas, Huston (2013) suggests that nurses must increasingly speak up and ask "how" and "why" technology should be implemented. What parameters need to be put into place to determine its ethical use? These questions and others related to the ethical use of technology should be reviewed by ethics committees prior to the technology implementation and nurses should have a voice in that discussion.

In addition, Mayhew (n.d.) suggests that agencies should provide all employees with ethics training that engages them in scenarios to learn how to address and resolve ethical dilemmas. Policies should be developed that hold employees accountable for their actions and alert them to their responsibilities in upholding professional standards. In addition, Mayhew suggests that an ombudsperson should be available to assist employees with workplace ethical concerns and that an ethics hotline be available to employees who encounter ethical dilemmas that put them or patients into uncomfortable or threatening positions.

In a recent speech, Thomas Baldwin, a professor of philosophy at Britain's York University, suggested that new technologies bring significant hopes of curing terrible diseases as well as fears about the consequences of trying to enhance human capability beyond what is normally possible (Kelland, 2012). Baldwin concluded that the blurring of the line between man and machine will continue to pose concerns about the ethics of emerging technologies in medicine and other fields. It is important for nurses to be a part of conversations to address these ethical concerns.

CONCLUSION

Huston (2014b) notes that evolving technologies offer great opportunities to improve the quality of patient care, but technology alone is not the answer. Regardless of the system that is deployed, health care organizations must consider what technology can best be used in each individual setting and how it should be used ethically. In addition, successfully adopting and integrating new technology requires care providers to understand that technology's limitations as well as its benefits.

Unfortunately, Wadhwa (2014) suggests that with the pace of technology growth, we have not been able to come to grips with what is ethical, let alone determine what laws or rules should be in place. Gabr (n.d.) agrees, suggesting that the ethical consequences associated with technological change must be further examined and that some institutionalization of health ethics should be required. In doing so, new, sensitive, reliable indicators as well as a vigilance system must be developed to monitor inequalities in health care and the abuse or neglect of human rights.

Rhodes (2013) agrees, suggesting that as patients, their families, and the public increasingly rely on health care professionals to assist in bioethical decision making, health care professionals must accept robust responsibilities for setting standards of competency and upholding those standards.

Critical Thinking Questions and Activities

1. In the chapter Case Scenario, can Julie's health care providers make appropriate health care assessments/treatment plans if they are not given access to Julie's genetic screening results?

2. What makes new technology worth the cost? What criteria should be used in making these value-based decisions?

3. Should health care technology be rationed by age? By ability to pay? By perceived potential contributions to society at large?

4. What emerging technologies are being introduced where you practice (as a student or as a nurse) that you believe need further ethical analysis/safeguards for patient use prior to their implementation?

5. Florence Nightingale said, "Rather, ten times, die in the surf, heralding the way to a new world, than stand idly on the shore" ("Florence Nightingale," 2015). How can you apply this quote to the use of technology in your current nursing practice?

6. What does the following quote mean to you in terms of your nursing practice?

   Ours is a world of nuclear giants and ethical infants. If we continue to develop our technology without wisdom or prudence, our servant may prove to be our executioner.
   Omar Bradley ("Quotations by author," 1977–2001)

7. What strategies could the professional nurse use to deemphasize the cold dehumanizing aspects of technological device use and reinforce the human caring (art of nursing)?

8. Consider the following information and questions from the John J. Reilly Center at the University of Notre Dame:

   Genetic testing has resulted in huge public health successes (diseases can now be prevented or helped by early intervention), but it also creates a new set of moral, legal, ethical, and policy issues surrounding the use of these tests. If the testing is useful, how do we provide equal access? What are the potential privacy issues and how do we protect this very personal and private information? Which genetic abnormalities warrant some kind of intervention? How do we ensure that the

(continued)

> **Critical Thinking Questions and Activities** *(continued)*
>
> information provided by genome analysis is correct (especially in the case of at-home tests)? Are we headed toward a new era of therapeutic intervention to increase quality of life, or a new era of eugenics? (John J. Reilly Center, 2015b, para 2).

REFERENCES

Agency. (2016). *Merriam-Webster's dictionary online*. Retrieved from http://www.merriam-webster .com/dictionary/agency

Allhoff, F., Lin, P., Moor, J., & Weckert, J. (2009, August 31). Ethics of human enhancement: 25 questions & answers. Prepared for: U.S. National Science Foundation. Retrieved from http:// ethics.calpoly.edu/NSF_report.pdf

Autonomy. (2016). *Merriam-Webster's dictionary online*. Retrieved from http://www.merriam-webster .com/dictionary/autonomy

Bajarin, T. (2015, January 12). This will be the most disruptive technology over the next 5 years. *Time*. Retrieved from http://time.com/3663909/technology-disruptive-impact/#3663909/technology -disruptive-impact

Bilton, N. (2013, May 19). Disruptions: Helper robots are steered, tentatively, to care for the aging. *The New York Times*. Retrieved from http://bits.blogs.nytimes.com/2013/05/19/disruptions -helper-robots-are-steered-tentatively-to-elder-care/?_r=0

Calzone, K. A., Cashion, A., Feetham, S., Jenkins, J., Prows, C. A., Williams, J. K. & Wung, S. F. (2010, January). Nurses transforming health care using genetics and genomics. *Nursing Outlook, 58*(1), 26–35.

Chan, D. K. (2015). The concept of human dignity in the ethics of genetic research. *Bioethics, 29*(4), 274–282. doi:10.1111/bioe.12102

Crisotomo, C. (2015). Robots: Japan's future elderly care workers. VR World Media. Retrieved from http://www.vrworld.com/2015/01/22/robots-japans-future-elderly-care-workers

da Silva, R. C., & de Assunção Ferreira, M. (2013). The practice of intensive care nursing: Alliance among technique, technology and humanization. *Revista Da Escola De Enfermagem Da USP, 47*(6), 1324–1331. doi:10.1590/S0080-623420130000600011

Dignity. (2016). *Merriam-Webster's dictionary online*. Retrieved from http://www.merriam-webster .com/dictionary/dignity

Do robots drive up prostate surgeries? (2011). FoxNews.com. Retrieved from http://www.foxnews .com/health/2011/07/20/do-robots-drive-up-prostate-surgeries.html

Dodds, S. (2015, February 11). 3D printing raises ethical issues in medicine. *ABC Science*. Retrieved from http://www.abc.net.au/science/articles/2015/02/11/4161675.htm

Dombo, E. A., Kays, L., & Weller, K. (2014). Clinical social work practice and technology: Personal, practical, regulatory, and ethical considerations for the twenty-first century. *Social Work in Health Care, 53*(9), 900–919. doi:10.1080/00981389.2014.948585

Ethical quotes. Daniel Dennet quotation. (2001–2015). Brainy Quote. Retrieved from http://www .brainyquote.com/quotes/keywords/ethical.html

European Commission. (2015). The walking robot set to help elderly people live an autonomous life. Retrieved from http://www.euronews.com/2015/04/24/the-walking-robot-set-to-help-elderly -people-live-an-autonomous-life

Florence Nightingale Quotes. (2015). Good Reads. Retrieved from http://www.goodreads.com/author/quotes/63031.Florence_Nightingale

Fox, M. (2015, May 20). Dramatic change for workforce ahead: Experts. Retrieved from http://www.cnbc.com/2015/05/20/dramatic-change-for-workforce-ahead-experts.html

Gabr, M. (n.d.). Health ethics, equity and human dignity. Retrieved from http://humiliationstudies.org/documents/GabrHealthEthics.pdf

Hansen, S. F., & Gee, D. (2014). Adequate and anticipatory research on the potential hazards of emerging technologies: A case of myopia and inertia. *Journal of Epidemiology & Community Health, 68*(9), 890–895. doi:10.1136/jech-2014-204019

Harris, S. E., & Robinson Kurpius, S. E. (2014). Social networking and professional ethics: Client searches, informed consent, and disclosure. *Professional Psychology: Research & Practice, 45*(1), 11–19. doi:10.1037/a0033478

Huston, C. (2013, May 31). The impact of emerging technology on nursing care: Warp speed ahead. *OJIN: The Online Journal of Issues in Nursing, 18*(2), Manuscript 1. doi:10.3912/OJIN. Vol 18No02Man01. Retrieved from http://nursingworld.org/MainMenuCategories/ANAMarket place/ANAPeriodicals/OJIN/TableofContents/Vol-18-2013/No2-May-2013/Impact-of -Emerging-Technology.html

Huston, C. (2014a). *Professional issue in nursing: Challenges and opportunities* (3rd ed.). Chapter 19: Assuring provider competence through licensure, continuing education, and certification. Philadelphia, PA: Lippincott, Williams, and Wilkins.

Huston, C. (2014b). *Professional issue in nursing: Challenges and opportunities* (3rd ed.). Chapter 14: Technology in the health care workplace: Benefits, limitations, and challenges. Philadelphia, PA: Lippincott, Williams, and Wilkins.

The International Federation of Social Workers. (2012, March 3). Statement of ethical principles. Retrieved from http://ifsw.org/policies/statement-of-ethical-principles

John J. Reilly Center. (2012). Emerging ethical dilemmas in science and technology. University of Notre Dame. Retrieved from http://www.sciencedaily.com/releases/2012/12/121217162440 .htm

John J. Reilly Center. (2015a). Human enhancements. Retrieved from http://reilly.nd.edu/outreach/emerging-ethical-dilemmas-and-policy-issues-in-science-and-technology/human-enhance ments

John J. Reilly Center. (2015b). Genetic testing & personalized medicine. University of Notre Dame. Retrieved from http://reilly.nd.edu/outreach/emerging-ethical-dilemmas-and-policy-issues-in -science-and-technology/personalized-medicine

Kamei, T. (2013). Information and communication technology for home care in the future. *Japan Journal of Nursing Science, 10*(2), 154–161. doi:10.1111/jjns.12039

Kelland, K. (2012, March 1). Super-human brain technology sparks ethics debate. *Reuters*. Retrieved from   www.reuters.com/article/2012/03/01/us-brain-neurotechnology-ethics-idUSTRE 82000F20120301

Krotoski, A. (2011, January 9). What effect has the internet had on healthcare? *The Guardian*. Retrieved from http://www.guardian.co.uk/technology/2011/jan/09/untangling-web-krotoski-health-nhs

Markkula Center for Applied Ethics. (n.d.). Unhealthy dilemmas. Santa Clara University. Retrieved from http://www.scu.edu/ethics/publications/iie/v3n3/homepage.html

Mayhew, R. (n.d.). How to handle ethical issues in the workplace. Retrieved from http://smallbusiness .chron.com/handle-ethical-issues-workplace-10157.html

Munro, D. (2012, August 2). Healthcare's often missing element—The human element. *Forbes/Business*. Retrieved from http://www.forbes.com/sites/danmunro/2012/08/02/healthcares-often -missing-element-the-human-element

Pickersgill, M. (2013). From "implications" to "dimensions": Science, medicine and ethics in society. *Health Care Analysis, 21*(1), 31–42. doi:10.1007/s10728-012-0219-y

Pols, J. (2015). Towards an empirical ethics in care: Relations with technologies in health care. *Medicine, Health Care & Philosophy*, *18*(1), 81–90. doi:10.1007/s11019-014-9582-9

Quotations by author: Omar Bradley. (1997–2001). Quoteland.com. Retrieved from http://www .quoteland.com/author/Omar-Bradley-Quotes/2478

Rhodes, R. (2013). Bioethics: Looking forward and looking back. *American Journal of Bioethics*, *13*(1), 13–16. doi:10.1080/15265161.2013.748318

Sharkey, A., & Sharkey, N. (2012). Granny and the robots: Ethical issues in robot care for the elderly. University of Sheffield. Retrieved from http://staffwww.dcs.shef.ac.uk/people/A.Sharkey/shar key-granny.pdf

Sivy, M. (2012, April 19). Facing up to the ethical dilemmas in the healthcare debate. *Time*. Retrieved from http://business.time.com/2012/04/19/facing-up-to-the-ethical-dilemmas-in-the-health care-debate

Stakman, E. V. To the 116th meeting of the American Association for the Advancement of Science, New York City (December 26–31, 1949), as quoted in *Life Magazine* (January 9, 1950), *28*(2), 17.

Technology. (1997–2001). Quoteland.com. Retrieved from http://www.quoteland.com/topic/Tech nology-Quotes/141/?pg=3

Van Manen, M. A. (2015). The ethics of an ordinary medical technology. *Qualitative Health Research*, *25*(7), 996–1004. doi:10.1177/1049732314554101

Wadhwa, V. (2014, April 15). Laws and ethics can't keep pace with technology. *MIT Technology Review*. Retrieved from http://www.technologyreview.com/view/526401/laws-and-ethics-cant -keep-pace-with-technology

Walcerz, M. (1999–2015). Legal & ethical issues in technology. Retrieved from http://www.ehow .com/list_7640133_legal-ethical-issues-technology.html

Ward, J. (2012, August 31). Ethics in nursing: Issues nurses face. Retrieved from http://www.nurse together.com/ethics-nursing-issues-nurses-face

ADDITIONAL BIBLIOGRAPHY

Andersen, L. R., & Rasmussen, S. (2015, February 12). Tomorrow's technology will lead to sweeping changes in society—It must, for all our sakes. The Conversation. Retrieved from http://thecon versation.com/tomorrows-technology-will-lead-to-sweeping-changes-in-society-it-must-for -all-our-sakes-36023

Cameron, N. S. (2014). Humans, rights, and twenty-first century technologies: The making of the Universal Declaration on Bioethics and Human Rights. *Journal of Legal Medicine*, *35*(2), 235–272. doi:10.1080/01947648.2014.913458

Fisher, G. S. (2014). Reflections on the information age, social norms, and professional ethics. *Administration & Management Special Interest Section Quarterly*, *30*(3), 1–4.

Knapp van Bogaert, D., & Ogunbanjo, G. A. (2014). Ethics in health care: Confidentiality and infor mation technologies. *South African Family Practice*, *56*(1), S3–S5.

Terry, N. P., Priest, C. S., & Szotek, P. P. (2015). Google glass and health care: Initial legal and ethical questions. *Journal of Health & Life Sciences Law*, *8*(2), 93–114.

Competent Ethical Practice as It Relates to Quality and Safety in Nursing Practice

12

Applying IntegratedEthics in Nursing Practice

BARBARA L. CHANKO

LEARNING OBJECTIVES AND OUTCOMES

Upon completion of this chapter, the reader will be able to:

- Describe what is meant by *ethics quality*
- Discuss the levels of ethics quality throughout an organization
- List the domains of ethics in health care
- Describe the IntegratedEthics model and its three core functions: ethics consultation, preventive ethics, and ethical leadership
- Indicate how IntegratedEthics can be applied in the work setting

As an RN, you may have felt a conflict over how you should weigh the values that are important to you as a person, as a professional, and as a member of the organization where you work in deciding about what is the right thing to do in a particular circumstance. Have you thought about the quality of ethics throughout the organization in which you are employed? As you read the following Case Scenario, think about how well your organization supports ethics and how you can actively participate in ethics activities by asking yourself the following questions.

- From whom in the organization can I seek guidance when faced with an ethical concern that I cannot answer?

- How can I help to close a practice gap involving an ethics standard?

- Do I see leaders supporting an ethical environment and culture that benefits patients and staff?

CASE SCENARIO RELATED TO AN OVERVIEW OF INTEGRATEDETHICS

Beatrice has been the nurse manager on the unit for 5 years. In that time she has evolved as a leader and it is clear that she takes her responsibility of creating a positive workplace very seriously. Personally, she attributes much of her growth to her conscious decision to implement the concepts and practices of IntegratedEthics® that she learned when she worked at a Department of Veterans Affairs medical center. The staff members on her unit know that while not perfect, it is a great place to work, and recognize that in large part it is because ethics matters to Beatrice.

Over the past few years, Beatrice has been working to integrate ethics into all aspects of the unit's operations. Beatrice demonstrates to all staff that ethics is a priority, communicates clear expectations for ethical practice, practices ethical decision making, and supports the hospital's overall ethics program. Staff members notice that she focuses on her responsibilities as a leader to promote a positive ethical environment and culture.

When anyone has an ethical concern about particular patient care situations or ethical concerns about general situations involving patient care or operations of the unit that he or she cannot resolve on his or her own, Beatrice is the first to suggest they call for an ethics consultation. Staff members have come to value the expertise that the ethics consultants bring to discussions about conflicts or uncertainty over values. They know that ethics consultants will analyze the situation; help foster consensus and resolve the conflict in an atmosphere of respect; honor participants' authority and values in the decision-making process; and identify actions that are consistent with high ethical standards. The consultants do all this and they can be counted on to educate staff so that staff can become more skilled at handling the current and future ethical concerns. Knowing that ethical concerns will be responded to by the ethics consultation service makes staff members feel confident that they will not need to struggle alone with the inevitable ethical dilemmas that occur when providing health care.

Lately, Beatrice has been talking during staff meetings about some recurring ethical issues that she sees on the unit that create real gaps between what she knows is ethically the right thing to do and what staff sometimes do—these are ethics quality gaps. For example, she has noticed that informed consent and advance care planning practices are not being carried out in ways that are consistent with the best ethics practices that have been established in hospital policy. She knows that the nurses try their best but also that the organization's systems and processes sometimes get in the way of doing what is right. Beatrice believes that there are ways to prevent these ethics quality gaps by looking upstream and fixing the systems problems that cause the concerns in the first place. She wants to get a group together to do "preventive ethics," that is, performance improvement activities that reduce ethics quality gaps on a systems level.

Beatrice is excited to share what she knows and practices from Integrated-Ethics so that everyone can participate and be a part of ensuring that the ethics

(continued)

CASE SCENARIO RELATED TO AN OVERVIEW OF INTEGRATEDETHICS *(CONTINUED)*

quality on the unit is top notch. Alex, a relatively new nurse on the unit, has had some quality improvement experience and is intrigued to learn about Beatrice's approach. Beatrice senses that Alex may be a budding ethics champion and encourages her to read about the IntegratedEthics Program at the Department of Veterans Affairs National Center for Ethics in Health Care (2015). The website contains publically available information that can be used to guide implementation of IntegratedEthics (IE), a comprehensive approach to managing ethics in health care organizations, as well as tools and resources that make it easy to move the program forward on the unit.

Nurses, along with other staff of a health care organization, have a duty to integrate values with the myriad rules that guide and direct actions meant to provide high-quality care to patients. Nurses promote quality in their everyday practice through leadership and quality improvement activities. The American Association of Colleges of Nursing (AACN) Quality and Safety Education in Nursing (QSEN) graduate competencies state, "Graduate nurses will be the future leaders in practice, administration, education, and research. . . . It is essential that these nurses understand, provide leadership by example, and promote the importance of providing quality health care and outcome measurement" (American Association of Colleges of Nursing, 2012, p. 2). QSEN competencies relevant to quality in nursing are presented in Table 12.1.

Nurses play a critical role in ensuring that high ethical standards are practiced and maintained as they are one of the core health professionals that work 24 hours a day, 7 days a week in many health care settings. Their work is most fruitful when it is done as part of an overall ethics program in an organization committed to ethics quality. Health care organizations that have strong ethics programs and staff committed to *ethics quality* reap many benefits for their patients, employees, and the organization itself. Box 12.1 lists examples from a brief business case for ethics that describe how doing the right thing is also the sensible and wise thing to do (National Center for Ethics in Health Care, 2014a).

Questions to Consider Before Reading On

1. How do I know when I have provided nursing care of high ethics quality?

2. How would I define *ethics quality*?

When most people in health care think of quality, they think of technical quality (e.g., clinical indicators that a procedure or action was properly

Table 12.1

Quality in Nursing

KNOWLEDGE	SKILLS	ATTITUDES
Describe strategies for improving outcomes at all points of care	Translate aims for quality improvement efforts Align the aims, measures, and changes involved in improving care	Commit to concepts of transparency, managing variability measurement and accountability
Describe nationally accepted quality measures and benchmarks in the practice setting	Use a variety of sources of information to review outcomes, compare benchmarks of care, and identify potential areas for improvement (e.g., National Database of Nursing Quality Indicators; Hospital Compare; Centers for Medicare/Medicaid Services [CMS] indicators, The Joint Commission: ORYX, National Public Health Performance Standards and others) Participate in analysis of databases as sources of information for improving patient care Use quality indicators and benchmarks for improving system processes and outcomes	Commit to achieving the highest level of processes and outcomes of care Inspire others to achieve benchmark performance Model behaviors reflective of a commitment to high-quality outcomes
Evaluate the relevance of quality indicators and their associated measurement strategies	Identify useful measures that can be acted on to improve outcomes and processes	Value the importance of the use of data in quality improvement

(continued)

Table 12.1

Quality in Nursing (continued)

KNOWLEDGE	SKILLS	ATTITUDES
Explain variance and its common causes in patient care process and outcomes including costs	Select and use quality improvement tools (e.g., run charts, control charts, root cause analysis, flow diagrams, and GANTT charts) to achieve best possible outcomes	Commit to reducing unwarranted variation in care
Analyze ethical issues associated with continuous quality improvement	Participate in the design and monitoring of ethical oversight of continuous quality improvement projects Maintain confidentiality of any patient information used in quality improvement efforts	Value ethical conduct in quality improvement efforts Value the roles of others, such as IRBs, in assessing ethical and patient rights/ informed decision making
Analyze the impact of context such as access, cost, environment, workforce, team functioning, or community engagement on improvement efforts	Lead improvement efforts, taking into account context and best practices based on evidence Demonstrate commitment to process improvement	Value context (e.g., work environment, team functioning, social determinants) as an important contributor in quality care
Understand principles of change management	Apply change management principles by using data to improve patient and systems outcomes	Appreciate that all improvement is change Demonstrate leadership in affecting the necessary change

(continued)

Table 12.1

Quality in Nursing *(continued)*

KNOWLEDGE	SKILLS	ATTITUDES
Evaluate the effect of planned change on outcomes	Design, implement, and evaluate small tests of change in daily work (e.g., using an experiential learning method such as Plan-Do-Study-Act)	Value planned change
Analyze the impact of linking payment to quality improvement	Use benchmarks that carry financial penalties (e.g., serious reportable events) to improve care	Consistent with the National Quality Strategy, commit to achieving the highest quality of care in the practice setting (e.g., national strategy's aims of better care, healthy people, and affordable care)
Describe the intent and outcomes of public reporting	Use public reporting information to advance quality improvement efforts Appreciate that consumers will be more empowered to make decisions based on quality information	Value community engagement in quality improvement decision making

Note: Quality improvement (QI) in the area of *ethics quality* focuses on ensuring that systems and processes regarding specific *ethical* standards are improved.
Source: American Association of Colleges of Nursing (2012).

performed according to standards) and service quality (e.g., patient satisfaction with the health care experience). But ethics quality is equally important in the care provided by the staff of a health care organization (Wynia, 1999, p. 296) including its nurses. For example, consider a patient who has had a peripherally inserted central venous catheter (PICC) line placed by the nurse. From a technical quality perspective, the care was perfectly executed by the nurse who maintained sterile technique, and from a service quality perspective, the patient experienced no pain and was perfectly satisfied with the

Box 12.1

A Brief Business Case for Ethics

Doing the right thing brings business benefits by:

Increasing patient satisfaction. When organizations support ethical health care practices—for example, by encouraging clinicians to actively involve patients in decisions about their health care—patients do better clinically and say they are more satisfied with the care they receive (Kaplan, Greenfield, & Ware, 1989; Tierney, 2001).

Improving employee morale. Organizations that support ethical decision making—especially organizations whose ethics programs focus on achieving high standards instead of simply complying with policy or law (Paine, 2003)—can expect to have happier, more dedicated employees (Bischoff, DeTienne, & Quick, 1999; 1999 National Business Ethics Study, 1999).

Enhancing productivity. A strong corporate ethics culture can improve not only employee morale but also performance, and help improve an organization's efficiency and productivity (Arthur Anderson Co., 1999; Biel, 1999; Verschoor, 1999). An effective ethics program also makes it easier to recruit and retain quality staff (Francis, 2001).

Conserving resources/avoiding costs. Effective ethics programs have been shown to improve quality of care and reduce length of stay and cost (Halloran, 1995). Supporting patients' rights to forgo life-sustaining treatment meets an important ethical standard, and at the same time can have the effect of avoiding costs (Dowdy, Robertson, & Bander, 1998; Heilicser, Meltzer, & Siegler, 2000; Schneiderman et al., 2003).

Improving accreditation reviews. As of January 2016, The Joint Commission includes 16 standards explicitly pertaining to ethics, patient rights, and organizational responsibilities (RI.01.01.01–RI.02.01.01 and LD.04.02.03). A strong ethics program can help ensure that the organization meets or exceeds those standards ("Joint Commission Manual," 2016).

Reducing risk of lawsuits. Organizations that make strong commitments to ethical health care practices, such as being honest with patients, can reduce the risk of litigation and liability (Kraman, & Hamm, 1999; Levinson, Roter, Mullooly, Dull, & Frankel, 1997; Vincent, Young, & Phillips, 1994).

Safeguarding the organization's future. Lack of an effective ethics program can seriously jeopardize an organization's reputation and even its survival (Gellerman, 2003). Creating structures and processes by which an organization can hold itself accountable to its core values and to ethical practices is an investment in the organization's future.

professional manner and efficiency of the nurse who provided the care. So, one may think that the care was of high quality, right? Well, not necessarily. Imagine that the nurse never really informed—or even misinformed—the patient about the purpose of the PICC line and the risks, benefits, and burdens of having it placed. As informed consent is a standard, a norm, and an expectation in health care and for nursing practice, this would indicate a problem with the *ethics quality* of the care provided by the nurse. The Integrated-Ethics model defines ethics quality in health care as, "Practices throughout an organization are consistent with widely accepted ethical standards, norms, or expectations for the organization and its staff" (National Center for Ethics in Health Care, 2013, p. 1).

LEVELS OF ETHICS QUALITY

Ethics quality should be evident, maintained, and improved throughout an ethical health care organization. The IntegratedEthics model developed by the U.S. Department of Veterans Affairs National Center for Ethics in Health Care (2007) uses the image of an iceberg (see Figure 12.1) to illustrate how ethical practices cut across three levels of the organization. In a highly ethical organization, there are strong practices at each of the three levels.

Figure 12.1, the IntegratedEthics iceberg, illustrates at the first level above the waterline, the *decisions or actions* of individual staff in their daily work at the bedside, in the clinic, in administration, or in the board room. The staff's everyday decisions and actions are driven by the organization's mission and values statements, policies and procedures, and personal and/or professional standards, and codes of ethics. When an individual or group has a question about what is the right thing to do in a given circumstance, they call upon the ethics consultation function for assistance in resolving the ethical concern.

At the second level just below the waterline in Figure 12.1, we can examine the *systems and processes* that guide behavior of the organizations' staff. It is through value- and rule-based policies and procedures that the organization's staff knows if they are doing the right thing in a consistent and measurable manner. When an individual or group notices or discovers that the systems and practices are not consistent with ethical standards, or there is a quality gap between what is being done and what should be done, they call upon the preventive ethics function to close the ethics quality gap.

At the third level, deep below the surface seen in Figure 12.1, nurses must carefully and consciously examine the *environment and culture* of the organization in which they practice nursing. Nurses must explore the values, understanding, assumptions, habits, and unspoken messages (what people in the organization know but rarely make explicit) as they are the foundation for everything else. What is it about some organizations that set them apart as a magnet or more desirable workplace for staff and care setting for patients?

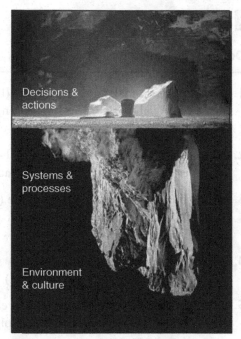

Figure 12.1 IntegratedEthics iceberg.
Image courtesy of Uwe Kills. Used with permission.

Each leader at every level of the organization has a responsibility to examine and improve the environment and culture. Leaders need to foster a positive environment and culture through what they say and do. The ethical leadership function supports leaders in this critical work.

Thus, ethics quality is the product of the interplay of factors at three levels: (a) decisions and actions, (b) systems and processes, and (c) environment and culture. Together, these three levels define the ethics quality of an organization. The IntegratedEthics iceberg model embraces a comprehensive approach to improving ethics quality by focusing on all three levels. The model is structured around three core functions, each of which targets a different level of ethics quality:

1. Ethics consultation—targets ethics quality at the level of decisions and actions

2. Preventive ethics—targets the level of systems and processes

3. Ethical leadership—targets the level of environment and culture

Questions to Consider Before Reading On

1. Which domains of health care (Box 12.2) are most prominent in my workplace?

2. How does the mission of my organization relate to each domain?

Box 12.2

Domains of Ethics in Health Care

1. Shared decision making with patients (how well the organization promotes collaborative decision making between clinicians and patients)

2. Ethical practices in end-of-life care (how well the organization addresses ethical aspects of caring for patients near the end of life)

3. Ethical practices at the beginning of life (how well the organization promotes ethical practices with respect to conception, pregnancy, and the perinatal period)

4. Patient privacy and confidentiality (how well the organization protects patient privacy and confidentiality)

5. Professionalism in patient care (how well the organization fosters behavior appropriate for health care professionals)

6. Ethical practices in resource allocation (how well the organization demonstrates fairness in allocating resources across programs, services, and patients)

7. Ethical practices in business and management (how well the organization promotes high ethical standards in its business and management practices)

8. Ethical practices in research (how well the organization ensures that its employees follow ethical standards that apply to research practices)

9. Ethical practices in the everyday workplace (how well the organization supports ethical behavior in everyday interactions in the workplace)

DOMAINS OF HEALTH CARE ETHICS

With the understanding that IntegratedEthics has three levels, let us think about the scope of the program. Within IntegratedEthics, the concept of ethics quality is very broad, crossing over clinical, organizational, and research ethics and encompassing the full range of ethical issues that all types of health care organizations including acute care hospitals, rehabilitation hospitals, outpatient facilities, nursing homes, home care organizations, and large health care systems encounter. IntegratedEthics defines for the organization domains of ethics in health care and specific topics within each content domain and recognizes that there may be additional domains that are relevant to an organization based on its particular mission (National Center for Ethics in Health Care, 2014b). For example, the Department of Veterans Affairs has special responsibilities by virtue of its role as a government organization, and for that reason has added the domain of "ethical practices in government service (how well the organization fosters behavior appropriate for government employees)." Additional domains derived from special mission-specific responsibilities might include, for example the following:

- Ethical practices in mission integration (how well the organization manages the relationship between individual values and the values of Catholic health care)

- Ethical practices in military medicine (how well the organization ensures that its employees follow ethical standards that apply to military medicine)

- Ethical practices in occupational medicine (how well the organization manages conflicting ethical responsibilities to workers, employers, and the public)

A listing of the domains of ethics in health care is found in Box 12.2.

WHAT IS THE GOAL OF THE INTEGRATEDETHICS PROGRAM?

IntegratedEthics is a transformational idea that redefines ethics as it is practiced in the health care arena. The goal of IntegratedEthics is to move ethics into the organizational mainstream and to ensure that there is high ethics quality at all three levels of the organization. To achieve this goal, staff must coordinate ethics-related activities throughout the organization. This requires more than simply implementing the three core functions in a single work unit as is described in this chapter. It also requires strong leadership support, involvement of multiple programs, and clear lines of accountability as well as policy and evaluation. (A description of these requirements is beyond the scope of this chapter but further information is available at www.ethics.va.gov/integratedethics/index.asp.)

Questions to Consider Before Reading On

1. Do we have an ethics consultation team or committee in my organization?

2. How have or could I use this team or committee to resolve an ethical concern?

THE FUNCTION OF ETHICS CONSULTATION: RESPONDING TO ETHICS QUESTIONS IN HEALTH CARE

Often nurses must weigh important and relevant values to guide decisions or before taking actions involving patient care. Sometimes a conflict or uncertainty about the values—an *ethical concern*—arises. Ethical concerns lead to ethics questions. Every ethics program must have an effective mechanism for responding to these concerns to help nurses and other staff members, patients, and families. That is the role of the IntegratedEthics ethics consultation function. *Ethics consultation in health care* has been defined as "a service provided by an individual ethics consultant, ethics consultation team, or ethics committee to help patients, staff, and others resolve ethical concerns in a health care setting setting" (Berkowitz, Chanko, Foglia, Fox, & Powell, 2015, p. vi).

The overall goal of ethics consultation is to "improve health care quality by facilitating the resolution of ethical concerns" (Berkowitz et al., 2015, p. vi). By providing a forum for discussion and methods for careful analysis, effective ethics consultation does the following:

- Promotes practices consistent with high ethical standards
- Helps foster consensus and resolve conflict in an atmosphere of respect
- Honors participants' authority and values in the decision-making process
- Educates participants to handle current and future ethical concerns

THE CASES APPROACH

The CASES approach is a practical, systematic, step-by-step approach to ethics consultation. The CASES steps were designed to guide ethics consultants through the complex process needed to effectively respond to ethical questions and concerns. Nurses who call for an ethics consult should expect that a consultant will work through a number of steps similar to those in the CASES approach as described in Box 12.3 (Berkowitz et al., 2015, p. 19).

Box 12.3

The CASES Approach

Clarify the consultation request
- Characterize the type of consultation request
- Obtain preliminary information from the requester
- Establish realistic expectations about the consultation process
- Formulate the ethics question

Assemble the relevant information
- Consider the types of information needed
- Identify the appropriate sources of information
- Gather information systematically from each source
- Summarize the case and the ethics question

Synthesize the information
- Determine whether a formal meeting is needed
- Engage in ethical analysis
- Identify the ethically appropriate decision maker
- Facilitate moral deliberation about ethically justifiable options

Explain the synthesis
- Communicate the synthesis to key participants
- Provide additional resources
- Document the consultation in the health record
- Document the consultation in consultation service records

Support the consultation process
- Follow up with participants
- Evaluate the consultation
- Adjust the consultation process
- Identify underlying systems issues

Case Scenario Related to the CASES Approach

Clare, a nurse on the unit, has an ethical concern about care decisions being made for her patient who cannot participate in decision making because he is sedated on a ventilator. She knows that the patient's surrogate is authorized to make decisions for the patient and his decision to keep the ventilator should be respected, but she also knows from reading the patient's living will that he would not want to be maintained on a ventilator if he had a terminal diagnosis and poor prognosis for ever coming off the ventilator, which is the current case. Staff and the surrogate seem to be at a standoff about what should be done.

(continued)

CASE SCENARIO RELATED TO THE CASES APPROACH (CONTINUED)

*With encouragement from Beatrice, Clare call an ethics consultation and the CASES process began. The consultant **clarified** the concerns by obtaining some preliminary information, let her and others on the unit know what to expect about the process, and formulated the ethics question as follows: Given that staff believe that they ought to follow the wishes of an authorized surrogate of a patient without capacity because the patient trusted this individual to make decisions for him, but the staff believe that they should follow the wishes of the patient as described in his living will because they are his own wishes expressed for just this circumstance, what decisions or actions are ethically justifiable? The consultant then **assembled** information from primary sources about the patient's medical facts, his preferences and interests, other party's preferences and interests, and ethics knowledge about advance directives and informed consent. The consultant **synthesized** the information and then engaged in ethical analysis and facilitated deliberation about what decisions or actions were ethically justifiable in a formal meeting with the nurse, the team, and the patient's surrogate. It was a very successful meeting and the ethics consultant clearly and concisely **explained** the synthesis to all the parties. He also provided some recommended reading for the staff and the surrogate. A few days later, the consultant **supported** the consultation process by calling Clare to as if the planned decisions and actions had been implemented and if the concern was resolved. He also asked that she complete a feedback tool about the experience so that the consultation process can be improved.*

In this case, the consultation process assisted all the parties but especially the surrogate who learned that he is called upon to make decisions when the patient lacks decision-making capacity and that he is responsible to make decisions based on the known wishes of the patient (i.e., substituted judgment [e.g., based on the patient's living will]) or in the patient's best interests. To this point, he had been somewhat overwhelmed with the numerous decisions being presented to him and could think only about keeping the patient alive at all costs so that he would not be burdened by the thought that his decision caused the patient's death. Once the role of surrogate and the medical facts were explained to him, he felt more at ease following the direction left to him by the patient in the living will. He was glad that the nurse recognized the tension and called for an ethics consultation.

Nurses who have an interest in ethics consultation should seek out the ethics consultation leader or coordinator at their organization to learn more about how they might participate in ethics consultations or become an ethics consultant.

THE FUNCTION OF PREVENTIVE ETHICS: ADDRESSING ETHICS QUALITY GAPS ON A SYSTEMS LEVEL

In addition to responding to individual ethics questions as they arise, it is essential that organizations address the underlying systems and processes that influence ethical behavior. Every ethics program needs a systematic approach for proactively identifying, prioritizing, and addressing concerns about ethics quality at the organizational level. That is the role of the IntegratedEthics preventive ethics function. *Preventive ethics* is defined as "activities performed by an individual or group on behalf of a health care organization to identify, prioritize, and address systemic ethics issues" (Cook, Foglia, Landon, & Bottrell, 2015, p. 1*)*. An *ethics issue* is an ongoing situation involving organizational systems and processes that gives rise to ethical concerns (i.e., that gives rise to uncertainty or conflicts about values). We use the term "ethics issue" to distinguish systemic ethical problems from the more familiar concept of "ethics cases." Ethics issues differ from ethics cases in that issues describe ongoing situations, while cases describe events that occur at a particular time; in addition, issues involve organizational systems and processes, while cases involve specific decisions and actions by individuals. To help illustrate the difference, imagine a conflict about whether to provide home oxygen to a patient who smokes. The patient wants the home oxygen because it improves his quality of life, but the team thinks he should not get the home oxygen because there is risk of fire and harm to the patient and others. The parties might request an ethics consultation to help them decide what to do about the individual patient case. But what if this were not the first time this sort of situation had come to the attention of the ethics consultation service? What if this consultation was typical of many consultations involving the home oxygen program? In such circumstances, responding specifically to questions about the particular situation (i.e., through ethics consultation) is not enough. What is needed is a systematic approach to addressing the underlying systems and processes that repeatedly give rise to similar ethical concerns. That is the role of preventive ethics.

It is important to note that preventive ethics is not restricted to ethics issues in clinical care but is relevant to a whole host of issues across the domains of ethics in health care. For example, it might be used to address ethics quality gaps in personnel practices (e.g., around fair hiring), fiscal management (e.g., how some vendors are paid more timely than others), or protection of research subjects (e.g., proper informed consent processes).

The overall goal of preventive ethics is to *improve quality by identifying, prioritizing, and addressing ethics quality gaps on a systems level*, where the ethics quality gap is the difference between what is (current ethics practices) and what ought to be (best ethics practices). Best ethics practices refer to ideal practices established on the basis of widely accepted standards, norms, or expectations for the organization and its staff. When current ethics practices deviate from best ethics practices, a measurable ethics quality gap results

(Cook et al., 2015, p. 4). The systems-level changes must generate measurable improvements in the organization's ethics practices by reducing the disparity between current practices and best practices in the relevant area. Preventive ethics applies quality improvement techniques to improve ethics quality.

Specific quality improvement interventions in preventive ethics may include the following:

- Redesigning work processes to better support ethical practice

- Implementing checklists, reminders, and decision support

- Evaluating organizational performance with respect to ethical practices

- Developing specific protocols to promote ethical practices

- Designing strategies for patients and/or staff to address system-wide knowledge deficits

- Offering incentives and rewards to motivate and acknowledge ethical practices among staff

The preventive ethics function encompasses two types of activities to address systemic ethics issues: (a) general maintenance activities and (b) quality improvement cycles. General maintenance activities are often carried out by standing committees and typically include the following:

- Periodically updating policies on various ethical practices

- Providing regular ethics education for staff

- Maintaining continuous readiness relating to ethics for surveys by The Joint Commission and other accreditation organizations

In contrast, quality improvement cycles are time-limited interventions targeted toward specific ethics quality gaps and are best carried out by small, dynamic workgroups that include one or more members trained in the ISSUES approach (described in Box 12.4) and one or more ad hoc members who have subject matter expertise in the particular ethics issue being addressed.

Bringing the two activities together helps ensure that they are effectively coordinated and system-level thinking is applied to each activity. Ethics maintenance activities can benefit from a quality improvement approach. For example, instead of carrying out an ethics educational program to meet a vague training requirement, a preventive ethics approach targets educational activities to address identified quality gaps (e.g., clinical staff have significant misconceptions about the optimal timing for and benefits of holding goals of care conversations with patients), sets specific goals (e.g., 90% of clinical staff will complete the training and score at least 85% on the posttest), and then evaluates the effectiveness of the activities in meeting those goals. A quality improvement mindset is similarly useful when developing or updating policy or ensuring that the health care organization maintains accreditation readiness with respect to ethics standards.

Box 12.4

The ISSUES Approach

Identify an issue
- Identify ethics issues proactively
- Characterize the type of issue
- Clarify each issue by listing the improvement goal

Study the issue
- Diagram the process behind the relevant practice
- Gather specific data about best practices
- Gather specific data about current practices
- Refine the improvement goal to reflect the ethics quality gap

Select a strategy
- Identify the major cause(s) of the ethics quality gap—do a root cause analysis
- Brainstorm about possible strategies to narrow the gap
- Choose one or more strategies to try

Undertake a plan
- Plan how to carry out the strategy
- Plan how to evaluate the strategy
- Execute the plan

Evaluate and adjust
- Check the execution and the results
- Adjust as necessary
- Evaluate your ISSUES process

Sustain and spread
- Sustain the improvement
- Disseminate the improvement
- Continue monitoring

THE ISSUES APPROACH

The ISSUES approach is a step-by-step method to help preventive ethics teams improve the systems and processes that influence ethics practices in a health care organization. While nurses are familiar with standard quality improvement (QI) methods, such as Plan-Do-Study-Act (PDSA), to address clinical or managerial quality issues, ISSUES is designed specifically to address *ethics quality* gaps (Cook et al., 2015). The steps of the ISSUES approach are summarized in

Box 12.4. For a more detailed description see Cook et al., 2015 http://www .ethics.va.gov/docs/integratedethics/pe_primer_2_edition_042015.pdf

Questions to Consider Before Reading On

1. What mechanisms are in place at my work place to address and close gaps between what I know to be the right thing to do and how the systems and processes are currently set up?

2. Do I use quality improvement techniques to improve ethics practices? Could I?

CASE SCENARIO RELATED TO THE ISSUES APPROACH

Two months ago, the ethics consultation coordinator came to the realization that the service had been called eight times over the past 6 months to consult in the intensive care and other units about ethical concerns regarding surrogate decision making. She summarized the overall ethics issue as a gap between the best ethics practice for surrogate decision making described in hospital policy and the actual current practice in the various care settings, and presented the issue to the preventive ethics team for review and consideration. She was just informed that the preventive ethics team agreed that they would be starting an ISSUES cycle.

*The preventive ethics team could easily **identify the issue** that having staff members and surrogates engaged in less than best practices around surrogate decision making was ethically problematic for the organization. The team also recognized that an improvement effort would likely have a real impact on the ethical practices and that increasing the agreement or consensus among parties caring for patients who had surrogate decision makers was a high priority for clinical and administrative leaders. The team began to **study the issue** by describing the best ethics practice articulated in ethical standards found in the hospital policy as well as the current ethics practices. Once the magnitude of the gap was quantified, the team was able to refine the improvement goal to reflect how much improvement could be achieved within a specific time period. Meetings were held to identify the major causes of the ethics quality gap. Included in the meetings were subject matter experts who assisted in completing cause-and-effect tools to identify the causes of the gap. They also helped identify and **select a strategy** that had the highest likelihood of success using the fewest resources. They decided to do some small-scale testing of the strategy on Beatrice's unit and Alex, who had become an IE champion, became the point of contact. Alex was able to assist the preventive ethics team and the unit staff to **undertake the plan** and evaluate if the strategy narrowed the gap. Weeks went by but eventually there were enough patients who lacked capacity but had a surrogate so that the team could **evaluate and adjust** the small-scale test. With only minor adjustments, a plan was put in place to **sustain and spread** the strategy to additional units.*

(continued)

CASE SCENARIO RELATED TO THE **ISSUES** APPROACH (*CONTINUED*)

Within 18 months, the units involved in the preventive ethics ISSUES cycle had increased the rate consensus among parties caring for patients who had surrogate decision makers and similar tools and strategies were being used across the entire hospital. Staff expressed confidence that the surrogates were clear about their role and responsibilities in decision making, and they were better skilled at both providing the surrogates with the information they needed to make informed decisions for the patients and supporting the surrogates in what is often a challenging situations.

Nurses who have an interest in preventive ethics should seek out the preventive ethics coordinator or quality improvement leader at their organization to learn more about how they might participate in quality improvement efforts designed to close ethics quality gaps.

THE FUNCTION OF ETHICAL LEADERSHIP: FOSTERING AN ETHICAL ENVIRONMENT AND CULTURE

The third core function of IntegratedEthics is ethical leadership, which addresses ethics quality at the level of organizational environment and culture. Leaders in any health care system have obligations as health care providers and as managers of resources. As health care providers, leaders have an obligation to meet the health care needs of individual patients and the community they serve. In addition, leaders are responsible for leading others by demonstrating their commitment to quality and safety by role modeling high expectations in this area. Ethics must also be considered in their management of resources (The Joint Commission, 2016, Standard LD.03.01.01).

To fulfill these roles, leaders must meet their own ethical obligations and ensure that employees throughout the organization are supported in adhering to high ethical standards. Because the behavior of individual employees is influenced by the culture in which they work, the goal of ethical leadership is to foster an ethical environment and culture.

There is a plethora of writing about ethics and leadership; however, practical, how-to advice for leaders who wish to improve ethics quality in their organizations is harder to come by. IntegratedEthics seeks to fill that void by drawing on and complementing scholarly discussions of ethical leadership in ways that can inform health care leaders' day-to-day practices. The National Center for Ethics in Health Care's approach combines insights from ethicists and managers to provide a practical model, including tools, rather than engaging in thorough conceptual explorations of ethics in health care or leadership. The ethical leadership function targets staff at the executive leadership to mid-manager levels, although leaders at all levels of health care organizations may find the approach useful.

In the IntegratedEthics model, *ethical leadership* is defined as "activities on the part of leaders to foster an ethical environment and culture" (Fox, Crigger, Bottrell, & Bauck, 2007, p. 13). Rarely is it the case that ethical lapses in organizations are due to rogue employees or bad apples who willfully misbehave. Instead, research shows that the ethical behavior of individuals is profoundly influenced by the environment and culture in which they work. In organizations with a strong ethical culture, the frequency of observed ethical misconduct is dramatically reduced. For this reason, fostering an organizational environment and culture that makes it easy for employees to do the right thing is the key to ethical leadership.

Questions to Consider Before Reading On

1. Do I work in an organization with an ethical environment and culture? Why? Why not?

2. What is an ethical environment and culture?

Research has shown that certain features of an organization's environment and culture predictably affect ethical practices in a positive way (Treviño, Weaver, Gibson, & Toffler, 1999). The IntegratedEthics model identifies specific features that characterize an organization with a positive or healthy ethical environment and culture as one in which everyone:

- Appreciates that ethics is important
- Recognizes and discusses ethical concerns
- Seeks consultation on ethics cases when needed
- Works to resolve ethics issues on a systems level
- Sees ethics as part of quality
- Understands what is expected of him or her
- Feels empowered to behave ethically
- Views organizational decisions as ethical

If leaders are to meet the challenge of fostering an ethical environment and culture, it is essential that they cultivate specific knowledge, skills, and habits required to demonstrate true ethical leadership.

The ethical leadership function of IntegratedEthics calls on leaders to observe four compass points, as described in Box 12.5. The ethical leadership compass applies insights and principles from organizational and business ethics to leadership in the context of health care ethics. It is specifically designed to help leaders orient themselves to their unique responsibilities in the terrain of ethics in health care, and to provide practical guidance to help

Box 12.5

The Four Compass Points

Demonstrate that ethics is a priority
- Talk about ethics
- Prove that ethics matters to you
- Encourage discussion of ethical concerns

Communicate clear expectations for ethical practice
- Recognize when expectations need to be clarified
- Be explicit, give examples, explain the underlying values
- Anticipate barriers to meeting your expectations

Practice ethical decision making
- Identify decisions that raise ethical concerns
- Address ethical decisions systematically
- Explain your decisions

Support your local ethics program
- Know what your ethics program is and what it does
- Champion the program
- Support participation by others

them address the challenges of fostering an environment and culture that support ethical practices across their organizations (Fox et al., 2007). A more detailed description of the four compass points is available at www.ethics.va .gov/integratedethics/elc.asp

Questions to Consider Before Reading On

1. What specific things have leaders in my organization done or said that support strong ethics practices by nurses and other staff?

2. Describe a time when leaders in my workplace guided the organization from an ethics perspective.

CASE SCENARIO RELATED TO ETHICAL LEADERSHIP

Recently other unit managers have become interested in Beatrice's leadership approach and they asked her to give a briefing at the nurse manager's semiannual meeting. She was honored to be asked and wanted to make the most of the opportunity to influence others to join her in integrating ethics into the

(continued)

CASE SCENARIO RELATED TO ETHICAL LEADERSHIP (*CONTINUED*)

workings of the organization. She focused her comments on the "four compass points" that she uses every day to guide her in fostering a positive ethical environment and culture and provided examples of her actions as follows:

Compass Point 1: Demonstrate that ethics is a priority

In my day-to-day interactions with staff and patients I make sure that those I relate to know that ethics is a priority for me. People see it in what I do and say, and I always encourage others to show their commitment to ethics, too. In staff meetings I spend a few minutes practicing with staff about how to communicating directly that ethics is important. I encourage staff to find time during their work to demonstrate that ethics is a priority. For instance, staff should say to one another, as the situation dictates, "If it's the right thing to do, we'll just have to figure out a way to do it" or "Now that we understand what we can do within the rules, or what's legal, let's talk about what we should do."

Compass Point 2: Communicate clear expectations for ethical practice

Expertise in this compass point takes some work and experience to build. For starters I have to recognize when expectations for ethical practice need to be clarified before I can be explicit about the underlying values and what should be done. Harder still sometimes is being able to anticipate barriers that might come up for staff to meet the expectations. The chance to communicate clear expectations comes up, for instance, when there is a department-wide requirement that staff thinks is not as important as other duties. A simple example may be an all staff competency check for infection control protocols or privacy and confidentiality. Sure, every staff member knows that infection control is important for the safety of staff and patients, or that confidentiality of patient information is critical to maintain the trust of our patients and the community, but when it comes to processing through the competency checks, it's pretty hard for the staff to stay committed with everything else they have to do. For that reason, I make the values explicit and anticipate barriers to full participation by the staff. I also ask staff to bring an unanticipated barrier to my attention so that I can do what I need to do as a leader to remove the barrier.

Compass Point 3: Practice ethical decision making

Whenever there is a decision to be made that involves values that might conflict or in an area that is highly charged from an ethics perspective, I am sure to break out the IntegratedEthics ethical decision-making rubric. For example, when I was developing a new overtime policy for my unit, I knew that the policy would need to balance patient care needs and the strong family values held by my staff. I was very systematic about making decisions about the policy. For example, I made sure to have all the important facts and involved everyone who should be part of the decision. I also ensured that the decision reflected organizational, professional, and social values and that the benefits of the decision

(continued)

CASE SCENARIO RELATED TO ETHICAL LEADERSHIP (*CONTINUED*)

outweighed any potential harms. Having done this, I found that staff members were able to more readily accept the policy.

Compass Point 4: Support your local ethics program
    While I do all I can personally to foster a positive environment and culture and champion ethics, I can't do it alone. That's why I support the various ethics activities that go on around the hospital and support the participation of others. For example, even if I need to relieve nurses at the bedside, I try to always be sure that at least someone can attend the hospital's ethics journal club. As staff members become interested in ethics, I have encouraged them to join a preventive ethics team working on the unit. I even have one staff member working toward becoming an ethics consultant. Staff and patients benefit from the positive ethical environment and culture that I and my staff work to achieve. I am always available to help others integrate ethics into their work. Please feel free to contact me at any time.

Nurses have a responsibility to display ethical leadership within the health care setting regardless of their individual scope of authority. By focusing on the four compass points of ethical leadership each nurse has the power to influence the environment and culture of the organization.

INTEGRATEDETHICS PROGRAM STRUCTURE

An IntegratedEthics program has two essential tasks. First, the program must move ethics into the organizational mainstream; second, it must coordinate ethics-related activities throughout the organization. This requires more than simply implementing the three core functions. It also requires strong leadership support, involvement of multiple programs, and clear lines of accountability. More information about the IE program structure and management is available at www.ethics.va.gov/integratedethics/program_management.asp.

CONCLUSION

This chapter presented a description of IntegratedEthics as a program comprising three functions—ethics consultation, preventive ethics, and ethical leadership—that are designed to improve ethics quality in health care. Nurses can and should adopt the concepts of IntegratedEthics and seek to participate in activities at all three levels of such a program in an effort to continuously ensure and improve ethics quality—an essential component of health care quality. Whether the nurse (a) needs assistance with an ethical concern and calls for an ethics consultation, (b) recognizes that there are systemic problems that cause an ethics quality gap between what is the right thing to do and what the current systems/processes allow and engages with others in a preventive ethics quality improvement cycle, or (c) appreciates that a positive environment and culture is important and demonstrates through words and actions that he or she is an ethical leader, there are IntegratedEthics resources to guide and improve his or her practices.

Critical Thinking Questions and Activities

1. Describe what staff can expect from an ethics consultant who is using the CASES approach.

2. Describe a situation from your nursing experience in which you believe you could have benefited from an ethics consultant.

3. Have you observed any ethical quality gaps in your workplace? Describe.

4. Use the four leadership compass points to describe ways to improve or foster an ethical environment in your current workplace.

5. Using the resources at http://www.ethics.va.gov/integratedethics/index.asp, choose one IntegratedEthics function (i.e., ethics consultation, preventive ethics, ethical leadership) to learn more about and make a plan to incorporate that learning into your practice.

REFERENCES

American Association of Colleges of Nursing. (2012). *Graduate level QSEN competencies: Knowledge, skills, and attitudes.* Washington, DC: Author. Retrieved from http://www.aacn.nche.edu/faculty/qsen/competencies.pdf

Arthur Anderson Co. (1999). *Ethical concerns and reputation risk management: A study of leading U.K. companies.* London, UK: London Business School.

Berkowitz, K., Chanko, B., Foglia, M., Fox, E., & Powell, T. (2015). *Ethics consultation: Responding to ethics questions in health care* (2nd ed.). Washington, DC: U.S. Department of Veterans Affairs. Retrieved from http://www.ethics.va.gov/docs/integratedethics/ec_primer_2nd_ed_080515.pdf

Biel, M. A. B. (1999). Achieving corporate ethics in healthcare's current compliance environment. *Federal Ethics Report, 6,* 1–4.

Bischoff, S. J., DeTienne, K. B., & Quick, B. (1999). Effects of ethics stress on employee burnout and fatigue: An empirical investigation. *The Journal of Health and Human Services Administration, 21,* 512–532.

Cook, R., Foglia, M., Landon, M., & Bottrell, M. (2015). *Preventive ethics: Addressing ethics quality gaps on a systems level* (2nd ed.). Washington, DC: U.S. Department of Veterans Affairs. Retrieved from http://www.ethics.va.gov/docs/integratedethics/pe_primer_2_edition_042015.pdf

Dowdy, M. D., Robertson, C., & Bander, J. A. (1998). A study of proactive ethics consultation for criti-cally and terminally ill patients with extended lengths of stay. *Critical Care Medicine, 26*, 252–259.

Fox, E., Crigger, B., Bottrell, M., & Bauck, M. (2007). *Ethics leadership: Fostering an ethical environ-ment and culture.* Washington, DC: U.S. Department of Veterans Affairs. Retrieved from http://www.ethics.va.gov/ELprimer.pdf

Francis, R. D. (2001). Evidence for the value of ethics. *Journal of Financial Crime, 9*(1):26–30.

Gellerman, S. (2003). Why good managers make bad ethical choices. *Harvard Business Review on Corporate Ethics,* 49–66. (Article originally published in *Harvard Business Review, 64*(4), 85–90, July–August 1986.)

Holloran, S. D., Starkey, G. W., Burke, P. A., Steele, G., & Forse, R. A. (1995). An educational inter-vention in the surgical intensive care unit to improve ethical decisions. *Surgery, 118*, 294–295.

Heilicser, B. J., Meltzer, D., & Siegler, M. (2000). The effect of clinical medical ethics consultation on healthcare costs. *The Journal of Clinical Ethics, 11*, 31–38.

The Joint Commission. (2016). Patient safety systems. *Comprehensive Accreditation Manual for Hos-pitals.* Retrieved from http://www.jointcommission.org/assets/1/18/PSC_for_Web.pdf

The Joint Commission Manual. (2016, January 1). Retrieved from https://e-dition.jcrinc.com/Main Content.aspx

Kaplan, S. H., Greenfield, S., & Ware, J. E., Jr. (1989). Assessing the effects of physician–patient interactions on the outcomes of chronic disease. *Medical Care, 27*, S110–S127.

Kraman, S. S., & Hamm, G. (1999). Risk management: Extreme honesty may be the best policy. *Annals of Internal Medicine, 131*, 963–967.

Levinson, W., Roter, D. L., Mullooly, J. P., Dull, V. T., & Frankel, R. M. (1997). Physician–patient communication. The relationship with malpractice claims among primary care physicians and surgeons. *Journal of the American Medical Association, 277*, 553–559.

1999 National Business Ethics Study, Walker Information in association with the Hudson Institute. (1999, September). Retrieved from http://www.bentley.edu/sites/www.bentley.edu.centers/files/centers/cbe/cbe-external-surveys/1999-national-business-ethics-study.pdf

National Center for Ethics in Health Care. (2007). Improving ethics quality: Looking beneath the surface. Retrieved from http://www.ethics.va.gov/docs/integratedethics/Improving_Ethics_Quality-Looking_Beneath_the_Surface_20070808.pdf

National Center for Ethics in Health Care. (2013). What is ethics quality? Retrieved from http://www.ethics.va.gov/docs/integratedethics/2013130_what_is_ethics_qual_art.pdf

National Center for Ethics in Health Care. (2014a). A brief business case for ethics. Washington, DC: U.S. Department of Veterans Affairs. Retrieved from http://www.ethics.va.gov/docs/integratedethics/brief_business_case_for_ethics_02182014.pdf

National Center for Ethics in Health Care. (2014b). Domains of ethics in health care. Washington, DC: U.S. Department of Veterans Affairs. Retrieved from http://www.ethics.va.gov/docs/integratedethics/domains_of_ethics_in_health_care_022515.pdf

National Center for Ethics in Health Care. (2015). IntegratedEthics. Retrieved from http://www.ethics.va.gov/integratedethics

Paine, L. S. (2003). Managing for organizational integrity. *Harvard Business Review on Corporate Eth-ics* (pp. 85–112). Cambridge, MA: HBS Publications. (Originally published in *Harvard Business Review,* March–April 1994.)

Schneiderman, L. J., Gilmer, T., Teetzel, H. D., Dugan, D. O., Blustein, J., Cranford, R., . . . Young, E.W. (2003). Effect of ethics consultations on nonbeneficial life-sustaining treatments in the intensive care setting. *Journal of the American Medical Association, 290*, 1166–1172.

Tierney, W. M., Dexter, P. R., Gramelspacher, G. P., Perkins, A. J., Zhou, X. H., & Wolinsky, F. D. (2001). The effect of discussions about advance directives on patients' satisfaction with primary care. *Journal of General Internal Medicine, 16*, 32–40.

Treviño, L., Weaver, G., Gibson, D., & Toffler, B. (1999). Managing ethics and legal compliance: What works and what hurts. *California Management Review, 41*(2), 131–151.

U.S. Department of Veterans Affairs. (2016). IntegratedEthics. Retrieved from http://www.ethics .va.gov/integratedethics

Verschoor, C. C. (1999). Corporate performance is closely linked to a strong ethical commitment. *Business and Society Review, 104,* 407–416.

Vincent, C., Young, M., & Phillips, A. (1994). Why do people sue doctors? A study of patients and relatives taking legal action. *The Lancet, 343,* 1609–1613.

Wynia M. (1999). Performance measures for ethics quality. *Effective Clinical Practice, 2*(6), 294–299.

13

Understanding the Relationship Between Quality, Safety, and Ethics

CATHERINE ROBICHAUX

LEARNING OBJECTIVES AND OUTCOMES

Upon completion of this chapter, the reader will be able to:

- Discuss the difference and relationship between quality health care and patient safety
- Explain the nursing profession's history in assessing quality care and articulating ethical responsibilities
- Identify how ethics principles, virtue ethics, and care ethics are manifested in the Institute of Medicine (IOM) domains
- Discuss how ethics principles, virtue ethics, and care ethics are manifested in patient/family care, practice, and leadership
- Analyze strategies to develop an ethical and just safety culture

As a registered nurse, you know that the language of quality and safety permeates health care today. As the providers who spend the most time with patients, nurses are critical to ensuring their safety through identifying, interrupting, and correcting potential errors that can result in adverse events (Henneman, Gawlinski, & Giuliano, 2012; Henneman et al., 2014). In fact, nurses have been involved in defining and assessing quality health care, the umbrella under which patient safety resides, since long before the current proliferation of quality/safety programs and initiatives (Robichaux & Sauerland, 2012).

This chapter provides a brief history of the nursing profession's concern with quality care, patient safety, and ethics. In addition, the relationship of ethics principles, virtue ethics, and care ethics and examples of how they are manifested in the Institute of Medicine's (IOM, 2001) quality domains are presented. Implications of the ethical principles, virtue ethics, and care ethics approaches for patient/family care, and nursing practice and leadership are discussed. To practice ethically and deliver safe, quality care, nurses must work in an ethical, supportive environment that reflects the same principles and qualities.

As you read the opening to the following Case Scenario, ask yourself:

- Which factors might contribute to a patient safety event?

- How could you prevent this potential patient safety event?

- Would you report this patient safety event? To whom?

CASE SCENARIO

Betsy has worked on a cardiovascular intermediate unit for 4 years and assumed a charge nurse position last month. This morning, the 26 monitored patients include those postcardiac surgery and intervention procedures in addition to two admitted for unstable angina and EKG changes, respectively. The unit generally has two monitor techs per shift but one has been floated to the coronary care unit (CCU) and Betsy is caring for two patients. One recently admitted patient, Mr. D., is taken for an exercise stress test at 10 a.m. and Betsy becomes busy with Mrs. S. whose newly inserted pacemaker is failing to capture. After Mrs. S. is taken to the cardiac catheterization lab, Betsy checks on Mr. D. who states that he has been back for 15 minutes because he experienced light-headedness during the stress test. Noticing that his telemetry unit low battery alarm light is on, Betsy calls for new batteries and obtains a blood pressure of 122/74. Joe, the monitor tech, informs her that Mr. D is in a sinus rhythm of 66 bpm, somewhat slower than his average rate of 75 to 80 bpm. Although Mr. D states that he feels "a lot better now," Betsy continues to monitor him and thinks, "That was a close call."

Question to Consider Before Reading On

1. How do you describe quality and safety in your current nursing practice?

QUALITY AND SAFETY

While both are essential, the difference between *patient safety* and *quality* has been debated for some time. Safety has to do with a lack of harm, while quality means efficient, effective, purposeful care that gets the job done at the right time for the right cost. Quality nursing care also means meeting and exceeding the expectations of the client. Safety focuses on avoiding bad events while quality focuses on doing things well (Hospital Safety Score, 2015).

The Institute of Medicine describes six domains (safe, effective, efficient, timely, equitable, and patient centered) that constitute overall, quality health care. These six attributes were identified in the 2001 publication, *Crossing the Quality Chasm: A New Health System for the 21st. Century* (IOM, 2001), a follow-up to *To Err is Human: Building a Safer Health System* (Kohn, Corrigan, & Donaldson, 2000). The latter document reported that, at the time, medical errors were estimated to cause 44,000 to 98,000 deaths annually and result in $17 to $29 billion dollars in *excess* medical expenses. Despite myriad international, national, and private endeavors to improve patient safety over the past 15 years, recent estimates indicate that 2 to 4 million serious adverse events still occur in the United States each year, with approximately 400,000 resulting in premature deaths (James, 2013).

Definitions of terms associated with patient safety and quality care also differ somewhat among agencies such as the National Quality Forum (NQF), the World Health Organization (WHO), and the Agency for Healthcare Research and Quality (AHRQ). NQF (2009) describes "error" as: "the failure of a planned action to be completed as intended or the use of a wrong plan to achieve an aim (commission). This definition also includes failure of an unplanned action that should have been completed (omission)." AHRQ (2012) identifies both "close calls" and "near misses" as: "an event or situation that did not produce patient injury, but only because of chance. This good fortune might reflect robustness of the patient (e.g., a patient with penicillin allergy receives penicillin, but has no reaction) or a fortuitous, timely intervention (e.g., a nurse happens to realize that a physician wrote an order in the wrong chart)." Similarly, the WHO (2009) defines "near miss" as a serious error or mishap that has the potential to cause an adverse event but fails to do so because of chance or because it is intercepted, as presented in the opening Case Scenario.

NURSING, QUALITY CARE, AND ETHICS: A BRIEF HISTORY

Florence Nightingale (1863) was a pioneer of quality care. Her persistent advocacy of quality care included systematic data collection and statistical analyses. Nightingale was responsible for perhaps the most significant hospital quality improvement project ever undertaken and, as demonstrated in her meticulous documentation, of the processes and outcomes of care. Using innovative, color-coded bar graphs and pie charts, her analysis of mortality data among British troops at Scutari Hospital in what is now Istanbul accomplished significant reductions in deaths through organizational and hygienic practices. Sheingold and Hahn (2014) observe that Florence Nightingale's three key contributions to the development of quality care evaluation and improvement are:

- The measurement of quality improvement in all of health care, which is the foundation upon which current international benchmarks for excellence are identified today

- The importance of proper documentation and presentation of measurement results

- The value of generating buy-in from others to support health care quality intervention (p. 21)

Nightingale also maintained that nurses should make independent judgments as opposed to unquestionably following the demands of physicians, thus providing the groundwork for modern nursing practice.

Aydelotte and Tener (1961) conducted one of the first studies exploring the relationship between the quality of the care provided by nurses and patient recovery or "welfare." It was hypothesized that the quality of nursing care would improve by increasing the number of nursing staff and offering an education program focused on elements of quality care. Patient outcome measures assessed were number of hospital days, postoperative days, fever, and number of doses of narcotics, sedatives, and pain medications administered. Aydelotte and Tener's findings indicated no significant improvement in patient recovery, perhaps due to insufficient reliability and validity of the instruments used (Griffith, 1995). The study served as a template for future investigations exploring the relationship of nurse staffing to patient outcomes (Aiken et al., 2012). Aydelotte identified the connection between quality care and ethics in her description of nursing: "Nursing encompasses an art, a humanistic orientation, a feeling of value of the individual, and an intuitive sense of ethics, and of the appropriateness of the actions taken" (*Scrubs Magazine*, 2015).

Phaneuf and Wandelt (1974) noted that "any profession that does not monitor itself becomes a technology" (p. 328) and encouraged nurses to develop and use methods of quality assessment that would assist in the improvement of nursing practice. Reflecting Provision 8 of the American Nurses Association (ANA) Code of Ethics (2015a), Phaneuf and Wandelt observed that "the availability of and access to health care for all are seen as human rights" and "the quality, quantity, and costs of care have become interrelated social and professional issues" (p. 329). The authors developed or shared in the development of several nursing quality care measures that remain in use today. These include the Slater Nursing Competencies Rating Scale (Wandelt & Stewart, 1975), the Quality Patient Care Scale (Wandelt & Ager, 1974), and the Nursing Audit (Phaneuf, 1972).

In 1975, Lang proposed a quality assurance model that included an assessment of values, observing "it is impossible to discuss quality without examining values of the professional" and "most of our conflicts arise from a difference of opinion regarding values" (p. 180). She also noted that the staff nurse is a major determiner of quality. Integrating societal and professional values in addition to the most current scientific knowledge, Lang's work and model predate the IOM's definition of quality by almost two decades and continues to be used today.

The ANA developed the Patient and Quality Safety Initiative (ANA, 1995), to evaluate linkages between nurse staffing and the quality of care through a series of pilot studies across the United States. An initial set of 10 nursing sensitive indicators were identified for use in evaluating patient care quality and implementation guidelines were published (ANA, 1996, 1999). The National Database of Nursing Care Quality Indicators (NDNQI) was established by ANA in 1998 to continue to collect data to evaluate and improve patient care. Originally managed at the University of Kansas School of Nursing under contract to ANA, the database was sold to Press Ganey, a patient experience improvement firm with a similar commitment to quality, patient-centered care in 2014. At present, more than 2,000 U.S. hospitals and 98% of Magnet® facilities participate in the NDNQI program to measure nursing quality, improve nurse satisfaction, strengthen the work environment, and improve current pay for performance policies (Press-Ganey, 2015).

The quality mandate is evident in foundational nursing documents such as Nursing's Social Policy Statement (ANA, 2010a), Code of Ethics (ANA, 2015a) and Scope Standards of Practice (ANA, 2015b). Standard 11 of the latter addresses the quality of practice and states, among other competencies, that the registered nurse uses indicators to monitor the quality, safety, and effectiveness of nursing practice. Graduate-level and advanced practice nurses are expected to use the results of quality improvement to initiate changes in nursing practice and the health care delivery system. Several chapters in the present book illustrate integration and application of relevant competencies developed by the Quality and Safety Education for Nurses (QSEN) initiative. This project aimed to provide nurses "with the knowledge, skills, and attitudes (KSAs) necessary to improve the quality and safety of the health care systems in which they work" (QSEN, 2015).

Question to Consider Before Reading On

1. How are you and other nurses involved in evaluating the quality of care?

As discussed in earlier chapters in this text, nurses have an extensive history of identifying and responding to ethical issues and taking seriously their moral responsibilities as health care providers. From the earliest nursing text by Eva Luckes (1886), through the 11th revision of the Code of Ethics (ANA, 2015a), nurses have sought to articulate how their roles and actions have been grounded in ethical principles. The essential, interdependent relationship between ethics and quality initiatives designed to measure, evaluate, and improve nursing practice is reflected in Provision 3 of the Code of Ethics, which states "The nurse promotes, advocates for, and protects the rights, health, and safety of the patient" (p. 9). Quality and patient safety are addressed specifically in provisions 3 and 6 and in many statements throughout the document (Box 13.1).

Question to Consider Before Reading On

Statement 3.4 in Box 13.1 identifies the nurse's role in establishing a "culture of safety."

1. How would you describe the culture of safety in your institution?

Box 13.1	

Quality Health Care, Patient Safety and Ethics: Relevant Provisions and Statements from the Code of Ethics (2015)

PROVISION 3
The nurse promotes, advocates for, and protects the rights, health, and safety of the patient.

INTERPRETIVE STATEMENT 3.4
Professional responsibility in promoting a culture of safety
    Nurses must participate in the development, implementation, and review of and adherence to policies that promote patient health and safety, reduce errors and waste, and establish and sustain a culture of safety. When errors or near misses occur, nurses must follow institutional guidelines in reporting such events to the appropriate authority and must ensure disclosure of events to patients. Nurses must establish procedures to investigate causes of errors or near misses and to address system factors that may have been contributory.
    When error occurs, whether it is one's own or that of a coworker, nurses may neither participate in, nor condone through silence, any attempts to conceal that error.

PROVISION 5
The nurse owes the same duties to self as to others, including the responsibility to promote health and safety, preserve wholeness of character and integrity, maintain competence, and continue personal and professional growth.

PROVISION 6
The nurse, through individual and collective effort, establishes, maintains, and improves the moral environment of the work setting and conditions of employment that are conducive to safe, quality health care.

Source: ANA (2015a).

ETHICS PRINCIPLES, VIRTUE ETHICS, CARE ETHICS, AND QUALITY/SAFETY

As presented in Chapter 1, the principles of autonomy, beneficence, nonmaleficence, and justice form the foundation of Western health care ethics. Quality care and patient safety are grounded in these principles and reflected in the IOM domains (Table 13.1). The principles also have implications for nursing practice and leadership in regard to intra/interprofessional collaboration

Table 13.1

Implications of Ethics Principles, Virtue Ethics, and Care Ethics to IOM Quality Domains and Patient Safety

ETHICS PRINCIPLES, VIRTUE ETHICS, AND CARE ETHICS	RELEVANT IOM QUALITY DOMAINS	APPLICATION TO QUALITY DOMAINS	APPLICATION TO PATIENT SAFETY
Autonomy	Patient centered, equitable	The obligation to recognize "the patient or designee as the source of control and full partner in providing compassionate and coordinated care based on respect for patient's preferences, values and needs" (Cronenwett et al., 2007, p. 123)	Adequate, informed consent; preventing unwanted care; supporting autonomy through relational understanding; reporting/disclosure of errors/near misses
Beneficence	Patient centered, effective, safe, timely, equitable, efficient	The obligation to provide benefit; the performance of good acts that benefit others	Establishing standard practices that promote benefit, maximize efficacy, in accordance with patient values/desires
Nonmaleficence	Safe, effective, timely, patient centered	The obligation to refrain from actions that cause harm and to actively protect the patient from actions that cause harm	Not offering treatment that lacks efficacy; establishing procedures/practices to prevent harm; reporting near misses, incompetence

(continued)

Table 13.1

Implications of Ethics Principles, Virtue Ethics, and Care Ethics to IOM Quality Domains and Patient Safety *(continued)*

ETHICS PRINCIPLES, VIRTUE ETHICS, AND CARE ETHICS	RELEVANT IOM QUALITY DOMAINS	APPLICATION TO QUALITY DOMAINS	APPLICATION TO PATIENT SAFETY
Justice	Equitable, efficient, patient centered	The obligation to ensure equitable health care access and treatment; fair distribution of the benefits/burdens related to health care delivery	Increasing awareness of racial/ethnic disparities; eliminating variations due to cost, reimbursement, insurance, ability to pay; cultural competence/safety
Virtue ethics	Patient centered, safe, equitable	The obligation to provide individualized, compassionate care	Demonstrating compassion, being honest with patient/family members; acting with courage
Care ethics	Patient centered, safe, timely, efficient, effective	The obligation to be attentive, responsible, competent, and responsive (Tronto, 1993)	Demonstrating relational and contextual understanding to provide individualized care

Sources: Egan (2014); Nelson, Gardent, Shulman, and Splaine (2010); Robichaux and Sauerland (2012).

and development of an ethical environment conducive to the provision of quality, safe nursing care. These implications were discussed in earlier chapters and are addressed further in this chapter.

Unlike principle-based ethics, virtue ethics does not emphasize specific rules of behavior but recognizes the significance of moral character and the role of emotions and experiences in providing safe, quality care. In addition, "Virtue is the tenet that a nurse has an obligation to maintain one's own integrity as well as the integrity of the profession" (see Chapter 1, p. 17). While ethical principles focus on "What should I do?" in a particular situation, virtue ethics asks, "What kind of nurse should I be?" (Armstrong, 2006; Robichaux & Sauerland, 2012). As Dans (1993) states, perhaps the greatest guarantee for safe, quality health care for the patient lies in the *character* of the provider both at the practice and leadership levels. Relevant virtues include honesty, compassion, prudence, and courage, among others.

An ethic of care has relevance for discussions of overall health care quality as it recognizes the inherent relational nature of nursing practice and, in particular, the IOM domain of patient/family-centered care (Chapter 6). Much research has been conducted to measure, evaluate, and improve the quality of care by means of objective measurements that focus on the IOM domains. In each domain, tools have been developed to measure and improve the performance of health care professionals and assess indicators such as number of readmissions, reoperations, and prevalence of pressure ulcers. Questionnaires are also used to evaluate patient outcomes and satisfaction as indicators of quality care. While objective measurements are vital to improvement in quality/safety, they may neglect one of the most important aspects of health care, the patient–provider relationship (Kuis, Hesselink, & Goosensenn, 2014). Milton (2011) has suggested that emphasis on quality and safety in the performance of tasks may diminish the nurse–patient caring relationship. She questions whether the "monitoring for potential error is the new standard for nursing practice rather than participating in the nurse–patient relationship with responsibility and accountability" (p. 110). Milton maintains that inattention to situational context with a focus on "doing things right" rather than "doing the right thing" (p. 110) has the potential to harm both the nursing profession and the recipients of care.

An ethic of care acknowledges nursing responsibility and accountability yet recognizes that care is not delivered to vulnerable others as a product. Clinical guidelines and standardized protocols are insufficient for facilitating the care that each unique patient needs, much like ethics principles alone are inadequate for ethical nursing practice. Supporting principles with elements of virtue ethics and care ethics may enable nurses to provide safe, quality care while integrating the essential humanistic and relational characteristics that consistently make nursing the most trusted profession. This integrated approach may contribute to developing an ethical environment in which nurses can practice quality care.

In the following section, the significance of each ethics principle in the provision of quality, safe care to the patient/family and in nursing practice

| Table 13.2 | | |

Implications of Ethics Principles, Virtue Ethics, and Care Ethics to Practice and Leadership

ETHICS PRINCIPLES, VIRTUE ETHICS, AND CARE ETHICS	PRACTICE	LEADERSHIP
Autonomy	Autonomous practice	Collaborative leadership, supportive governance structures
Beneficence	Treat one another with care and concern; assist our coworkers	Develop and sustain benevolent ethical climate
Nonmaleficence	Refrain from bullying, lateral violence; develop communication/ conflict competencies	Model professional behaviors; develop policies to address disruptive behaviors; support systemic mindfulness value system
Justice	Treat coworkers equally and fairly	Support a just, nonpunitive culture; encourage reporting of errors/near misses
Virtue	Demonstrate compassion and fairness	Develop/maintain a just culture; understand and support of second victims
Care	Maintain collaborative, caring relationships with coworkers	Demonstrate empathy and caring concern

Source: Robichaux and Sauerland (2012).

and leadership is discussed. Aspects of virtue ethics and care ethics relevant to each principle are addressed. Table 13.1 presents a summary of the implications of ethics principles, virtue ethics, and care ethics to the IOM quality domains and patient safety. Table 13.2 presents a summary of the implications of each principle and those of virtue ethics and care ethics to practice and leadership.

AUTONOMY

Patient/Family Care

Individual autonomy is highly valued in Western culture. In bioethics, respect for autonomy is associated with supporting patients in making decisions about which treatments or interventions they will or will not receive. The IOM domain and QSEN competency of patient-centered care reflect this ethical principle and provide an expanded understanding intended to correct entrenched tendencies of health care to be too disease focused or system or provider centric. Patient-centered care (PCC) or, to use the more inclusive term, patient/family-centered care (PFCC, Chapter 6), has been shown to result in improved health outcomes, including survival, greater patient satisfaction and well-being, improved communication between patients and health care professionals, and reductions in health care resource needs and costs (Berghout, van Exel, Leensvaart, & Cramm, 2015; Rathert, Wyrwich, & Boren, 2013). Elements of virtue ethics and care ethics also contribute to a relational understanding of autonomy that may enhance the overall quality of patient care.

Associating respect for autonomy *solely* with autonomous decision making and independence in choosing may neglect the idea that people are located within personal relationships, environments, and cultural systems. Simply offering and allowing patient/family choices about health care options or interventions and then standing back will isolate them in their decision-making and would be contrary to PFCC and the Code of Ethics (Box 13.1). A relational understanding of autonomy encourages us to consider these factors and recognize our interdependence in collaborative decision making (Ells, Hunt, & Chambers-Evans, 2011; Entwistle, Carter, Cribb, & McCaffney, 2010). Respectful, caring communication elicits and considers patient/family perspectives and promotes understanding of them as persons with guiding values, including those that are cultural and spiritual in nature (Epstein & Peters, 2009; Robichaux & Sauerland, 2012). As Houghton (Chapter 3) observes, nurses must be aware that many other factors such as race, level of education, and trust in the provider influence decision making.

While self-determination without undue provider influence may be associated with patients' perceptions of quality care, it is enhanced by provider prudence. Understood as practical wisdom, prudence is the ability to make decisions, often in the face of uncertainties (Marcum, 2011). Larrabee (1996) described one of the first models of health care quality as viewing patients and families as equal partners, and included the virtue of prudence, described as "good judgment in setting realistic goals . . . and skill in using resources to achieve those goals" (p. 356). Nurses and other providers can provide information regarding the availability, suitability, and cost of care. Prudence acknowledges, however, that patients/families may need help in understanding what they believe and want in complex medical situations, including the use of technological interventions.

Respect for autonomy embodies the virtues of honesty and trust and thus includes the duty to report and disclose errors and near misses to patients and appropriate authorities (Egan, 2014). Despite an emphasis on transparency in developing a patient safety culture, research indicates that fear of retaliation and subsequent underreporting persists. This is especially true in regard to near misses or close calls. Additional factors identified for lack of error/near-miss disclosure and underreporting include personal sense of responsibility, cumbersome documentation, and lack of feedback on reports (Lederman, Dreyfus, Matchan, Knott, & Milton, 2013; Ulrich & Kear, 2014). Individual accountability or responsibility for nursing actions and decisions is addressed throughout the Code of Ethics (ANA, 2015a) but perhaps best exemplified in the statement: "To be accountable, nurses follow a code of ethical conduct that includes such moral principles as fidelity, loyalty, *veracity*, beneficence and respect for the dignity, worth and self-determination of patients. . . ." [emphasis added] (p. 15). This accountability is more fully realized in a just, patient safety culture.

Questions to Consider Before Reading On

1. Can you describe a patient/family situation(s) in which you believe the principle of autonomy was compromised and/or supported?

2. What is the process for identifying and reporting errors/near misses in your facility?

Nursing Practice and Leadership

In nursing practice, Weston describes "autonomy" as the freedom to make decisions within the domain of the profession and to act accordingly (Weston, 2010). Professional autonomy and self-regulation are necessary for implementing nursing standards and guidelines and for ensuring *quality care* (ANA, 2015a, p. 28). Similarly, professionalism is described as the ability to make autonomous decisions based on knowing the patient/family, clinical knowledge, experience, and evidence (Papathanassoglou et al., 2012). The ability to exercise autonomy in nursing practice is directly related to job satisfaction and perceptions of quality patient care (Twigg & McCullough, 2014; Van Bogaert, Kowalski, Weeks, Van Huesden, & Clarke, 2014). In contrast, limited nurse autonomy, lack of interprofessional collaboration and ethical leadership contribute to moral distress and turnover (Chapters 4 and 10).

Nursing leaders can actively support nurse autonomy through praise and recognition and inclusion of staff nurses on unit and organizational committees. These strategies, among other supporting governance structures, strengthen the professional practice environment and contribute to a just, patient safety culture. Positive patient safety outcomes, including a decrease

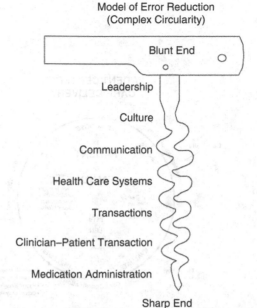

Figure 13.1 Systemic mindfulness model of proactive safety.
Source: Rich (2008).

in medication errors and overall adverse events, have been associated with collaborative leadership (Regan, Laschinger, & Wong, 2015). Leaders who create opportunities for meaningful dialogue with nurses to resolve care issues that risk patient safety and then follow through on staff suggestions for improvement role model their commitment to patient care (Wong, 2015). One such leader is Victoria Rich, who has developed several national and international patient safety initiatives for health care systems ("Patient Safety Movement," 2015). Rich (2008) created a Model of Error Reduction, the Systemic Mindfulness Model of Proactive Patient Safety (Figure 13.1). This figure, which resembles a corkscrew, illustrates the complex, circular, and collaborative pathway to an ethical patient safety culture. The model is discussed in more detail in the section on Justice.

Stallings-Welden and Shirey (2015) demonstrated how development and implementation of a professional practice model (PPM) can significantly improve patient care quality and safety, among other factors. Figure 13.2 is the PPM created by staff nurses at Deaconess Health System in Evansville, Indiana. The Deaconess FIRST acronym (**F**antastic people **I**ncreasing quality **R**esulting in growth **S**uperior service and **T**op financial performance) demonstrates how nursing practice (mission, vision, values, and philosophy) is in alignment and integrated within the organization. Nursing values (not inclusive) are listed below the PPM pillars (Stallings-Welden, personal communication, June 9, 2016). The PPM reflects elements of nursing's foundational documents such as the Social Policy Statement (ANA, 2010a) as it emphasizes

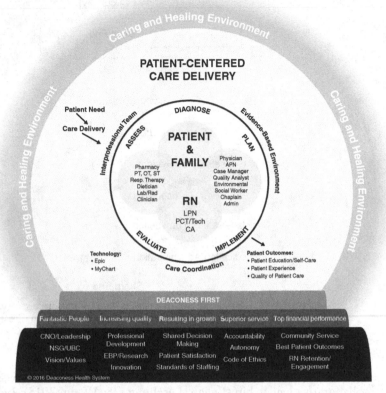

Figure 13.2 Professional practice model of nursing. The professional practice model (PPM) is a schematic description that articulates how Deaconess nurses provide patient-centered care using evidence-based practice and by establishing patient/family and interprofessional partnerships to achieve optimal outcomes in a caring and healing environment. The model describes how nurses have a comprehensive understanding of their role and exercise professional autonomy through the fundamental responsibilities and accountabilities of nursing that illustrate their education, training, legal, social, and ethical obligations. The PPM is in alignment with the mission and values of the organization and illustrates this alliance by denoting nursing philosophy and values in conjunction with the acronym of Deaconess FIRST. © 2016 Deaconess Health System. Printed with permission.

the provision of safe, quality care to all. In addition, the PPM provides a framework for an accountable and autonomous practice of nursing supported by a just culture in accordance with the Code of Ethics (ANA, 2015).

CASE SCENARIO (*CONTINUED*)

Returning to the chapter Case Scenario, Betsy continues to think about Mr. D. and the possible outcome(s) if she had not intervened in time. She realizes that a "near miss" such as this has happened previously to her and other nurses but has not

(continued)

CASE SCENARIO (*CONTINUED*)

reported them because of fear of management reprisal. Betsy decides to speak with her friend and former nurse manager, Vicki, who is now a nursing director in a different facility. Vicki tells her that a similar atmosphere of distrust existed in the institution when she initially assumed the director position. After researching and discussing the issue with other administrators, Vicki determined that implementation of a Professional Practice Model (PPM) for nursing was indicated. In addition, as the institution was beginning the Magnet journey, development and evaluation of a PPM were required for designation. Staff nurses created the model to illustrate the education, legal, social, and ethical obligations of nurses as they coordinate patient/family care. Vicki stated that the PPM provides a framework for an accountable and autonomous practice of nursing supported by establishment of a just culture.

Questions to Consider Before Reading On

1. Does your facility utilize a PPM? If so, how is ethics integrated in the model?

2. If not, using the Deaconess PPM as an example, what would you include in a model?

BENEFICENCE

Patient and Family Care

Beneficence is the principle of acting for the benefit of others and promoting their welfare. Provider actions associated with beneficence include protecting the rights of the patient, preventing harm, rectifying conditions or situations that may cause harm, and aiding those in need of rescue. This principle is often discussed in conjunction with nonmaleficence, the obligation to avoid actions that would cause harm to others or oneself. Although both are important, the duty to "first, do no harm," is viewed as the stronger obligation in health care and nursing practice. As seen in Table 13.1, the relationship of beneficence and nonmaleficence to the IOM quality domains is similar. The distinction between beneficence and nonmaleficence is that the former is a moral obligation to take positive actions to help others, not to simply prevent harm.

At times, there may be an inherent conflict between the principles of beneficence and autonomy (Moriates, Arora, & Shah, 2015; Thompson, 2007). Patients and/or family members may request a treatment or procedure that a provider believes will be of limited benefit or even result in physical or financial harm. On the other hand, patients and family members may refuse treatment that the provider deems beneficial. Although beneficence is an ancient concept found in the works of Aristotle (Irwin, 1999), autonomy and the participation of the patient/family in the decision-making process are central to PFCC. Paternalism, a subtype of beneficence in which someone with more knowledge, experience, or authority determines what actions are in another's best interest, has a limited role in this collaborative model (Egan, 2014). To resolve such dilemmas, nurses and other health care professionals need to listen to the patient/family and explore their rationale for the request or refusal. When the situation cannot be resolved, it is important to acknowledge that patient autonomy may not be limitless, and providers should not consider a patient request that would result in greater harm than good to the patient (Moriates et al., 2015). The principle of justice must also be considered in relation to autonomy. The community perspective or factors outside the patient–provider relationship such as use of scarce resources and services may be pertinent. Complex ethical dilemmas in which various ethical principles appear to be at odds may require the skills of an ethics consultant or team.

Practice and Leadership

In nursing practice, beneficence means that we treat one another with care and concern and, as with patients and families, take positive steps to help our health care team members. Given the current, complex, and often chaotic practice environments, this can prove an exceptional challenge for nurses and all health care providers. Personal dislikes and differences of opinion are understandable; however, we are professionally obligated to assist and interact with team members in a respectful, caring manner (ANA, 2015a). Units and facilities with benevolent ethical climates report improved quality of care, better clinical outcomes, increased patient/family satisfaction, decreased mortality, and less nurse turnover (Rathert et al., 2013; Vanderheide, Moss, & Lee, 2013). A benevolent, caring ethical climate or environment enhances nurses' organizational commitment and interpersonal cohesiveness unlike those that are egoistic (self-interested) or principled (rule based). In addition, nurses and others are more likely to speak up and report errors/near misses in this nonpunitive climate or "just culture."

The impact of ethical leadership on nursing practice and the work environment has been addressed in Chapter 8. Supportive leadership at the management and administration levels is also associated with a just culture (discussed in the section on Justice), improved patient safety and related factors such as reduced absenteeism. Leaders who demonstrate benevolent, caring behaviors are trusted by nurses who are then more likely to engage in questioning and reporting unsafe practices and events (Merrill, 2015; Wong, 2015). The Deaconess PPM depicted in Figure 13.2 illustrates how nurses envision practice within a caring and healing environment.

NONMALEFICENCE

Patient and Family Care

As a component of quality care, patient safety is primarily rooted in the principle of nonmaleficence. Patient safety focuses on eliminating preventable harm but recognizes that the decision of what is acceptable risk in pursing health is made by the competent patient and his or her family (Egan, 2014). Reflecting the IOM domains of safe, effective, timely, and patient centered, nonmaleficence also includes the obligation not to offer treatment that lacks efficacy. This obligation can become an issue and conflict with principles of autonomy and justice in the provision of marginal or expensive treatments. In these instances, such as provision of end-of-life interventions deemed of minimal benefit or even harmful, elements of virtue ethics and caring ethics support the advocacy role of the nurse. Adams, Bailey, Andersen, & Doughterty (2011) provide a comprehensive review of the proactive strategies used by nurses in these challenging circumstances, including information broker (to patient/family and physicians), mediator, and supporter.

Nurses are also involved in developing and implementing safeguards to prevent foreseeable harm to patients. Among others, these include hand washing/infection control measures, use of checklists, structured communication techniques such as Situation, Background, Assessment, Recommendation (SBAR) and Concerned, Uncomfortable, Safety issue (CUS), and multidisciplinary rounds. The Comprehensive Unit-Based Safety Program (CUSP) is multifaceted strategy for culture change that includes interventions such as team training and use of evidence-informed guidelines. Preliminary research on the efficacy of these approaches suggests that use of a combination of components may more effectively promote patient safety and quality care (Weaver et al., 2013).

Working with providers who are perceived as incompetent is a persistent finding in studies of moral distress across disciplines (Sauerland et al., 2015). The Code of Ethics (ANA, 2015a) states that "nurses must take appropriate action in all instances of incompetent, unethical, illegal, or impaired practice or actions that place the rights or best interests of the patient in jeopardy" (p. 12). These actions, such as initially expressing concern to the provider involved and reporting to higher authorities when indicated, may require skills associated with moral courage.

Practice and Leadership

Although the obligation to "do no harm" extends to our coworkers at all levels, bullying, lateral violence, and incivility characterize many interactions and health care environments, threatening patient safety and quality care. At the practice level, developing individual communication and conflict competencies to address such behaviors is essential. Nursing leaders are obligated to model appropriate behaviors and hold others accountable to do the same. In addition, they are responsible for developing and implementing policies and protocols that address concerns such as provider incompetence or incivility, unsafe staffing, and disruptive patient/family behavior (Edmonson, 2015).

The establishment of a patient safety culture is interdisciplinary in nature and, as illustrated in Figure 13.1, complex, circular, and interactive. From the blunt end (leadership) through the many layers to the sharp end (direct care providers), risk and safety are embedded in each level of and transaction in the health care system. Reducing errors, such as in medication administration, requires a systemic mindfulness value system that holds both the sharp and blunt ends personally and professionally accountable (Rich, 2008; Schifalaqua, 2013). As discussed in Chapter 4, mindfulness meditation exercises have been shown to decrease moral distress and increase resilience (Gauthier, Meyer, Grefe, & Gold, 2015; Rushton, Batcheller, Schroeder, & Donohue, 2015). In regard to patient safety, mindfulness has been associated with reduction in errors/near misses and improved patient outcomes. Brown et al. (2015) reported a decrease in medication errors in an ICU setting and Hallman, O'Connor, Hasenau, & Brady (2014) noted a reduced need for 1:1 staff episodes in a high-acuity child/adolescent psychiatric unit after implementation of mindfulness strategies. It has also been proposed that these strategies or techniques may result in fewer clinical reasoning and diagnostic errors (Sibinga & Wu, 2010). Being mindful is "paying attention in a particular way; on purpose, in the moment and non-judgmentally" (Kabat-Zinn, 1994, p. 4)." Additional skills include being open, trusting, and letting go (Kabat-Zinn, 2013). More than just paying attention, mindfulness can be challenging in chaotic practice settings. One nurse relates how practicing mindfulness helps him in the clinical area:

> Using mindfulness techniques, I realized I was much more aware of the present, rather than being aware of the numerous work-related, negative thoughts we can become subject to and which can overwhelm us. I wasn't overwhelmed and was more effective at delegating to other professionals, resolving conflict and actively listening. By using mindfulness, I found I was more focused on the patient in front of me and could concentrate better. Because I was calm and present, the patient was more relaxed. Client safety was prioritized and achieved, leading to effective health-care outcomes. (Philbrick, 2015, pp. 32–33)

Organizational culture is defined as the norms, values, and basic assumptions of a given organization or unit. Individual unit cultures, such as in the chapter Case Scenario, have unwritten expectations where nurses learn what is or is not permissible. It is difficult to prioritize patient safety in a culture where communication between the blunt and sharp ends of the system is poor and providers are ignored or reprimanded for reporting near misses or errors. Ethical nursing leaders are responsible for developing and sustaining a non-punitive, just culture, and reward system for identifying unsafe practices (AONE, 2015). To do so, they must be visible and trustworthy, among other characteristics and behaviors. Leadership WalkRounds (WR) is an effective strategy to improve communication and patient safety at both the system and unit levels. The formatting and frequency of WR varies and can include specific questions Institute for Healthcare Improvement (IHI, 2016) or informal conversations that occur weekly or monthly. Members of the WR can include nursing and/or administrative executive leaders, nurse managers, and unit safety champions. Research indicates that WR is associated with immediate resolution of staff-identified safety issues, decreased provider burnout, and improved organization/unit safety culture (Schwendimann et al., 2013).

Questions to Consider Before Reading On

The Nonmaleficence section described several unit/institution safety strategies including use of checklists, communication techniques, WR, and CUSP.

1. Discuss strategies used at your facility with a class peer or colleague—what has worked?

2. What additional strategies could be implemented?

CASE SCENARIO (CONTINUED)

Returning to the chapter Case Scenario, Betsy thinks about her conversation with Vicki and the strategies she proposed about developing a PPM and the potential positive effects on patient safety and quality care. To gain staff and administrative awareness and support for creating a PPM, Vicki suggested that Betsy assess provider perceptions of the current safety culture using a survey developed by the AHRQ (2016). This survey assesses several dimensions of patient safety culture including feedback and communication about error, team work, and nonpunitive response to error. The survey takes about 10 to 15 minutes to complete and results can be compared with those of other hospitals. After exploring the survey questions and supportive material available on the AHRQ website (links provided as follows) with her manager, Stephanie, they make an appointment with the Chief Nursing Officer (CNO) to discuss distributing the survey.

http://www.ahrq.gov/professionals/quality-patient-safety/patientsafety culture/hospital/index.html

JUSTICE

Patient and Family Care

Many terms are used to describe the ethical principle of justice, including *fairness* and *equitable entitlement* in the distribution of resources, goods, and services. There are also several theories and types of justice such as distributive justice that are concerned with who receives which resources when they are limited or scarce. Daily patient care issues are affected by the principle of distributive justice. Nurses may ration care activities or report missed/omitted care because of inadequate staffing or insufficient time. Identified care activities that are rationed or missed include ambulation, timely medication administration, discharge teaching, and comforting. The effects of such rationing on quality care and patient outcomes are many, including increased adverse events and decreased nurse-reported care quality (Jones, Hamilton, & Murry, 2015; Orique, Patty, & Woods, 2016). Despite such negative outcomes, the reality of daily practice may require the rationing of care activities. The virtue of prudence or practical wisdom, gained through experience, enables nurses to balance complex and competing care demands while maintaining patient safety.

Justice is reflected in the IOM quality domains as equitable, efficient, and, as with all aims, patient centered. In regard to patient/family care, nurses are required to provide fair and equal treatment that respects "the inherent dignity, worth, unique attributes, and human rights of all individuals. The need for and right to health care is universal, transcending all individual differences" (ANA, 2015a, p. 1). Further, the just provision of care requires these factors be considered, as they influence the need for care and the allocation of resources. This idea expands what is addressed in the IOM quality domains, because the notion of social justice is recognized. Nurses are obligated to consider elements of social justice that focus on a broader analysis and critique of policies, structures, and customs that disadvantage or harm vulnerable or stigmatized groups (ANA, 2015a). The objective of this analysis is to develop strategies that would seek to redress unjust conditions such as the social determinants of illness, poverty, hunger, and illiteracy, among others (Fowler, 2015).

Practice and Leadership

As with patients and family members, nurses are required to treat all coworkers with justice and dignity. Justice issues affecting practice include perceived unfair treatment and/or distribution of workload or unacknowledged individual contribution. Bullying, lateral violence, and incivility also have justice implications. Supporting and encouraging our peers, demonstrating compassion, and treating all equally and fairly contribute to a just culture and patient safety.

In 2010, a pediatric patient at Seattle Children's Hospital died from a calcium chloride overdose. Kimberly Hiatt, the nurse caring for the infant at the time, was suspended, then terminated from a position she had held for 27 years. Her license was reinstated after satisfying state disciplinary requirements including paying a fine and agreeing to a 4-year probationary status. Hiatt could not find a job and her health and psychological well-being deteriorated. She committed suicide 7 months after the infant's death, at age 50. The critically ill infant's death could later not be attributed to her actions (Newland, 2011). Nursing leaders at all levels are responsible for developing and maintaining a just culture in which individuals are held accountable for their behavior but are not victimized. Hiatt was a "second victim" of an unjust culture of perfection in which mistakes are unacceptable and attributed to a failure of character (Santamauro, Kaukman, & Dekker, 2014). A term introduced by Wu in 2000, "second victims" are defined as:

> Healthcare team members involved in an unanticipated patient event, a medical error and/or patient related injury and become victimized in the sense that they are traumatized by the event. Frequently, these individuals feel personally responsible for the patient outcome. Many feel as though they have failed the patient, second guessing their clinical skills and knowledge base. (Center for Patient Safety, 2015)

Second victim responses are not limited to incidents that result in patient harm. In one multi-institutional study, approximately one-third of participants who had been involved in near-miss events reported symptoms such as insomnia and anxiety about future potential errors (Burlison, Scott, Browne, Thompson, & Hoffman, 2014). Lucian Leape, MD, a longtime leader in patient safety, observes that one of the biggest barriers to preventing errors/near misses in health care is our history of punishing people for making mistakes and not looking deeper into other contributing systemic factors. This approach results in provider reluctance to report such events and compromises patient safety. Over half of all health care providers have had a second victim experience during their careers. As a result, many have left their profession and some have turned to suicide to end their suffering. Although progress on just treatment of second victims in health care has been made, it lags behind other safety critical worlds such as aviation and nuclear power (Burlison et al., 2014).

Similar to medication administration safety, Denham (2007) proposes that caregivers and leaders consider the five rights of second victims as part of a fair and just culture. These rights have served as the basis of several health care institutions' second victim support programs (Scott et al., 2010; Wu & Steckelberg, 2012). Using the acronym, TRUST, these rights include:

- **T**reatment that is just—a caring and nonpunitive approach that may lead to improving the system in which the error/near miss occurred.

- **R**espect—all health care team members are susceptible to errors/near misses. A blame-shame culture denies the provider his/her right to respect and dignity.

- **U**nderstanding and compassion—second victims need support and compassionate help to heal. Leaders must understand the psychological emergency that occurs when a patient is unintentionally harmed or a near miss occurs.

- **S**upportive care—second victims are entitled to support services delivered in a professional and organized manner.

- **T**ransparency and opportunity to contribute—in a just organization, second victims have the right to participate in the learning gathered about the error/near miss and share in potential causal information. The opportunity to contribute to an improved safety climate and quality care helps second victims to heal.

CASE SCENARIO (CONTINUED)

Returning to the chapter Case Scenario, Betsy and Stephanie present the results of the hospital safety culture survey to the CNO and other members of the administration. They discuss the less-than-acceptable findings in several areas including staffing, unit teamwork, and openness to communication. For example, less than one-third of the staff rated the question "Staff freely speak up if they see something that may negatively affect a patient and feel free to question those in authority" as satisfactory. In addition, staff reported poor collaboration and lack of respect, reflecting an unsupportive ethical environment. At the conclusion of the meeting, the CNO and administrators agree to work with Betsy, Stephanie, and members of other disciplines to develop a just, caring patient safety culture built on ethics principles.

CONCLUSION

This chapter presented a brief overview of the nursing profession's concern with quality care and ethics. The relationship of ethical principles, virtue ethics, and care ethics as well as examples of how they are manifested in the IOM quality domains were discussed. Implications of the principles and virtue/care approaches for patient/family care, nursing practice, and leadership were addressed. Strategies to develop a just patient safety culture were presented.

Critical Thinking Questions and Activities

Explore the following websites that provide additional information on a just, caring safety culture and strategies to assist second victims. How would you use this information to implement/improve the safety culture in your facility?

http://www.mitsstools.org/tool-kit-for-staff-support-for-healthcare-organizations.html

http://www.ihi.org/resources/pages/ihiwhitepapers/respectfulmanagementseriousclinicalaeswhitepaper.aspx

http://www.centerforpatientsafety.org/second-victims/

http://nursingworld.org/psjustculture

http://www.nursingworld.org/MainMenuCategories/ANAMarketplace/ANAPeriodicals/OJIN/TableofContents/Vol-16-2011/No3-Sept-2011/Patient-Safety-Culture-and-Nursing-Unit-Leader.html

http://www.hopkinsmedicine.org/armstrong_institute/training_services/cusp_offerings/cusp_guidance.html

REFERENCES

Adams, J., Bailey, D., Andersen, R., & Doughterty, S. (2011). Nursing roles and strategies in end-of-life decision making in acute care: A systematic review of the literature. *Nursing Research and Practice*, Article ID 527834, 1–15. doi:10.1155/2011/527834. Retrieved from http://www.hindawi.com/journals/nrp/2011/527834

Agency for Healthcare Research and Quality. (2012). Improving patient safety systems for patients with limited English proficiency: Background on patient safety and LEP populations. Washington, DC: Author. Retrieved from http://www.ahrq.gov/professionals/systems/hospital/lepguide/lepguide1.html

Agency for Healthcare Research and Quality. (2016). *Hospital Survey on Patient Safety Culture*. Rockville, MD. Retrieved from http://www.ahrq.gov/professionals/quality-patient-safety/patientsafetyculture/hospital/index.html

Aiken, L., Sermeus, W., Van den Heede, K., Sloane, D., Busse, R., McKee, M., . . . Kutney-Lee, A. (2012). Patient safety, satisfaction, and quality of hospital care: Cross sectional surveys of nurses and patients in 12 countries in Europe and the United States. *British Medical Journal, 344*, e1717. doi:10.1136/bmj.e1717. Retrieved from http://www.bmj.com/content/344/bmj.e1717

American Nurses Association. (1995). *Nursings report card for acute care*. Washington, DC: American Nurses Publishing.

American Nurses Association. (1996). *Nursing quality indicators: Guide for implementation*. Washington, DC: American Nurses Publishing.

American Nurses Association. (1999). *Nursing quality indicators: Guide for implementation* (2nd ed.). Washington, DC: American Nurses Publishing.

American Nurses Association. (2010a). *Nursing's social policy statement: The essence of the profession.* Silver Spring, MD: Nursebooks.org. Retrieved from http://www.nursingworld.org/social-policy -statement

American Nurses Association. (2010b). *Position statement: Just Culture.* Retrieved from http://nursing world.org/psjustculture

American Nurses Association. (2015a). *Code of ethics for nurses with interpretive statements.* Silver Spring, MD: Nursebooks.org.

American Nurses Association. (2015b*). Nursing scope and standards of practice* (3rd ed.). Silver Spring, MD: Nursebooks.org.

American Organization of Nurse Executives. (2015). Nurse executive competencies. Washington, DC: Author. Retrieved from http://www.aone.org/resources/nec.pdf

Armstrong, A. (2006). Toward a strong virtue ethics for nursing practice. *Nursing Philosophy, 7,* 110–24.

Armstrong Institute for Patient Safety. (2016). CUSP guidance for hospitals. Retrieved from http:// www.hopkinsmedicine.org/armstrong_institute/training_services/cusp_offerings/cusp_guid ance.html

Aydelotte, M., & Tener, M. (1961). An investigation of the relation between nursing activity and patient welfare. *Nursing Research, 10*(2), 115.

Barnsteiner, J. (2011). Teaching the culture of safety. *The Online Journal of Issue in Nursing, 16*(3). doi:10.3912/OJIN.Vol16No03Man05

Berghout, M., van Exel, J., Leensvaart, L., & Cramm, J. (2015). Healthcare professionals' views on patient-centered care in hospitals. *BMC Health Services Research, 15,* 385. doi:10.1186/s12913-015-1049-z

Brown, L., Kilrain, B., Hohmeister, S., Stoeff, S., McGrath, R., Linnett, M., . . . Wisdom, M. (2015). Reducing intravenous medication errors in critical care by managing distraction. *Critical Care Nurse, 35*(2), e35.

Burlison, J., Scott, S., Browne, E., Thompson, S., & Hoffman, J. (2014). The second victim experience and support tool: Validation of an organizational resource for assessing second victim effects and the quality of support resources. *Journal of Patient Safety,* Advance online publication. Retrieved from http://www.ncbi.nlm.nih.gov/pmc/articles/PMC4342309/

Center for Patient Safety. (2015). The second victim experience. Retrieved from http://www.center forpatientsafety.org/second-victims

Conway, J., Federico, F., Stewart, K., & Campbell, M. (2011). *Respectful management of serious clinical adverse events* (2nd ed.). IHI Innovation Series white paper. Cambridge, MA: Institute for Healthcare Improvement. Retrieved from www.IHI.org

Cronenwett, L., Sherwood, D., Barnsteiner, J., Disch, J., Johnson, J., Mitchell, P., . . . Warren, J. (2007). Quality and safety education for nurses. *Nursing Outlook, 55*(3), 122–131.

Dans, P. (1993). Clinical peer review: Burnishing a tarnished icon. *Annals of Internal Medicine, 118,* 566–568.

Denham, C. (2007). TRUST: The 5 rights of the second victim. *The Journal of Patient Safety, 3*(2), 107–119.

Edmonson, C. (2015). Strengthening moral courage among nurse leaders. *The Online Journal of Issues in Nursing, 20*(2). Retrieved from http://www.nursingworld.org/MainMenuCategories/ ANAMarketplace/ANAPeriodicals/OJIN/TableofContents/Vol-20-2015/No2-May-2015/ Articles-Previous-Topics/Strengthening-Moral-Courage.html

Egan, E. (2014). Clinical ethics and patient safety. In A. Agrawal (Ed.), *Patient safety: A case-based comprehensive guide.* New York, NY: Springer.

Ells, C., Hunt, M., & Chambers-Evans, J. (2011). Relational autonomy as an essential component of patient-centered care. *International Journal of Feminist Approaches to Bioethics, 4*(2), 79–101.

Entwistle, V., Carter, S., Cribb, A., & McCaffney, K. (2010). Supporting patient autonomy: The importance of clinical relationships. *Journal of General Internal Medicine, 25*(7), 741–745.

Epstein, E., & Peters, E. (2009). Beyond information: Exploring patients' preferences. *Journal of the American Medical Association, 302*(2), 195–197.

Fowler, M. (2015). *Guide to the code of ethics for nurses with interpretive statements* (2nd ed.). Silver Spring, M.D: Nursebooks.org.

Gauthier, T., Meyer, R., Grefe, D., & Gold, J. (2015). An on-the-job mindfulness-based intervention for pediatric ICU nurses: A pilot. *Journal of Pediatric Nursing, 30*(2), 402–409.

Griffiths, P. (1995). Progress in measuring nursing outcomes.. *Journal of Advanced Nursing, 21*(6), 1092–1100.

Hallman, I., O'Connor, N., Hasenau, S., & Brady, S. (2014). Improving the culture of safety on a high acuity inpatient child/adolescent psychiatric unit by mindfulness-based stress reduction training of staff. *Journal of Child Adolescent Psychiatric Nursing, 27*(4), 183–189.

Henneman, E., Cunningham, H., Fisher, D., Plotkin, K., Nathanson, B., Roche, J., . . . Henneman, P. (2014). Eye tracking as a debriefing mechanism in the simulated setting improves patient safety practices. *Dimensions of Critical Care Nursing, 33*(3), 129–135.

Henneman, E., Gawlinski, A., & Giuliano, K. (2012). Surveillance: A strategy for improving patient safety in acute and critical care units. *Critical Care Nurse, 32*(2), e9–e18. Retrieved from http://ccn.aacnjournals.org/content/32/2/e9.long

Hospital Safety Score. (2015). What is patient safety? Retrieved from http://www.hospitalsafe tyscore.org/what-is-patient-safety_m

Institute for Healthcare Improvement (IHI). (2016). Retrieved from http://www.ihi.org/resources/Pages/Changes/ConductPatientSafetyLeadershipWalkRounds.aspx

Institute of Medicine. (2001). *Crossing the quality chasm: A new health system for the 21st century.* Washington, DC: National Academies Press. Retrieved from http://iom.nationalacademies.org/~/media/Files/Report%20Files/2001/Crossing-the-Quality-Chasm/Quality%20Chasm%202001%20%20report%20brief.pdf

Irwin, T. (1999). *Aristotle: Nicomachean ethics* (2nd ed.). Indianapolis, IN: Hackett Publishing.

James, J. (2013). A new, evidence-based estimate of patient harms associated with hospital care. *Journal of Patient Safety, 9*(3), 122–128.

Jones, T., Hamilton, P., & Murry, N. (2015). Unfinished nursing care, missed care, and implicitly rationed care: State of the science review. *International Journal of Nursing Studies, 52,* 1121–1137.

Kabat-Zinn, J. (1994). *Wherever you go, there you are: Mindfulness meditation in everyday life.* New York, NY: Hyperion.

Kabat-Zinn, J. (2013). *Full catastrophe living: Using the wisdom of your body and mind to face stress, pain, and illness.* New York, NY: Bantam Dell Publishing Group.

Kohn, L., Corrigan, J., & Donaldson, M. (Eds.), *To err is human: Building a safer health system.* Washington, DC: National Academies Press. Retrieved from http://iom.nationalacademies.org/Reports/1999/To-Err-is-Human-Building-A-Safer-Health-System.aspx

Kuis, E., Hesselink, G., & Goosensenn, A. (2014). Can quality from a care ethical perspective be assessed? A review. *Nursing Ethics, 21*(7), 774–793.

Lang, N. (1975). Quality assurance in nursing. *Association of Operating Room Nurses Journal, 22*(4), 180–186.

Larrabee, J. (1996). Emerging model of quality. *Image: The Journal of Nursing Scholarship, 28*(4), 353–358.

Lederman, R., Dreyfus, S., Matchan, J., Knott, J., & Milton, S. (2013). Electronic error reporting systems: A case study into the impact on nurse reporting of medical errors. *Nursing Outlook, 61,* 417–446.

Luckes, E. (1886). *Hospital sisters and their duties.* Philadelphia, PA: P. Blakiston Son & Co.

Marcum, J. (2011). The role of prudent love in the practice of clinical medicine. *Journal of Evaluation in Clinical Practice, 17*, 877–882.

Medically Induced Trauma Support Services. (2015). Tools for building a clinician and staff support program. Retrieved from http://www.mitsstools.org/tool-kit-for-staff-support-for-healthcare-organizations.html

Merrill, K. (2015). Leadership style and patient safety: Implications for nurse managers. *The Journal of Nursing Administration, 45*(6), 319–324.

Milton C. (2011). An ethical exploration of quality and safety initiatives in nursing practice. *Nursing Science Quarterly, 24(2)*, 107–10.

Moriates, C., Arora, V., & Shah, N. (2015). *Understanding value-based healthcare*. New York, NY: McGraw Hill.

National Quality Forum. (2009). Patient safety terms and definitions. Retrieved from https://www.qualityforum.org/Topics/Safety_Definition.aspx

Nelson, W., Gardent, P., Shulman, E., & Splaine, M. (2010). Preventing ethics conflicts and improving healthcare quality through system redesign. *Quality and Safety in Health Care, 19*, 526–530.

Newland, J. (2011). Medical errors snare more than one victim. *The Nurse Practitioner, 36*(9), 5. Retrieved from http://journals.lww.com/tnpj/Fulltext/2011/09000/Medical_errors_snare_more_than_one_victim.1.aspx

Nightingale, F. (1863). *Notes on hospitals* (3rd ed.). London, UK: Longman, Green, Longman, Roberts, and Green.

Orique, S., Patty, C., & Woods, E. (2016). Missed nursing care and unit-level workload in the acute and post-acute settings. *Journal of Nursing Care Quality, 31*(1), 84–89.

Papathanassoglou, E., Karanikola, M., Kalafati, M., Giannakopoulou, M., Lemonidou, C., & Albarran, J. (2012). Professional autonomy, collaboration with physicians, and moral distress among European intensive care nurses. *American Journal of Critical Care, 21*(2), e41–e52. Retrieved from http://ajcc.aacnjournals.org/content/21/2/e41.full

Patient Safety Movement. (2015). Victoria Rich, RN, PhD, FAAN. Retrieved from http://patientsafetymovement.org/speakers-panelists/victoria-rich

Phaneuf, M. (1972). *The nursing audit: Profile for excellence*. New York, NY: Appleton-Century-Crofts.

Phaneuf, M., & Wandelt, M. A. (1974). Quality assurance in nursing: "-any profession that does not monitor itself becomes a technology." *Nursing Forum, 13*(4), 328–345.

Philbrick, G. (2015). Using mindfulness to enhance nursing practice. *Kai Tiaki Nursing New Zealand, 21*(5), 32–33.

Press-Ganey. (2015). Nursing quality (NDNQI). Retrieved from http://www.pressganey.com/solutions/clinical-quality/nursing-quality

QSEN. (2015). Retrieved from http://qsen.org/about-qsen

Rathert, C., & Fleming, D. (2008). Hospital ethical climate and teamwork in acute care: The moderating role of leaders. *Healthcare Management Review, 33*(4), 323–331.

Rathert, C., Wyrwich, M., & Boren, S. (2013). Patient-centered care and outcomes: A systematic review of the literature. *Medical Care Research Review, 70*(4), 351–379.

Regan, S., Laschinger, H., & Wong, C. (2015). The influence of empowerment, authentic leadership, and professional practice environments on nurses' perceived interprofessional collaboration. *Journal of Nursing Management, 24*(1), e54–e61.

Rich, V. (2008). Clinical vignette: Creation of a patient safety culture. In R. Hughes (Ed.), *Patient safety and quality: An evidence-based handbook for nurses*. Rockville, MD: AHRQ Publication No. 08-0043. Retrieved from http://archive.ahrq.gov/professionals/clinicians-providers/resources/nursing/resources/nurseshdbk/RichV_VCPSC.pdf

Robichaux, C., & Sauerland, J. (2012). Health care quality and ethics: Implications for practice and leadership. *Perioperative Nursing Clinics, 7*(3), 333–342.

Rushton, C., Batcheller, J., Schroeder, K., & Donohue, P. (2015). Burnout and resilience among nurses practicing in high intensity settings. *American Journal of Critical Care, 24*(5), 412–420. Retrieved from http://ajcc.aacnjournals.org/content/24/5/412.full.pdf+html?sid=b8128317 -ce1b-4c3d-a94e-38c943956836

Santamauro, C., Kaukman, C., & Dekker, S. (2014). Second victims, organizational resilience and the role of hospital administration. *Journal of Hospital Administration, 3*(5), 95–103. Retrieved from http://www.sciedu.ca/journal/index.php/jha/article/view/4328

Sammer, C., & James, B. (2011). Patient safety culture: The nursing unit's leader role. *The Online Journal of Issues in Nursing, 16*(3), Manuscript 3. Retrieved from http://www.nursingworld.org/ MainMenuCategories/ANAMarketplace/ANAPeriodicals/OJIN/TableofContents/Vol-16- 2011/No3-Sept-2011/Patient-Safety-Culture-and-Nursing-Unit-Leader.html

Sauerland, J., Marotta, K., Peinemann, M., Berndt, A., & Robichaux, C. (2015). Assessing and address-ing moral distress and ethical climate Part II: Pediatric and neontatal nurses' perspectives. *Dimensions of Critical Care Nursing, 34*(1), 33–46. Retrieved from http://journals.lww.com/dccn journal/Fulltext/2015/01000/Assessing_and_Addressing_Moral_Distress_and.8.aspx

Schifalaqua, M. (2013). Victoria Rich, PhD, RN, FAAN. *Nurse Leader, 11*(3), 15–18. Retrieved from http://www.nurseleader.com/article/S1541-4612(13)00083-9/fulltext

Schwendimann, R., Milne, J., Frush, K., Ausserhofer, D., Frankel, A., & Sexton, J. (2013). *American Journal of Medical Quality, 28*(5), 414–421.

Scott, S., Hirschinger, L., Cox, K., McCoig, M., Hahn-Cover, K., Epperly, K., . . . Hall, L. (2010). Caring for our own: Deploying a systemwide second victim rapid response team. *The Joint Commission Journal on Quality and Patient Safety, 36*(5), 233–240.

Scrubs Magazine. (2015). Inspirational quotes every nurse should read, May 7, 2014. Retrieved from http://www.scrubsmag.com/inspirational-quotes-every-nurse-should-read

Sheingold, B., & Hahn, J. (2014). The history of healthcare quality: The first hundred years 1860– 1960. *International Journal of Africa Nursing Sciences, 1*(1), 18–22.

Sibinga, E., & Wu, A. (2010). Clinician mindfulness and patient safety. *Journal of the American Medical Association, 304*(22), 2352–2353.

Stallings-Welden, L., & Shirey, M. (2015). Predictability of a professional practice model to affect nurse and patient outcomes. *Nursing Administration Quarterly, 39*(3), 199–210.

Thompson D. (2007). Principles of ethics: In managing a critical care unit. *Critical Care Medicine, 35*, S2–S10.

Tronto, J. (1993). *Moral boundaries: A political argument for an ethic of care.* New York, NY: Routledge.

Twigg, D., & McCullough, K. (2014). Nurse retention: A review of strategies to create and enhance positive practice environments in clinical settings. *International Journal of Nursing Studies, 51*(1), 85–92.

Ulrich, B., & Kear, T. (2014). Patient safety and patient safety culture: Foundations of excellent health care delivery. *Nephrology Nursing Journal, 41*(5), 447–505.

Van Bogaert, P., Kowalski, C., Weeks, S., Van Huesden, C., & Clarke, S. (2014). The relationship between nurse practice environment, nurse work characteristics, burnout and job outcome and quality of nursing care: A cross-sectional survey. *International Journal of Nursing Studies, 50*(12), 1667–1677.

Vanderheide, R., Moss, C., & Lee, S. (2013). Understanding moral habitability: A framework to enhance the quality of the clinical environment as a workplace. *Contemporary Nurse, 45*(1), 101–113.

Wandelt, M., & Ager, J. (1974). *Quality patient care scale.* New York, NY: Appleton-Century-Crofts.

Wandelt, M., & Stewart, D. (1975). *Slater nursing competencies rating scale.* New York, NY: Appleton-Century-Crofts.

Weaver, S., Lubomksi, L., Wilson, R., Pfoh, E., Martinez, K., & Dy, S. (2013). Promoting a culture of safety as a patient safety strategy: A systematic review. *Annals of Internal Medicine, 158*(5), 369–374. Retrieved from http://annals.org/article.aspx?articleid=1656428

Weston, M. (2010). Strategies for enhancing autonomy and control over nursing practice. *The Online Journal of Issues in Nursing, 15*(1), Manuscript 2. Retrieved from http://www.nursing world.org/MainMenuCategories/ANAMarketplace/ANAPeriodicals/OJIN/TableofCon tents/Vol152010/No1Jan2010/Enhancing-Autonomy-and-Control-and-Practice.html

Wong, C. (2015). Connecting nursing leadership and patient outcomes: State of the science. *Journal of Nursing Management, 23*, 275–278.

World Health Organization. (2009). Glossary of patient safety concepts and references. Retrieved from http://www.who.int/patientsafety/taxonomy/icps_technical_annex2.pdf

Wu, A. (2000). Medical error: The second victim. *British Medical Journal, 320*, 726–727.

Wu, A., & Steckelberg, R. (2012). Medical error, incident investigation and the second victim: Doing better but feeling worse? *BMJ Quality and Safety, 21*(4), 267–270. Retrieved from http://qualitysafety.bmj.com/content/21/4/267.full

Index

reality shock, 79–80
Registered Nurse Safe Staffing Act (2014), 187
research integrity, 170–171
research misconduct, 170
respect for potential and enrolled subjects, 169–170
Rest, James, 11, 19
Rest's model, defined, 11–12, 19, 24, 58, 302
Right to Self Determination, 35
rigor, 93
risk–benefit ratio, 160, 163, 165–166. *See also*
    Nuremberg Code
Robot Kingdom, 260
robotic walkers, 260
Robotics Institute's Quality of Life Technology
    Center, 261

scientific validity, 164–165
self-care competencies, 93–96
self-determination, 256
self-governance, 17
self-reflection, 40
self-soothing, 36
sensitivity, 12
Silver Tsunami, 245
Slater Nursing Competencies Rating Scale, 306
social justice, 220–222
social value, 163–164
Spectrum Health in West Michigan, 91
substituted judgment standard, 168
support services, 97–105. *See also* organizational
    policies
supportive leadership, 96–97
surrogate, role in decision making, 54–55
Systemic Mindfulness Model of Proactive Patient
    Safety, 315

TeamSTEPPS, 91
technology
    competence in workforce, 267–268
    devices, 263–264

ethical use, 268–269
and human element, 259
Internet, 262–263
robots as caregivers, 260–262
telenursing, 268
terminal values, 25
theories, ethical, 13–14
transformational leadership, 184
TRUST, 323–324

University of California at San Francisco, 122
University Health System in San Antonio, 90, 97,
    103, 193
University of Kansas School of Nursing, 307
University of Kentucky, 90
University of Nebraska, 122
University of Reading in England, 261
University of Virginia Health System, 103
U.S. Department of Veterans Affairs National
    Center for Ethics in Health Care, 278, 279,
    284, 287, 295
Utilitarianism, 16, 216

values
    defined, 24
    and ethical skills, 24–26
    instrumental, 25
    strategies to elicit patient's preferences, needs, and,
        149–152
    terminal, 25
Vanderbilt University Wellness Center, 95–96, 97
Veterans Health Administration, 194
virtue, nurse, 17
vulnerability, 168

WalkRounds (WR), leadership, 320
WHO. *See* World Health Organization
workforce, technology competence, 267–268
workplace violence, 82, 86–89, 99
World Health Organization (WHO), 220

Printed in the United States
By Bookmasters